'Catrina Brown and colleagues have once again debunked a tin god in the world of therapy and shown it to operate in the service of neoliberalism, individualism and the social control of those struggling with mental health. This rigorous and path-breaking volume is critical of the widespread pathologizing and biomedicalizing of trauma, and shows instead the efficacy and hopefulness of feminist and narrative approaches to violence and human distress, operating within well-resourced community-based prevention and supports. An excellent book for practitioners and students, and all those working for more socially just futures.'

**Donna Baines**, *Professor and Former Director of the UBC School of Social Work, The University of British Columbia, Canada*

'Reflective of classic feminist trauma analyses, ala Judith Herman, Christine Courtois, Laura Brown and Bonnie Burstow, this inspirational multidisciplinary volume celebrates resistance to the pathologizing biomedical and neoliberal framing of trauma. In contrast, this innovative book reframes trauma as social justice, deconstructs how discursive/institutional practices and structural systems of power/oppression are co-implicated in people's struggles, and advocates alternative feminist practices and approaches that are structural, preventative and community-/care-based. In doing so, this book helps to enhance capacity to better serve and support survivors, sustain practitioners as active witnesses to trauma, build healthier communities, and fulfill professional objectives to achieve social justice.'

**Dr. Susan Hillock**, *Professor of Social Work, Trent University, Canada*

'This book refreshingly moves away from pathologizing constructions of trauma to critically analyzing how aspects such as hierarchically embedded medicalized discourses, gendered power relations and socially constructed scenarios frame and reframe interactions, understandings and knowledge reproduction. It not only presents a compelling critique but also offers grassroots ways forward that emphasize a range of viable and diverse policy and practice options. It is essential reading for policymakers, practitioners and students. All of whom have substantial capacity to engage in transformational change.'

**Barbara Fawcett**, *Professor of Social Work at the University of Strathclyde, UK. She specializes in research methodologies, post-structural feminist analyses and associated research in the arenas of mental health, disability and older age*

'In this excellent collection, the authors use their varied locations and experiences to reflect on how the suffering of women and men in neoliberal societies has been reframed in ways that are extremely damaging to them and to the pursuit of social justice. Whose knowledge counts and whose voices can be heard are key concerns throughout with a critical intersectional lens applied to the processes of silencing and invalidating. Very valuable practice alternatives are offered, drawing from the authors' engagement with intergenerational and culturally embedded stories of healing and restoration.'

**Brid Featherstone**, *Professor of Social Work, University of Huddersfield, UK*

T0384849

'This much needed volume rebuts the pathologizing of trauma as individual inadequacy and provides a counter-narrative reaching into feminist analyses of subjugation by biomedical industries. Turning trauma-informed therapy on its head, symptoms are reframed from personal deficiency into coping skills in an unjust world and attention is redirected to the violent sources of trauma. Multiple contributing authors offer perspectives out of the wealth of their own personal experiences, cultural contexts, practice settings and qualitative research, while consistently returning to the central theme of making sense of what is labelled as 'disorders' and moving us toward respect, trust and healing.'

**Joan Pennell,** *Professor Emerita, North Carolina State University, USA, and long-term feminist activist and proponent of restorative approaches*

'*Reframing Trauma through Social Justice: Resisting the Politics of Mainstream Trauma Discourse* is a welcome antidote to the proliferation of neurocentric perspectives on trauma, which reinforce neoliberal and postfeminist individualistic understandings. Grounded firmly in the rich history of feminist responses to trauma, this collection uses intersectional and postmodern frameworks to surface the ways in which trauma is intimately tied with social and structural inequities. Designed with practitioners in mind, contributing scholars provide alternative responses to trauma grounded in narrative and relational approaches that upend psychiatric hegemony. The result is a handbook of 'discursive resistance' to mainstream trauma talk, which can guide practice and wider societal responses.'

**Marina Marrow,** *Professor and Chair of the School of Health Policy and Management, York University, Canada*

'Brown and her colleagues call into question taken-for-granted, pathologizing discourses and assumptions about trauma based on individualized understandings and practices, and instead band together in a collective resistance the understanding of trauma as a social justice issue. They offer powerful alternative possibilities for moving away from demoralizing practices toward remoralizing practices. A must read for those involved in working with people who have experienced the consequences of trauma.'

**Jim Duvall,** *Co-editor, JST Institute;* *Editor,* Journal of Systemic Therapies

# REFRAMING TRAUMA THROUGH SOCIAL JUSTICE

This cross-disciplinary volume examines and reframes trauma as a social and political issue in the context of wider society, critiquing the widely accepted pathologizing of trauma and violence in current discourse.

Rooted in critical social theory, this insightful text reinvokes the critiques and analysis of the women's movement and the "personal is political" framing of trauma to unpack the mainstreaming of trauma discourse that has emerged today. Accomplished contributors address the social construction of femininity and masculinity in relation to trauma and violence, and advocate for a broader framing of trauma away from the constrained focus on pathologizing and diagnosing trauma, individual psychologizing and therapy. Instead, the book offers a fresh and compelling look at how discursive resistance, alternative feminist and narrative approaches to emotional distress and the mental health effects of violence can be developed alongside community-based, preventive, political and policy-based actions to create effective shifts in discourse, practice, policy and programming.

This is fascinating reading for upper-level undergraduate and postgraduate students, researchers and academics in a broad range of fields of study, including psychology, social work, gender and women's studies and sociology, as well as for professionals, including policymakers, clinical psychologists and social workers.

**Catrina Brown** is Professor at the School of Social Work and is cross-appointed as Professor in Gender and Women's Studies, Dalhousie University, Nova Scotia. As the graduate coordinator at the School of Social Work for 15 years, until recently she focused on integrating critical theory and critical practice. Both her academic and clinical work focuses on social justice approaches to women's health and mental health issues, including trauma, post-trauma, relational injury, substance-use problems, depression and "eating disorders" within a feminist postmodern/narrative lens.

# Women and Psychology

Series Editor: Jane Ussher

*Professor of Women's Health Psychology, University of Western Sydney*

This series brings together current theory and research on women and psychology. Drawing on scholarship from a number of different areas of psychology, it bridges the gap between abstract research and the reality of women's lives by integrating theory and practice, research and policy.

Each book addresses a 'cutting edge' issue of research, covering topics such as postnatal depression and eating disorders, and addressing a wide range of theories and methodologies.

The series provides accessible and concise accounts of key issues in the study of women and psychology, and clearly demonstrates the centrality of psychology debates within women's studies or feminism.

**Other titles in this series:**

**Domestic Violence and Psychology**
*Paula Nicolson*

**Women, Sex, and Madness**
*Breanne Fahs*

**The Maternal Experience**
*Margo Lowy*

**Postfeminism and Body Image**
*Sarah Riley, Adrienne Evans and Martine Robson*

**Trans Reproductive and Sexual Health: Justice, Embodiment and Agency**
*Damien W. Riggs, Jane M. Ussher, Kerry H. Robinson, Shoshana Rosenberg*

**Reframing Trauma Through Social Justice: Resisting the Politics of Mainstream Trauma Discourse**
*Catrina Brown*

For more information about this series, please visit: https://www.routledge.com/Women-and-Psychology/book-series/SE0263

# REFRAMING TRAUMA THROUGH SOCIAL JUSTICE

Resisting the Politics of
Mainstream Trauma Discourse

*Edited by Catrina Brown*

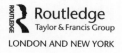

Routledge
Taylor & Francis Group

LONDON AND NEW YORK

Cover Image: Getty Images © Vicente Méndez

First published 2025

by Routledge
4 Park Square, Milton Park, Abingdon, Oxon OX14 4RN

and by Routledge
605 Third Avenue, New York, NY 10158

*Routledge is an imprint of the Taylor & Francis Group, an informa business*

*British Library Cataloguing-in-Publication Data*
A catalogue record for this book is available from the British Library

*Library of Congress Cataloging-in-Publication Data*
Names: Brown, Catrina, editor.
Title: Reframing trauma through social justice: resisting the politics of mainstream trauma discourse/edited by Catrina Brown.
Description: Abingdon, Oxon; New York, NY: Routledge, 2024. |
Series: Women and psychology | Includes bibliographical references and index.
Identifiers: LCCN 2023054509 (print) | LCCN 2023054510 (ebook) |
ISBN 9781032459899 (paperback) | ISBN 9781032459912 (hardback) |
ISBN 9781003379591 (ebook)
Subjects: LCSH: Women–Violence against. | Children–Violence against. |
Feminism. | Post-traumatic stress disorder–Social aspects. | Social justice.
Classification: LCC HV6250.4.W65 R437 2024 (print) | LCC HV6250.4.W65 (ebook) |
DDC 362.88082–dc23/eng/20240131
LC record available at https://lccn.loc.gov/2023054509
LC ebook record available at https://lccn.loc.gov/2023054510

ISBN: 978-1-032-45991-2 (hbk)
ISBN: 978-1-032-45989-9 (pbk)
ISBN: 978-1-003-37959-1 (ebk)

DOI: 10.4324/9781003379591

Typeset in Times New Roman
by Deanta Global Publishing Services, Chennai, India

*To all those who have struggled to speak of their suffering.*

*To my mother – who was able to move from silence to speech.*

# CONTENTS

# CONTRIBUTORS

## Editor

**Catrina Brown, BA, MA, MSW, PhD, RSW**, is professor at the School of Social Work and is cross-appointed to Gender and Women's Studies at Dalhousie University, Nova Scotia. She served as graduate coordinator at the School of Social Work for 15 years, until recently. Her work focuses on social justice approaches to women's health and mental health issues, including trauma, post-trauma, relational injury, substance-use problems, depression and "eating disorders", within a feminist postmodern/narrative lens. Her current research focus has included the impact of neoliberalism and biomedicalism on the provision of mental health care in Canada. A similar Nova Scotia study on mental health is documented in a recent report entitled, *Repositioning Social Work Practice in Mental Health in Nova Scotia*. Another study is underway on the provision of effective services for family violence in rural and remote areas of Atlantic Canada. Overall, her work centers on integrating critical theory into direct critical practice, which is illustrated in her three co-edited books, *Consuming Passions: Feminist Approaches to Weight Preoccupation and Eating Disorders* (with Karin Jasper, 1993, Second Story Press), *Narrative therapy: Making Meaning, Making Lives* (with Tod Augusta-Scott, 2007, Sage) and *Critical Clinical Social Work: Counterstorying for Social Justice* (with Judy MacDonald, Canadian Scholars Press). She has contributed to a number of significant edited collections including *Social Justice and Counseling* (2018), edited by D. Pare and C. Audet; *Doing Anti-oppressive Practice: Social Justice Social Work*, edited by D. Baines (2011, 2017); *Doing Anti-oppressive Practice: Rethinking Theory and Practice*, edited by D. Baines, N. Clark and B. Bennett, 2022) and *Women Voicing Resistance. Discursive and Narrative Exploration*, edited by M. Lafrance and S. McKenzie-Mohr (2014), which received the Distinguished Publication Award of the Association for Women and Psychology. Catrina has also served on the Editorial Boards of *Narrative Work: Issues, Investigations, and Interventions* and *Journal of Systemic Therapies*. She is a private practice psychotherapist, adopting a feminist, narrative, discursive and collaborative approach. She is active with the Dalhousie Faculty Association, Dalhousie Senate, Nova Scotia College of Social Workers and the national Family Violence Knowledge Hub and Community of Practice.

## Contributors

**Tod Augusta-Scott, MSW, RSW,** is known internationally for his work with gender-based violence, restorative justice and narrative therapy. He has worked for a trauma-based, community organization for over 25 years. For the past 15 years he has also worked for the Canadian Armed Forces. He has presented his work across Canada and internationally (Asia, Europe, British Isles, America). He is the co-founder of the Canadian Domestic Violence Conference. He has also taught in the Department of Social Work, Dalhousie University, Nova Scotia, and continues as a guest speaker on a regular basis. Tod is the co-editor and contributor to *Narrative Therapy: Making Meaning, Making Lives* (Sage, 2007) and *Innovations in Interventions to Address Intimate Partner Violence: Research and Practice* (Routledge, 2017). He was awarded the Distinguished Service Award from the Canadian Association of Social Workers. His work is featured in the documentary *A Better Man* (2017), a film about domestic violence and restorative justice. He serves on the Advisory Council for the Status of Women, Canada. He received an Award of Excellence from the Deputy Minister of National Defence for his work addressing sexual violence in the Canadian Armed Forces (2019).

**Laura Boileau, MA, RPsych,** Registered Psychologist (NWT, AB). Since 2012 Laura Boileau (she/her) has worked on the front lines to help address, prevent, and heal racialized and gender-based violence. First, she served clients in the Northwest Territories helping intergenerational survivors of the Indian Residential School system take responsibility to stop their use of abusive behaviour and repair its effects. Next, she chose to help victims directly address the effects of sexualized violence in Alberta. Now in Ontario, after the birth of her first child, she was surprised by the general lack of understanding of the potential traumatic impacts of birth and seeks to bring her intersectional trauma-focused narrative and somatic therapy skills to help others heal.

**Jean Carruthers, PhD,** is a lecturer and course coordinator in Social Work and Human Services at the School of Public Health and Social Work, Faculty of Health, Queensland University of Technology, Australia. Before starting her career in academia, Jean practiced in diverse areas within social work, including domestic and family violence, sexual assault, community development in rural communities, and family law. Further to her work in direct practice, Jean has been heavily involved in social activism, community education and research, working collaboratively with community groups such as the Justice Dance Project and Applied Theatre Project. In her academic work, Jean has used the arts, specifically performance art, as a means for embodied critical learning in social work education. Her PhD titled "Performance as a platform for critical pedagogy in social work education" outlines the use of critical performance pedagogy, a critical and creative educational approach used in social work education. Her current research program is focused on using the arts, particularly drama, to expose novel and innovative directions in teaching critical social work practice.

**Amanda Dupupet, MA, MTA, RCT, CCC**, is a registered counseling therapist with the Nova Scotia College of Counselling Therapists and a registered music therapist with the Canadian Association of Music Therapists. Amanda began her work as a counseling therapist using narrative therapy approaches to help support people when they have caused harm and when they have been harmed by family violence. She is also currently engaged in research in the field of family violence. In addition, Amanda runs a private practice focusing on perinatal mental health in Halifax, Nova Scotia. Her private practice focuses on supporting individuals through the transition to parenthood and potential associated obstacles such as fertility challenges, grief and loss, birth trauma, perinatal mood and anxiety disorders, attachment and bonding with baby, and navigating identity changes.

**Heather Gaskill, MSW, RSW**, involvement with rape crisis work began in 1998 as a volunteer. She spent the following ten years working mostly in sexual assault centers doing feminist advocacy, public education and crisis work. Heather has a master's degree in social work from Dalhousie University, Nova Scotia, and began counseling in 2006. She worked for nearly a decade as a psychotherapist in community mental health and addiction, almost exclusively with women survivors of sexual assault and abuse, until 2018 when she took up a position at an inpatient addiction treatment center for men. Heather most recently worked as a therapist on a military base, again with a specialization in addictions and trauma. She is now in private practice on Vancouver Island.

**Samantha Good, BSc, MSc candidate**, is completing her Master of Science in Experimental Psychology at Dalhousie University, Nova Scotia. She previously completed a BSc in Psychology with a minor in Social Justice and Inequality, as well as a certificate in Indigenous Studies. Sam's primary field is cognitive psychology, where she focuses on processes such as attention and memory. However, Sam is an interdisciplinary researcher, involved in many diverse research projects, including topics such as COVID-19, youth homelessness and sexual health.

**Ami Goulden, PhD candidate**, is an assistant professor at the School of Social Work, Memorial University, Newfoundland, and doctoral candidate at the

Factor-Inwentash Faculty of Social Work, University of Toronto, Ontario. She is a Social Sciences and Humanities Research Council doctoral fellow and previous recipient of the Ontario Graduate Scholarship and Royal Bank of Canada Graduate Fellowship in Applied Social Work Research. Ami has been practicing social work for over ten years in various settings, including pediatric and adult health care settings and child welfare services. Her most recent experience includes working in multidisciplinary health care clinics serving clients with chronic health conditions and their families during the coronavirus pandemic.

**Barb Hamilton-Hinch, BSc, MA, BEd, PhD**, is from the historical African Nova Scotian communities of Beechville and Cherry Brook. Barb is currently employed at Dalhousie University, Nova Scotia, as the assistant vice provost of equity and inclusion and an associate professor in the School of Health and Human Performance at Dalhousie University. Her work examines the impact of structural, systemic and institutional racism on diverse populations, particularly people of African descent. She holds a BSc in Recreation Management, an MA (from Dalhousie University), a BEd (from Mount St. Vincent University, Nova Scotia) and a PhD (from Dalhousie University). She is reputed to be the first African Nova Scotian to graduate with a PhD from Dalhousie University. Barb's current research projects include: Closing the Opportunity Gap for African Nova Scotian Learners; Optimizing Services for Families Living in Communities that have been Marginalized; Examining the Impact of Racism on the Health and Wellbeing of People of African Descent; The Benefits and Challenges of Culturally Relevant Programs for Post-secondary Students; Recreation for Individuals Living with Mental Health Challenges; Racialized Bodies and Elite Sports; and Mobilizing Supports and Programs for Incarcerated Individuals Integrating Back into the Community; and Exploring Support for Care Givers of Individuals with Dementia. At Dalhousie University, Barb holds a number of positions. She is: the co-team lead for the Health of People of African Descent Research Cluster with Healthy Populations Institute; one of the founders of Imhotep Legacy Academy (a program that is developed to increase the number of students in Science, Technology, Engineering and Math); co-chair of Promoting Leadership in Health for African Nova Scotians (a program to increase the number of students of African descent in health).

**Jean Hughes, PhD**, is professor with the School of Nursing at Dalhousie University, Nova Scotia. She is also a research scientist with the Department of Psychiatry at the IWK Health Centre for Women, Children and Families, Nova Scotia; a senior research scholar with Healthy Populations Institute, Nova Scotia; and former senior editor (2010–2015) for *Canadian Journal of Community Mental Health*. Jean's research and publications concentrate on marginalized populations with a focus on mental health issues and are funded by a number of federal and provincial sources. Several other of her studies have examined the effects of early psychosis programs – one examining the effects of an art therapy program and another examining the effectiveness of peer support on transitions back to community mental health care. She also has conducted several studies exploring the effects of a proven mental health intervention designed to build social and emotional skills (PATHS – Promoting Alternative Thinking Strategies) in elementary school children. She is currently exploring ways to optimize support and services for families with public school students from marginalized communities. Dr. Hughes's research is closely linked to her advocacy work with the highly marginalized North Dartmouth community of Nova Scotia to secure a community health home and the Mental Health Coalition of Nova Scotia.

**Marjorie Johnstone, PhD,** is associate professor in the School of Social Work at Dalhousie University, Nova Scotia, a position she has held since 2017. She has had over 30 years' social work field experience, predominantly in the area of mental health services with adults and families and youth. Her research interests are the history of Canadian social work with a particular focus in the influences of colonial imperialism and transformative radicalism. In addition, she has conducted community-based research on mental health services in Nova Scotia as well as analyses of mental health service delivery using the conceptual framework of epistemic injustice.

**Jeff Karabanow, PhD,** is professor and associate director in the School of Social Work at Dalhousie University, Nova Scotia, and cross-appointed with International Development Studies, College of Sustainability and The School of Health and Human Performance. He has worked with homeless populations in Toronto, Montreal, Halifax and Guatemala. His research focuses primarily upon housing stability, service delivery systems, trauma and homeless youth culture. He has completed a film documentary looking at the plight of street youth in Guatemala City and several animated shorts on Canadian street youth culture. He has numerous academic publications, including *Being Young and Homeless: Understanding How Youth Enter and Exit Street Life* (Peter Lang, 2004), *Leaving the Streets: Stories of Canadian Youth* (Fernwood, 2010) and *Homeless Youth and the Search for Stability* (WLU Press, 2018). Jeff is one of the founding members of Halifax's Out of the Cold Emergency Shelter, Nova Scotia, and is the co-director of the Dalhousie School of Social Work Community Clinic, Nova Scotia. He was awarded the Dalhousie Faculty of Health Senior Research Award (2014) and the William Webster Excellence in Interprofessional Education Award (2019). He is also a recent awardee of the Senate of Canada 150 Medal (2019).

**Eunjung Lee, PhD,** is a full professor and associate dean, academic, at the Factor-Inwentash Faculty of Social Work at the University of Toronto in Ontario, which she joined in 2007. She has over 20 years' clinical social work practice in various mental health fields, serving marginalized populations with trauma and violence experiences. She has worked as a clinical supervisor, currently keeping a small clinical consultation. Eunjung's research focuses on cross-cultural clinical practice in community mental health and how policy and its underlying politics construct dominant discourses that impact immigrants and refugees in a global neoliberal era.

**Judy E. MacDonald, PhD**, identifies as a (dis)Abled woman who has lived with chronic pain for over 30 years. She is professor, director of the School of Social Work, and assistant dean (equity and inclusion) within the Faculty of Health, Dalhousie University, Nova Scotia. Her areas of research are disability rights, inclusion and access. She had been co-chair of the Persons with Disability Caucus of CASWE (Canadian Association for Social Work Education) for over 20 years, and is founder of the newly constituted Staff and Faculty (dis)Ability Caucus at Dalhousie University. She continues to support students with (dis)Abilities through their research and life story writings. Together with Catrina Brown she co-edited *Critical Clinical Social Work: Counterstorying for Social Justice* (Canadian Scholars Press). Judy has influenced an Employee Accommodation Policy at Dalhousie University, a student accommodation policy at the School of Social Work, which identified an accommodation officer within the school, and she is currently on the Dalhousie Accessibility Advisory Committee, which is crafting plans to respond to the new provincial legislation on accessibility. She has contributed to numerous collections, including *Connecting Social Policy to Practice* (4th edition), edited by B. McKenzie and B. Wharf; *Canadian Social Policy for Social Workers*, edited by R. Harding and D. Jeyapal; *Canadian Perspectives on Community Development*, edited by S. Todd and S. Savard; and *Doing Anti-Oppressive Practice: Social Justice Social Work* (4th edition), edited by D. Baines, N. Clark and B. Bennett. Judy is also a consultant offering professional expertise on best practices related to disability policy and services and social work.

**Colin James Morrison, MSW, RSW,** has worked for over 25 years in child and adolescent mental health, and he currently serves as a social worker with IWK Child and Adolescent Mental Health and Addictions in Halifax, Nova Scotia, as well as working as a part-time sessional instructor with the School of Social Work at Dalhousie University, Nova Scotia. Colin completed an MSW from Dalhousie University in 2020 following the successful defense of his thesis work, "Toxic Masculinity, Male Childhood Sexual Trauma, and the Challenges to How Young Men Heal." Colin is a social justice and mental health advocate, and his research interests include the impact of trauma on men and boys, male violence and issues impacting the 2SLGBTQIA+ community.

**Nicole Moulding, PhD**, is professor and researcher and educator with special interests in gendered violence, mental health and social work. Nicole has published three books: *Gendered Violence, Mental Health and Recovery in Everyday Lives: Beyond Trauma* (Routledge, 2023); *The Sexual Politics of Gendered Violence and Women's Citizenship*, co-authored with S. Franzway, S. Wendt, C. Zuffery and D. Chung (2019); and *Contemporary Feminisms in Social Work Practice*, co-edited with S. Wendt (Routledge, 2018). She has also published over 40 journal articles in research into gendered violence, mental health and social work. Nicole is director of the Safe Relationships and Communities research group (SRC), an interdisciplinary research group with members from diverse disciplines across the University of South Australia and industry partners. She is involved in a number of ongoing research projects, including a national Australian Research Council (ARC) research project investigating the sociological dimensions of childhood emotional abuse, and a research project focusing on how young people forge positive intimate relationships after growing up in domestic violence. She was also a chief investigator on another ARC-funded nationwide study into the long-term impact of domestic violence on women's citizenship, with a focus on mental health, housing, employment and social participation, as well as a number of other research studies on gendered violence and mental health.

**Sarah E. Norris, PhD candidate**, is a PhD student in Health at Dalhousie University, Nova Scotia. Sarah has over 20 years of experience supporting vulnerable children, families and students within community, academic and hospital settings. She has contributed to scholarly research projects related to women's health, gender-based violence, trauma, disability and climate justice. In 2021, Sarah completed a Master of Social Work at the University of Victoria, Canada, where she held the position of graduate student representative for the Society of Students with a Disability. Sarah's master's thesis, titled *Where are Persons with Disabilities: A Reflexive Thematic Analysis of Canadian Federal Government Climate Change Strategies*, explored the consequential impacts of ableism and exclusion in climate change policies and strategies. Her research highlighted the urgent need to reduce disproportionate harms (dis)Abled people face in a changing climate, as exacerbated by existing societal inequities. Sarah's areas of interest include critical disability studies, social determinants of health, climate change trauma and grief.

**Norma Jean Profitt, BA, MSW, PhD**, has a long history of activism in feminist movements in Nova Scotia and Costa Rica, with a focus on patriarchal violence against women and girls. She developed the first course on international perspectives on violence against women at the Muriel McQueen Fergusson Centre for Family Violence Research, University of New Brunswick, Canada, and the first course on lesbian, gay, bisexual and Two-Spirit peoples in the School of Social Work, St. Thomas University, New Brunswick. In 2016, she received a Governor General's Award in Commemoration of the Persons Case for her work in advancing gender equality. In 2017, she was awarded the Diane Kays Memorial Award from the Nova Scotia College of Social Workers for her practice in the area of violence against women and her demonstration of exceptional professional and ethical standards with service users, colleagues and communities. Since leaving academia, she co-edited with Cyndy Baskin *Spirituality and Social Justice: Spirit in the Political Quest for a Just World* (Canadian Scholars Press, 2019). She recently published an article on the ethical and political dimensions of spirituality in *La Revista Costarricense de Trabajo Social* (*Costa Rican Social Work Journal*).

**Nancy Ross, PhD**, is assistant professor in the School of Social Work, Dalhousie University, Nova Scotia. Her prior work in Mental Health and Addiction Services motivates her research interest in exploring better responses to gender-based violence, in trauma and in prevention. She applies a feminist peacebuilding and trauma-responsive lens that acknowledges structural and cultural violences are linked to direct forms of violence. She has produced a short film titled *Women of Substance* (2012) that profiled stories of women meeting challenges of substance use. She has also co-produced a second film titled *I Work for Change* (co-produced with C. Hall, 2017), which explored the complexity of social work while celebrating the profession.

**Ann Schumacher, PhD**, completed trauma training at the International Trauma Studies Program in New York, and completed her PhD at Wayne State University, Michigan, with a focus on restorative justice and peace and conflict studies. In 2010, she established and has continued to facilitate a Talking Circle Program for teen girls in Detroit, Michigan, centered on developing social emotional literacy and conflict resolution skills. She has had further trauma training through her work over the last ten years with trauma specialist Thomas Hubl.

**Rose C.B. Singh, PhD candidate**, is a PhD candidate at Memorial University, Newfoundland, and a sessional lecturer at Dalhousie University, Nova Scotia. Rose is also a practicing social worker and brings over two decades of experience working in the social services sector, with a focus on supporting youth and adults living with disabilities, mental health concerns and substance use. Rose teaches courses on direct practice, theory, social justice and critical approaches to social work practice and policy in the areas of disability, mental health and addiction. Rose's research and scholarship interests center on critical social work education, social justice, disability justice, disabilities, mental health, online learning and teaching and emerging technologies.

**Nachshon Leger Siritsky, MSSW, D.Min., BCC, RSW**, is a second-generation holocaust survivor and identifies as transgender and non-binary. As a social worker, board-certified interfaith chaplain, and ordained Reform rabbi, they are committed to doing all that they can to bring healing to this world by working on decolonizing the spaces where they exist. In addition to serving as the professional practice and advocacy consultant with the Nova Scotia College of Social Workers, they are also the founding rabbi of Reform Judaism in Atlantic Canada: Decolonizing Judaism in Mi'kma'ki and Beyond. Previously, they served as a rabbi in several Reform Jewish communities and worked in hospice, palliative care and community mental health, as well as leading community organizing efforts with Interfaith Paths to Peace. Nachshon also served as vice president of Mission for Kentucky One Health, which included several hospitals in Louisville, Kentucky, including Our

Lady of Peace, which was the largest free-standing, non-profit psychiatric hospital in the United States.

**Mareese Terare, PhD**, is Bundjalung Goenpul – a woman, mother and grandmother. Her traditional country extends from the north coast of New South Wales to southeast Queensland, Australia. She is currently employed with the Faculty of Social Sciences, School of Education and Social Work, University of Sydney.Mareese has a BA in Welfare Studies, and a master's degree in Indigenous Studies. Her doctoral thesis explored the use of worldview by First Nations workers in the trauma field and is titled, *It hasn't worked for us so we have to change what we're doing: First Nations' worldview and human service practice*. Mareese teaches across social work areas, emphasizing human rights and cultural safety. Her teaching and practice work includes First Nations, healing, frameworks and ways, interpersonal trauma, counseling, clinical and cultural supervision, social justice, children's rights and human rights. Mareese has 40+ years of frontline work experience, providing client support, and training and community education with Aboriginal and non-Aboriginal workers in the trauma field. She has consulted, developed, implemented and evaluated the Australian Skills Qualification Authority accreditation for community services and health training, targeting both the First Nations and non-Aboriginal workforce. Mareese is strongly committed to human rights, and this is reflected in her research, curriculum development, teaching, community engagement and practice. Mareese's focus includes ongoing cultural and safety commitments to training, teaching, research, curriculum development and frontline client engagement.

**Andrea Titterness, PhD**, completed a doctorate in neuroscience at the University of British Columbia, Vancouver, where she studied the effect of prenatal stressors on learning and memory. She has served on the board of directors for the Victoria Women's Sexual Assault Center in Victoria, British Columbia. Andrea is an academic research associate for the Centre for Research & Education on Violence Against Women & Children at Western University, Ontario.

**Emma Tseris, PhD**, is a senior lecturer in social work and policy studies at the University of Sydney, where she is involved in research and teaching that aims to create space for alternative understandings of distress, difference and 'madness' beyond the constraints of the biomedical model. This includes a strong interest in the intersections between gender inequality and biomedical understandings of human experience.

**Tanya Turton, MSW**, is an award-winning entrepreneur, storyteller, wellness educator and mental health advocate. Graduating from Toronto Metropolitan University, Ontario, with a bachelors degree in Social Work, Tanya's work uses an intersectional lens to explore the relationship between narrative, mental wellness and care. As a graduate from the master's of Social Work Program at Dalhousie

University, Nova Scotia, Tanya's work cultivates frameworks for collective care rooted in practical approaches to equity. As a wellness world-builder, Tanya takes steps to tell intersectional stories, and construct a world for Black and queer communities to feel heard, seen and witnessed. Tanya is the author of *Jade Is a Twisted Green*, a coming-of-age story about Jamaican Canadian identity, love, passion, chosen family and rediscovering life's pleasures after loss. She is the founder and executive director of Adornment Stories Collective, a mental health, grassroots, non-profit for Black women, femmes, queer, trans and non-binary communities collective where people can tell their stories through a plurality of creative means while building their capacity. The lead educator and founder of NiaZamar, an intersectional education platform, a love-centered community and a space for reclaiming freedom via self-care and collective-care. Her work centers early engagement mental health initiatives and intersectional frameworks of engagement. Mixing wellness, narratives, education and mental health advocacy, she offers a unique blend of engaging tools to meet people where they are.

**Haorui Wu, PhD**, is Canada Research Chair (Tier 2) in Resilience and assistant professor in the School of Social Work at Dalhousie University, Nova Scotia. His interdisciplinary practice research explores human and non-human settlements' redevelopment through the lens of environmental and social justice in the global context of climate change, disaster and other crises.

Xime estrum faccusae od mi, ad et omnistibus voloribust, que corepedis mo berio. Nequis et, corionsero velicil iumquae pa volorae quatempore por sin preriam facepel iquatio molupta tiorend antest quid ma sitatem que pe re nis cus rae conecab imus, conestrum as dignatem rem. Nam que con nonsequatia aceperit molor moluptates dolut venihilleni cuptio. Accabo. Ibus nonsernatur?

Volum apere veni cone sam, sim et maiorep erferum facea numquid exceped endem ligenet volorerum ad mosa nis se nus am re doles videl et a conseque plaudi unt dolum rem. Ducimagnias ipsum, conestem fuga. Xim quis eumquaes dita iusam qui aut ant, quid quatiuntet ut mo vel inulpa et et maio. Et quo quibus sus, sedio volut magnatatur aut eos audanduciet vendis ea corero optate etur? Loribeaque venduciis modis rem idelign itinihictur, aute omnis ma sequi dolupta tiaturite nem resti dolor molor sam, sim es velignime quam lacerat quatiissequi nimaxim lab in corem auda prat accusam faceria velestrum quati illant et antia samustis volute con cuptas nonet as nulla iustia volor autem arum volut volupta audiation plit aut a volum faceri optaquaes volorep reprovitiore ex excest, cum conest, nos inci cor maximet, core nimillab idi quid ut essunditis sus aut dolupis millatet es aut qui rem quossitatia debit ligenih iliquunt peria nonsed ut et excerum etur, ipiduci entiur, cum fugia sitatus alibus.

Rem sequi aliqui ius nonem et qui te natatibusam sinveliti alis accum, occuptatur?

# INTRODUCTION

## Catrina Brown

### Talking Trauma Talk: Resisting the Politics of Mainstream Trauma Discourse

Beginning in the early 1970s, the women's movement made a significant socio-historical contribution by identifying the gendered, social and political context of violence against women and children, which included rape, battery, incest, sexual abuse and sexual harassment. Feminists worked to shift violence from the private to the public sphere, creating an impact on policy and law while broadly communicating how common violence is toward women and children in patriarchal society and how significantly it impacts upon their lives (Brownmiller, 1975; Butler, 1978; Courtois, 1988; Herman, 1981, 1992; Pizzey, 1974; Russell, 1986; Terr, 1990). The *"personal is political"* approach that was adopted situated women's experiences in the context of society, seeking to make sense of rather than pathologize women's responses to trauma and violence (Brown, L., 1992; Burstow, 2003; Burstow & Weitz, 1988; Chesler, 1972; Gavey & Schmidt, 2011; Levine, 1982; Penfold & Walker, 1983; Smith & David, 1975; Webster & Dunn, 2005). Subsequently, an intersectional feminist lens of power and subjugation has been essential to understanding the trauma of violence (Marecek, 2016). Reinvoking the critiques and analysis of the women's movement and the "personal is political" framing alongside contemporary intersectional and postmodern analysis will allow this collection to unpack the dominant depoliticized and conservatizing trauma discourse that has emerged today (Lafrance & McKenzie-Mohr, 2013; Marecek & Gavey, 2013; McKenzie-Mohr & Lafrance, 2011; Ussher, 1991, 2010). This book will critique both the mainstreaming of trauma discourse and the corresponding neoliberal/biomedicalized practices in the contemporary "postfeminist" era that shape these mainstream approaches to understanding and working with trauma.

DOI: 10.4324/9781003379591-1

Postfeminist and neoliberal social philosophies work together to create an impoverished system of social service delivery and analysis (Carney, 2008). The ideologies of postfeminism and neoliberalism conflate to produce deeply individualized and responsibilized expectations of the social citizen, which reinforce the simultaneously fiscally constrained and reduced social welfare system (Brown, C., 2021; Brown, C., Johnstone, & Ross, 2021; Brown, C., Johnstone, Ross, & Doll, 2022; Liebenberg, Ungar, & Ikeda, 2013). The *"personal is political"* foundation of feminist trauma work has been replaced by the mainstreaming of trauma-informed discourse, which is based upon the *"political is personal"* views of the rationalized citizen. Postfeminist neoliberal social, economic and individual rationalism work together to produce a tightly managed and constrained society that relies significantly on the psychological rationalization and management of individuals and is further legitimized and considered evidence-based through biomedicalizing trauma (Braedley & Luxton, 2010; Chen, 2013; Gill & Orgad, 2018). Subsequently, this volume will highlight the dangers and limitations of the "postfeminist", biomedical, neoliberal framing of trauma and will engage in discursive resistance as well as alternative practices through the critiques offered.

A feminist, discursive and narrative lens will advocate for a broader framing of trauma away from the diluted and constrained focus on pathologizing, diagnosing, individual psychologizing and therapy (Tseris, 2013). Through discursive resistance, alternative feminist and narrative approaches to emotional distress, relational injury, and the mental health effects of violence can be developed alongside community-based, preventive, political and policy-based actions (McKenzie-Mohr & Lafrance, 2014; Morley & Dunstan, 2016; Morrow & Malcoe, 2017; Morrow & Weisser, 2012). As histories of trauma and violence are significant social and relational determinants of mental health issues there is a critical need for social programming and funding in the area of trauma and violence that address the effects of trauma and violence on people's mental health and the associated subsequent coping strategies used to address trauma, including substance use (Brown, C., Johnstone & Ross, 2021; Moulding, 2015; Tseris, 2019). Coping strategies for dealing with trauma, including substance use, need to be understood as making sense rather than framed as deficits and pathology (Brown, C., 2020).

The overall critique offered in this collection is two-fold: (1) a challenge to the epistemological assumptions and framing of the discourses of trauma, violence and mental health as individual problems rather than issues of social justice and the subsequent epistemic injustice produced (Morrow & Weisser, 2012; Rimke, 2016), and (2) the context of neoliberalism (Cosgrove & Karter, 2018), biomedicalism (Lemke, 2001; Nathan & Webber, 2010), and "postfeminism" (Gill, 2008) in which these depoliticizing, individualizing and pathologizing discourses flourish (Marecek & Gavey, 2013; Lafrance & McKenzie-Mohr, 2013; LeFrançois, Menzies, & Reaume, 2013; McKenzie-Mohr & Lafrance, 2011; Rose, 2014; Ussher, 1991, 2010). Taken in tandem, the reduced welfare state, limited community resources, the intensified focus on biomedical discourse (e.g., neuroscience and the brain) and the lack of focus on the sociopolitical context of women's lives produces a decontextualized and depoliticized focus on the individual in trauma work. Further, the systemic, clinical and ethical violence, revictimization and retraumatization within existing services/trauma responses (e.g., psychiatric, medical, legal) needs to be challenged and changed. Adequate services to address complex trauma and co-occurring trauma, mental health issues and substance use need to be developed and made widely accessible. While those experiencing trauma often feel hopeless, vulnerable and out of control, those who work with trauma feel increasingly desperate as they struggle to find the time and resources they need to do this work within the current constrained and limited context of their work environments (Baines, Brown, C., & Cabahug, 2024; Brown, C., Doll, Baines, & Johnstone, 2024; Brown, C., Johnstone, & Ross, 2021).

Together the authors in this collection are engaged in discursive resistance and in subsequently reframing trauma as social justice. In Chapter 1, "Speaking the Unspeakable: Discursive and Political Resistance to Dominant Trauma Discourse and Trauma Work", Catrina Brown and Emma Tseris provide a theoretical foundation for this book. They elaborate on the need to deconstruct oppressive dominant social discourse on trauma and their relationship to dominant discourses on mental health and addictions, which together pathologize and medicalize daily life and individual struggle. They provide a history of the development of trauma discourse and how it has become more commonly part of everyday mainstream conversation, suggesting we need to reinvigorate earlier feminist analyses that centered the social context of trauma and violence including relations of power, oppression, exclusion, discrimination and marginalization. The conservatizing effects of mainstream approaches to being "trauma-informed" has depoliticized and degendered trauma work and the re-storying or creation of alternative stories of their identities and their lives will be offered. The focus today has become very individualized, shifting away from a "personal is political" to a "political is political" framing. They provide an analysis of how the current conflation of postfeminism, neoliberalism and biomedicalism has shaped the dominant trauma discourse and subsequent approaches to practice. Brown and Tseris argue that we need to resist this dominant discourse and offer alternative understandings and approaches alongside the integration of analyses of how discursive and institutional practices and structural systems of power and oppression are often co-implicated in people's struggles. Unhelpful dominant stories are unpacked, helping to produce a counterviewing of people's stories of struggle and the development of counterstories that participate in social resistance.

This discussion is followed by Marjorie Johnstone and Eunjung Lee, who reposition the trauma diagnosis through an examination of the biomedicalization of trauma and the epistemic injustice that results. In Chapter 2, Johnstone and Lee apply the theoretical frameworks of epistemic injustice and epistemic resistance and critical mental health studies with a feminist perspective to the current mobilization of trauma-informed services. However, in creating a typology of the psychological effects of trauma, the *Diagnostic and Statistical Manual of Mental Disorders* (5th edition) (DSM-5) (American Psychiatric Association, 2013) describes the symptoms of trauma as decontextualized psychological occurrences, thus presenting a template for individual victim-based interventions, and invisibilizing the triggering event(s). Hegemonic psychiatric discourses often disqualify the marginalized voices of the victims through both systemic and testimonial epistemic injustice. Johnstone and Lee draw on the work of Miranda Fricker (2007) who investigates the power and ethics of knowing. When some positions are given less authority and considered less credible and valid, this is described as an epistemic form of injustice. Johnstone and Lee acknowledge the contribution of the increased recognition of the harm experienced by trauma and its impact on mental health but critique the application of decontextualized psychiatric hegemony where trauma and violence are recast as a disorder rather than as phenomenon often rooted in patriarchy, misogyny and rape culture. Epistemic gaps occur when testimony is blocked or silenced, which further oppresses those experiencing this form of epistemic injustice. By tracing the effects of the biomedicalization of trauma in traditional mental health services, where the understanding of trauma has been severed from its contextual origins and repositioned as a psychopathology, they argue a multi-pronged approach, which blends psychological, sociological and political analysis.

In Chapter 3, Emma Tseris builds on Johnstone and Lees' critique through an examination of the myth of trauma-informed mental health services. She explores psychiatric coercion and institutional violence, and the retraumatizing and revictimizing effects of these practices, through interviews with women survivors of psychiatric coercion and social workers with experience in acute mental health settings. In this chapter, Tseris explores the substantial disconnect between what mental health services say they do, and the actual experiences of women receiving mental health services. Emma Tseris argues that mental health services involve a continuum of coercion, which at one end involves policing the thoughts and emotions of women (including their responses to gendered violence) within cognitive behaviour therapy, and at the other involves the continued use of practices such as seclusion and restraint, despite their well-documented harms. This work demonstrates the limitations of the mainstreaming of trauma and rhetorical claims of being trauma-informed, while adopting a paradigm of medicalized coercion. In this way, mainstream trauma discourses largely contribute to, rather than alleviate, the continuation of intersecting patriarchal violence and psychiatric harm.

Both Norma Jean Profitt and Heather Gaskill reflect on work they have done working in mental health and addictions services. In Chapter 4, Norma Jean Profitt continues the critique offered in the preceding chapters through reflecting on her work at a provincial rural mental health and addictions centre with women affected by gender violence and other forms of oppression. Profitt argues for an ethical approach that recognizes oppression, gender violence and trauma as root causes of women's mental health and addictions struggles. Consistent with this book's critique of dominant biomedical discourse and practice, Norma Jean argues this discourse fails to recognize women as social beings who make meaning of their experience of distress and as agents who engage in advocacy and social action to influence systems and institutions. Like Emma Tseris's research, which demonstrates psychiatric violence, Norma Jean Profitt questions the ethical conceptualization of emotional distress and substance use currently in place in mental health and addictions arguing mainstream practices are a form of epistemic and institutional violence against women. She argues the current biomedical model of psychiatric diagnosis obscures and individualizes gender violence, trauma and oppression such as misogyny, racism and income inequity.

Alongside Norma Jean Profitt, in Chapter 5, Heather Gaskill draws on her experience working as a feminist therapist in the public mental health care system, observing that clinicians who provide these services are often working with the most complex and most poorly resourced clientele in the country. In addition to experiences of violence and trauma, this population struggles with many difficulties that are often socially situated within multiple layers of oppression, including sexism, racism and poverty. Mainstream therapeutic responses to trauma continue to view feminist approaches as clinically weak, not as "serious" or "effective" therapy: Heather Gaskill describes this as a "missed opportunity of heartbreaking proportions". She critiques the dominant biomedical framing, which simplifies trauma to a "misfiring nervous system" while adopting a myth of neutrality. Like all of the writers in this book, Heather Gaskill rejects the decontextualization of this mainstream approach, which fails to consider gender, race, ability, sexual orientation or social position. The mainstream biomedical dominance pursues formula and technique at the expense of developing strong, effective therapeutic relationships that explore the meanings associated with trauma and violence. This approach then fails to connect with people and take seriously the meaning they attach to their trauma experiences. She suggests it is ironic that the system is disdainful of any approaches not considered "evidence-based", yet continues to overload complex trauma cases onto clinicians working in feminist, relational and meaning-centered ways.

In Chapter 6, Catrina Brown illustrates integrating critically based practice with a focus on gender and mental health counselling through applying a feminist narrative lens to a complex trauma case example. Women with histories of trauma are often pathologized and given an unhelpful diagnosis. In this chapter she emphasizes a critical discursive feminist practice which integrates discursive resistance to psychiatric medicalized and pathologizing approaches to trauma and critically based feminist practice which equalizes power in the therapeutic context by stressing safety, client power and control over their own choices, alongside transparency and collaboration throughout the work. A feminist narrative lens challenges pathologizing diagnoses and re-focuses the therapeutic conversations, adopting an ethical stance of unpacking the meaning and construction of women's stories of trauma, the influence of the stories on their lives, and the creation of more helpful, less harmful counterstories. This approach allows both for critical hope and for the exploration of possible selves (Dunkel & Kerpelman, 2006; Marcus & Nurius, 1986). As stories emerge in social, cultural, political and historical contexts they can challenge or reify harmful and unhelpful ideas. Trauma stories are often partial and uncertain and are often spoken through coping strategies which help people find some relief. Trauma stories are often difficult to tell, in part because they are often painful and pathologized, and because existing frameworks often fail to capture people's experiences. Catrina Brown explores the constraints and dangers of telling trauma stories and the importance of double listening for the absent but implicit in trauma stories – for the yet to be spoken. Moving from silence to speech often requires 'fearless speech' (Foucault, 2001) as speaking too often involves risk to oneself. Trauma work is contextualized and the collaborative approach emphasizes clients' strengths and agency alongside their vulnerability, marginalization, and pain. The therapeutic conversation relies on a strong therapeutic alliance when there is relational injury, unpacking the experience of being in relationships within trauma work and the movement from silence to speech when trauma has been unspeakable.

In Chapter 7, Judy MacDonald, Rose Singh, Ami Goulden and Sarah Norris explore trauma, (dis)Ability and chronic pain. Their approach is to value the experiences and knowledge of those who suffer from chronic pain in contrast to the inequities and oppression (dis)Abled people have experienced both historically and in the current neoliberal context. The dominant biomedical model prioritizes an individualized trauma discourse, which fails to recognize the structural elements of compounded trauma experienced through repeated ableist encounters and many barriers within health care systems. The writers highlight how these systemic barriers exacerbate experiences of isolation and minimize the voices and experiences of (dis)Abled people. Individualistic, decontextualized approaches negate social responsibility for accessibility and inclusion. They deconstruct ableism as it pertains to trauma, offering a holistic and anti-oppressive model of (dis)Ability practice that incorporates the social model of (dis)Ability, and acknowledges the impact of impairment and personal trauma concerning structural inequities (Hanes, Carter, & MacDonald, 2022; MacDonald, 2008; MacDonald, Brown, M., & Jones, 2023). Reflecting this approach, "disability is written as (dis)Ability: "(dis)" to respect the person's social and physical connection with disability, and "Ability" to highlight the creative and innovative ways of dealing with societal barriers" (MacDonald & Friars, 2010, p. 140). A case is provided to illustrate a way to situate chronic pain sufferer experiences and apply trauma-based practices while suggesting affirming approaches when working with sufferers of chronic pain.

In Chapter 8, Amanda Dupupet and Laura Boileau draw on their own birthing experiences to explore the impact of birth trauma on women's well-being. They explore birth trauma through unpacking the biomedical, social and discursive factors that contribute to a woman's experience of trauma while giving birth and afterward. They acknowledge that although both biomedical and obstetric violence fields make contributions to mitigating birth trauma, they also have limitations. They build on previous feminist work critiquing patriarchal medical practices in reproductive care, which have often rendered birth trauma invisible. Taken together, the current dominant discourses in both the biomedical model and among the obstetric violence critics tends to negate women's knowledge of their bodies and experiences. Dupupet and Boileau ask critical questions about the social construction of motherhood both in the dominant patriarchal medical model and in the idealized versions of motherhood sometimes advanced within midwifery and the obstetric violence movement. Ultimately, they conclude that collaborative engagement is needed to prevent birth trauma. This collaborative engagement encourages birthing mothers to make informed choices about what they believe is best for them without the pressure of feeling they have failed as women and mothers if they seek medical help or, equally, if they do not.

Jeff Karabanow, Andrea Titterness, Jean Hughes, Haorui Wu and Samantha Good explore the relationships between trauma and youth homelessness in Chapter 9. In this chapter, the voices of young people on the streets, taken from Canadian research, provide a powerful and compelling illustration of their often traumatic and violent home experiences that lead them to make the difficult choice of living on the streets – which is also often traumatic and violent. They face abuse and violence from the public and police who are often shaming and critical. Other youth may be supportive, but they may also be violent and abusive to each other. The voices in this chapter provide a context for understanding why it makes sense the youth make the difficult choice to live on the streets and show how devastating such a life often is. The chapter illustrates the ongoing compounding of trauma for these young people, and the difficult life journey that often lies ahead. Further, it illustrates the need for a comprehensive policy approach to youth homelessness, with immediate crisis services and counseling available alongside supports to enable youth to exit the streets.

Several of the chapters argue that an intersectional lens often benefits from considering the historical and intergenerational components of trauma and the impact of colonization. The personal experiences of Nachshon Siritsky, Barb Hamilton-Hinch, Mareese Tarere and Tanya Turton shape the contribution of these chapters. An exploration of the meaning of intergenerational trauma, through an intersectional lens is offered by Nachshon Siritsky in Chapter 10. Siritsky reflects upon their personal connection to this topic, and the reasons this matters as transgender, non-binary and second-generation holocaust survivor. The approach is grounded in social work ethics and values, with a focus on social justice (which often benefits from considering the intergenerational components of trauma and the impact of colonization). A critical analysis of ways that intergenerational trauma has been approached is provided along with reflections on the traumatic history of "evidence-based" medicine that has failed to adequately respond to systemic and historical intergenerational trauma. Nachshon Siritsky suggests we need to deepen our understanding of, and capacity to work with, intergenerational trauma within a decolonizing framework of social work practice.

In Chapter 11, Barb Hamilton-Hinch and Catrina Brown also explore intergenerational trauma and the impact of racism and gender on the health and well-being of African Nova Scotian women. Barb Hamilton-Hinch situates herself as an African Nova Scotian woman and has a first-hand understanding and connection to the women's stories, specifically their experiences of being silenced and silencing themselves. The theme of being silenced and keeping oneself silent among people who have experienced violence and trauma is a major theme throughout this book. This chapter connects silence, power and subjugation. Catrina Brown shares briefly her own mother hiding her Jewish identity and living with this secret. Silence is very often associated with the dangers of speaking. The African Nova Scotian women spoke explicitly about racism and its implications on their health, the health of their families and their community with a focus on their experiences of being silenced and silencing themselves, as well as supportive influences on their survival, success, health and well-being. Through the African Nova Scotian women's voices and stories, strategies for addressing inequities in health and well-being include challenges to ongoing systemic racism and the need for system-level changes.

In Chapter 12, Mareese Terare emphasizes the importance of establishing human rights within trauma work by reclaiming First Nations worldviews. When working in the trauma sector, this involves significant responsibilities, including ensuring First Nations people have access to services that emphasize both cultural humility and safety. The significance of cultural humility and safety, when working with First Nations peoples affected by interpersonal trauma, domestic/family violence, sexual assault and child maltreatment, extends to understanding the powerful impact of institutional trauma. Cultural safety and cultural humility practice as principles can support workers to have better knowledge and understanding of the sociopolitical and historical context that limit First Nations people's ability to access justice and health and community services. Mareese Terare argues this extends beyond generalist, face-to-face contact to a broader holistic community development process.

In Chapter 13, Tanya Turton expresses concern that conversations on trauma have centered on individualistic solutions, neglecting the valuable role of collective care. She suggests that practitioners who hope to be impactful should consider collective care as a valid approach for engaging in trauma talk. Tanya Turton recognizes that, for many marginalized communities, collective care was the only option when medical spaces either abandoned them or provided inadequate care. She emphasizes the importance of a love ethic that translates to care rooted in the community, actively reducing isolation. When working with intersectional communities, primarily those who have not only experienced personal trauma, but collective trauma over the course of multiple generations, she argues there is a need for validating the wisdom rooted in the collective understanding. Talking trauma within these communities and providing adequate care will require engaging with care as a collective initiative, incorporating not only the individual seeking care, but also their communities. Communities have used collective methods to survive trauma, but these methods have been delegitimized in professional clinical spaces, leaving communities such as Black queer women further marginalized and the individualist care provided ultimately becomes inaccessible. Addressing this mistrust and engaging with collective care is a vital step in working with folks who have navigated race-, gender- or sexuality-based traumas. Care that promotes agency, dignity and interdependence and is grounded in mutual trust can only be built with an understanding of the role of collective care as a survival tool.

In Chapter 14, Nicole Moulding notes the persistence of violence against women has not decreased despite improvements in gender equality and women's rights. However, much of the research and intervention in this field combines feminist understandings with psychological trauma or cognitivist psychosocial theories, leaving questions about the affective aspects of violence perpetration underexplored. Gendered violence is a profoundly visceral experience, yet the body – its emotions and sensations and their political effects – has been relatively absent from theorization, research and practice. Nicole Moulding argues that exploring the role of emotion and affect in gendered violence can help to better understand the intersubjective power relations driving violence and coercive control in the everyday, and their political effects on individuals and communities. Nicole Moulding considers how turning attention to the role of situated, intersubjective emotion in gendered violence can contribute to the development of new, more effective approaches to prevention and trauma-informed support.

In Chapter 15, Nancy Ross and Ann Schumacher argue for a paradigm shift in responding to family violence, replacing the adversarial approach with a restorative, just response that is trauma- and violence-informed. They demonstrate the limitations of the adversarial pro-arrest, pro-charge and pro-prosecution policies' response to family violence through a case study. Despite these policies, 60 percent to 70 percent of the people who experience violence in their intimate partnership wish to stay in the relationship (Ross & Ryan, 2021), but typically do not have adequate resources to support this preference. They draw on two models of family group circles and family group decision making introduced in Canada that address family domestic violence in a non-adversarial manner.

Tod Augusta-Scott discusses dominant masculinity, trauma and use of violence and pathways for repairing harm and ending violence in Chapter 16. He explores the interface between experiences of masculinity and trauma in the lives of men who abuse their female partners. The community-based domestic violence field has focused primarily on the influence of dominant masculinity and the politics of gender on men's choices to abuse their female partners. In this chapter he explores how symptoms of trauma can be masked as dominant masculinity, and how experiences of trauma and dominant masculinity serve to reinforce each other. Community-based practices have been uncertain about how to address men's experiences of violence and harm while also ensuring that men are held accountable and responsible for their own use of violence. This chapter offers strategies for addressing men's experiences of trauma and dominant masculinity to help men stop their abuse, repair harm in their relationships, and take greater responsibility for their choices. To address these expressions of masculinity, men are better served if they can attend to their experiences of trauma and the ideas that stem from both experiences that support their continued use of abuse.

In Chapter 17, Colin James Morrison investigates male childhood sexual trauma while challenging, deconstructing and re-storying dominant discourses. Through a discursive analysis, this chapter argues that men's stories are constrained by the limited discourses available that describe or fit their experience, and therefore male childhood sexual abuse is silenced and suppressed because it opposes dominant discourses that say men cannot be victims and that sexual abuse is something that happens only to women and girls. Although there are many commonalities in the psychological and social aftermath of these experiences, one significant difference for young male survivors is the specific way that victimization intersects with gender socialization and sexual identity formation within the context of a patriarchal and heteronormative society. This can influence male sexual trauma survivors' competency in making sense of their experiences within dominant social narratives that promote oppressive discourses such as disbelief and shame. The chapter also examines the influence of misogyny and homophobia, noting how survivors intuitively recognize the associated social stigma and therefore seek to disassociate themselves from anything that symbolizes femininity or homosexuality and serves to threaten the dominant discourse of masculinity. The chapter concludes by considering, through a narrative lens, how we must deconstruct and re-story the dominant discourses surrounding masculinity and male experiences of trauma to address the potential harms and to allow men and boys the chance to heal.

In the final chapter of the book, Chapter 18, Jean Caruthers offers a creative example of critical clinical performance pedagogy to support feminist social work in the context of gendered violence. The chapter recognizes that social work education needs to be able to address gendered violence in a way that is consistent with social justice, rather than relying on conservative neoliberal approaches, in order to support students thinking critically about gendered violence and how they respond critically in practice. In this chapter, Jean Caruthers illustrates critical performance pedagogy, which is an educational approach, used in a critical social work program in Australia designed to support critically reflexive practice in education. Critical and collaborative engagement to develop students' capacity for critical praxis is enabled through using performative strategies (e.g., performing arts). A performance assessment used in an introductory social work course demonstrates how this performative storytelling approach assists students to prioritize feminist social work when responding to domestic and family violence.

These chapters offer discursive resistance, consistently revealing the simultaneous inadequacies and injustices of the dominant discourses shaping trauma and trauma work today. Together the chapters in this book highlight the epistemic injustice that prevails in the area of violence against women where their experiences not only do not fit dominant available frameworks, but they also continue to be minimized and, too often, not believed (Gilmore, 2017; McKenzie-Mohr & Lafrance, 2011; Medina, 2013). Across the chapters there is a critique of the epistemic injustice of hegemonic "evidence-based" biomedical paradigms of trauma and the many failings of its translation into adequate trauma services and work. The focus on individual deficit, or the failings of the body rather than the overall historical, political and social context of people's lives, depoliticizes trauma and violence. The patriarchal violence against women, historical impact of intergenerational trauma, discrimination and violence against people who are queer-identified, and the limited stigmatizing approaches to care for those living with (dis) Ability all point to the need to situate people's experiences within the context of their lives. People who have experienced violence, trauma and intergenerational trauma need to be able to tell their stories, to be heard and to have access to non-pathologizing, culturally appropriate services, yet available services continue to be both limited and increasingly cut back (Avalon Sexual Assault Centre, 2019; Dale, Maki, & Nitia, 2021; Ending Violence Association of Canada, 2021).

The contributors in this book all bring a complex analysis with implications for social services delivery, practice and policy changes. Taken together, the dominant discourses of trauma are reflected in institutional and psychiatric violence and coercion. Given this, those who have experiences of trauma and violence have very few helpful resources of support. The dominant frameworks typically are not a good fit for their experiences, making it difficult for people to risk telling their stories. When those services available are short-term, one-size-fits-all, decontextualized and biomedicalized, they are often retraumatizing and revictimizing. The current system sustains and reinforces silence rather than hearing collective voices. Herman (1992) argued that in the aftermath of experiencing sexual violence women must face the "task of creating a future" (p. 196). Despite efforts on the part of feminist advocates, researchers and policymakers to position this "task" as one that must be taken up by the collective to build systems that ensure better outcomes for those who experience sexual violence, the growing emphasis on neoliberal/biomedicalized responses to violence and trauma has had the effect of downloading the work of "creating a future" onto individuals. It is imperative that approaches to social policy and social change reflect a collectivist understanding of the responsibility of "the task of creating a future" free from violence and trauma.

## References

American Psychiatric Association. (2013). *Diagnostic and Statistical Manual of Mental Disorders* (5th ed.). American Psychiatric Publishing.
Avalon Sexual Assault Centre. (April 15, 2019). Avalon unable to accommodate new counselling requests. https://avaloncentre.ca/wp-content/uploads/2019/04/Avalon-Sexual -Assault-Centre-Unable-to-Accommodate-New-Counselling-Requests-April-15.pdf.

Baines, D., Brown, C., & Cabahug, F. (2024). The shifting labour process in professional care: Recreating dominance and the managerialised mental health social worker. *The British Journal of Social Work*, 54(1) 475–493. https://doi.org/10.1093/bjsw/bcad210.

Braedley, S., & Luxton, M. (2010). Competing philosophies. Neo-liberalism and challenges of everyday life. In S. Braedley & M. Luxton (Eds.), *Neo-liberalism and everyday life* (pp. 3–21). McGill-Queen's University Press.

Brown, C. (2020). Feminist narrative therapy and complex trauma: Critical clinical work with women diagnosed as "borderline". In C. Brown & J. MacDonald (Eds.), *Critical clinical social work: Counterstorying for social justice* (pp. 82–109). Canadian Scholars Press.

Brown, C. (2021). Critical clinical social work and the neoliberal constraints on social justice in mental health. Special Issue on Social Justice. *Research on Social Work Practice*, 1–9. doi: 0.1177/1049731520984531.

Brown, C., Doll, K., Baines, D., & Johnstone, M. (2024 forthcoming). All dressed up and nowhere to go: The impact of neoliberalism on social justice-based practice with mental health and substance use. *Canadian Review of Social Work*.

Brown, C., Johnstone, M., & Ross, N. (2021). *Repositioning social work practice in mental health in Nova Scotia*. Report.

Brown, C., Johnstone, M., Ross, N., & Doll, K. (2022). Challenging the constraints of neoliberalism and biomedicalism: Repositioning social work in mental health. *Qualitative Health Research*, *32*(5), 771–787. https://doi.org/10.1177/10497323211069681.

Brown, L. (1992). A feminist critique of personality disorders. In L.S. Brown & M. Ballou (Eds.), *Personality and psychopathology: Feminist reappraisals* (pp. 206–228). Guilford Press.

Brownmiller, S. (1975). *Against our will. Men, women, and rape*. Simon and Schuster.

Burstow, B. (2003). Toward a radical understanding of trauma and trauma work. *Violence Against Women*, 19, 1293–1317.

Burstow, B., & Weitz, D. (1988). *Shrink resistant. The struggle against psychiatry in Canada*. New Star Books.

Butler, S. (1978). *The conspiracy of silence. The trauma of incest*. Volcano Press.

Carney, T. (2008). The mental health service crisis of neoliberalism – An antipodean perspective. *International Journal of Law and Psychiatry*, 31, 101–115.

Chen, E. (2013). Neoliberalism and popular women's culture: Rethinking choice, freedom and agency. *European Journal of Cultural Studies*, 16(4) 440–452. https://doi.org/10.1177%2F1367549413484297.

Chesler, P. (1972). *Women & madness*. Avon.

Cosgrove, L., & Karter, J.M. (2018). The poison in the cure: Neoliberalism and contemporary movements in mental health. *Theory & Psychology*, 28(5), 669–683.

Courtois, C. (1988). *Healing the incest wound*. Norton.

Dale, A., Maki, K., & Nitia, R. (2021). *Expert engagement to address and prevent gender-based violence final report*. Women's Shelters Canada. https://nationalactionplan.ca/wp-content/uploads/2021/06/NAP-Final-Report.pdf.

Dunkel, C., & Kerpelman, J. (2006). *Possible selves: Theory, research and applications*. Nova Science Publishers.

Ending Violence Association of Canada. (2021). *Building a national action plan to end gender-based violence: Identifying priorities for addressing sexual violence*. https://endingviolencecanada.org/wp-content/uploads/2021/03/EVA-Canada-SV-Engagement-Final-Report.pdf.

Foucault, M. (2001). TO FOLLOW

Fricker, M. (2007). *Epistemic injustice. Power and the ethics of knowing.* Oxford University Press.

Gavey, N., & Schmidt, J. (2011). "Trauma of rape" discourse: A double-edged template for everyday understandings of the impact of rape? *Violence Against Women,* 17(4) 433–456. doi: 10.1177/1077801211404194.

Gill, R. (2008). Culture and subjectivity in neoliberal and postfeminist times. *Subjectivity,* 25, 432–445. doi: 10.1057/sub.2008.28.

Gill, R., & Orgad, S. (2018). The amazing bounce-backable woman: Resilience and the psychological turn in neoliberalism. *Sociological Research Online,* 23(2), 477–495. https://doi.org/10.1177%2F1360780418769673.

Gilmore, L. (2017). *Tainted witness. Why we doubt what women say about their lives.* Columbia University Press.

Hanes, R., Carter, I., & MacDonald, J.E. (2022). Getting to the heart of the matter: A social-oppression model of disability. In D. Baines, N. Clark, & B. Bennett (Eds.), *Doing anti-oppressive social work: Rethinking theory and practice* (4th ed.) (pp. 244–266). Fernwood.

Herman, J. (1981). *Father-daughter incest.* Harvard University Press.

Herman, J. (1992). *Trauma and recovery. The aftermath of violence – from domestic abuse to political terror.* Basic Books.

Lafrance, M., & McKenzie-Mohr, S. (2013). The DSM and its lure of legitimacy. *Feminism and Psychology,* 23(1), 119–140. https://doi.org/10.1177%2F0959353512467974.

LeFrançois, B., Menzies, R., & Reaume, G. (Eds.) (2013). *Mad matters. A critical reader in Canadian mad studies.* Canadian Scholars Press.

Lemke, T. (2001). The "birth of bio-politics": Michel Foucault's lecture at the Collège de France on neo-liberal governmentality. *Economy and Society,* 30(2), 190–207. doi: 10.1080/03085140120042271.

Levine, H. (1982). The personal is political: Feminism and the helping professions. In G. Finn & A. Miles (Eds.), *Feminism in Canada: From pressure to politics* (pp. 175–210). Black Rose Books.

Liebenberg, L., Ungar, M., & Ikeda, J. (2013). Neo-liberalism and responsibilisation in the discourse of social service workers. *British Journal of Social Work,* 45(3),1006–1021.

MacDonald, J. (2008). Anti-oppressive practice with chronic pain suffers. *Social Work and Health Care,* 47(2),135-156.

MacDonald, J., Brown, M., & Jones, S. (2023). Social policy across social identities. In B. McKenzie & B. Wharf (Eds.), *Connecting Policy to Practice in the Human Services* (5th ed.) (pp. 272–290). Oxford University Press.

MacDonald, J., & Friars, G. (2010). Structural social work from a (dis)Ability perspective. In S. Hicks, H. Peters, T. Corner, & T. London (Eds.), *Structural social work in action* (pp. 138–156). Canadian Scholars Press.

McKenzie-Mohr, S., & Lafrance, M. (2011). Telling stories without the words: "Tightrope talk" in women's accounts of coming to live well after rape or depression. *Feminism & Psychology,* 21(1), 49–73.

McKenzie-Mohr, S., & Lafrance, M. (Eds.). (2014). *Women voicing resistance. Discursive and narrative explorations.* Routledge.

Marcus, H., & Nurius, P. (1986). Possible selves. *American Psychologist,* 41(9), 954–969. https://doi.org/10.1037/003-066X.41.9.954.

Marecek, J. (2016). Invited reflection: Intersectionality theory and feminist psychology. *Psychology of Women Quarterly*, 40(2), 177–181.

Marecek, J., & Gavey, N. (2013). DSM-5 and beyond: A critical feminist engagement with psychodiagnosis. *Feminism & Psychology*, 23(1) 3–9.

Medina, J. (2013). *The epistemology of resistance. Gender and racial oppression, epistemic injustice, and resistant imaginations.* Oxford University Press.

Morley, C., & Dunstan, J. (2016). Putting gender back on the agenda in domestic and family violence policy and service responses: Using critical reflection to create cultural change. *Social Alternative*, 35(4), 43–48.

Morrow, M., & Malcoe, L. (Ed.) (2017). *Critical inquiries for social justice in mental health.* University of Toronto Press.

Morrow, M., & Weisser, J. (2012). Towards a social justice framework for mental health recovery. *Studies in Social Justice*, 6(1), 27–43.

Moulding, N. (2015). *Gendered violence, abuse and mental health in everyday lives: Beyond trauma.* Routledge.

Nathan, J., & Webber, M. (2010). Mental health social work and the bureaubio-medicalisation of mental health care: Identity in a changing world. *Journal of Social Work Practice*, 24(1), 15–28. https://doi.org/10.1080/02650530903415672.

Penfold, S., & Walker, G. (1983). *Women and the psychiatric paradox.* Eden Press.

Pizzey, E. (1974). *Scream quietly or the neighbours will hear.* Penguin. https://doi.org/10.1192/bjp.126.3.295.

Rimke, H. (2016). Introduction. Mental and emotional distress as a social justice issue: Beyond psychocentrism. *Studies in Social Justice*, 10(1), 4–17.

Rose, D. (2014). The mainstreaming of recovery. *Journal of Mental Health*, 23(5), 217–218. https://doi.org/10.3109/09638237.2014.928406.

Ross, N., & Ryan, C. (2021). *A review of pro-arrest, pro-charge, and pro-prosecution policies: Redefining responses to domestic violence. A report.* https://dalspace.library.dal.ca//handle/10222/80242.

Russell, D. (1986). *The secret trauma: Incest in the lives of girls and women.* Basic Books.

Smith, D., & David, S. (Eds.). (1975). *Women look at psychiatry: I'm not mad, I'm angry.* Press Gang Publishing.

Terr, L. (1990). *Too scared to cry: Psychic trauma in childhood.* Harper & Row.

Tseris, E. (2013). Trauma theory without feminism? Evaluating contemporary understandings of women. *Affilia: Journal of Women and Social Work*, 28(2), 153–164.

Tseris, E. (2019). *Trauma, women's mental health, and social justice. Pitfalls and possibilities.* Routledge.

Ussher, J. (1991). *Women's madness: Misogyny or mental illness?* Harvester Wheatsheaf.

Ussher, J. (2010). Are we medicalizing women's misery? A critical review of women's higher rates of reported depression. *Feminism and Psychology*, 20(1), 9–35. https://doi.org/10.1177%2F0959353509350213.

Webster, D., & Dunn, E. (2005). Feminist perspectives on trauma. *Women & Therapy*, 28(3–4), 111–142.

# 1

# SPEAKING THE UNSPEAKABLE

Discursive and Political Resistance to Dominant
Trauma Discourse and Trauma Work

*Catrina Brown and Emma Tseris*

## Introduction

While on the one hand, it is encouraging that we are acknowledging and talking about trauma today, we can also see a mainstreaming of trauma talk. What
happened to words like rape, battery, incest, sexual abuse, and violence? Are
these words too much? Where is the violence, pain, suffering, impact, injustice,
exploitation and oppression? As feminists we know that language matters. What
we call things matters. Trauma talk today is too often minimized, sanitized and
stripped of particular meaning – DV, IPV, GBV, VAW, ACE. This shorthand talk
is a disservice to the importance of these issues. Reflecting the current "postfeminist", neoliberal conservative turn, violence is increasingly individually
and biomedically framed in terms of being trauma-informed and legitimized by
claims of "evidence-based" diagnoses. Biomedical frameworks such as neuroscience emphasizing brain chemistry now routinely enter trauma talk. Alongside
this is the notable responsibilization of people who have experienced violence
and trauma. They must cope, manage, self-regulate and recover, while, at best,
they seek help in an inadequately resourced and blaming system. Taken together,
the discursive influence of postfeminism, neoliberalism and biomedicalism has
shaped contemporary approaches to trauma.

Once believed to be rare human experiences – rape, battery, sexual abuse,
domestic violence and military trauma are now seen to be common. According
to Herman (1992), "[t]raumatic events are extraordinary, not because they occur
rarely, but rather because they overwhelm the ordinary human adaptions to life"
(p. 33). These experiences often involve threats to life or bodily integrity and
can be "close personal encounters with violence or death" (p. 33). Psychological
trauma is often characterized by "a feeling of intense fear, helplessness, loss of

DOI: 10.4324/9781003379591-2

control, and threat of annihilation"; "action is of no avail"; "resistance or escape is not possible"; and "the human system of self-defence becomes overwhelmed and disorganized" (Herman, 1992, pp. 33–34).

In addition to sexualized violence, domestic abuse, rape, sexual abuse/incest, physical violence, bullying and stalking, we also recognize other types of violence and trauma including medical-/health-related experiences, involuntary hospitalization, psychiatrization, obstetric violence and procedures, accidents, policing, incarceration, military, war, death, immigration, being a refugee, colonization, intergenerational trauma, racism, sexism and homophobia.

The effects of trauma are often labeled, pathologized and psychiatrized. This chapter critiques conservative, psychologized, individualized, pathologized, biomedicalized, therapeutized, decontextualized approaches to trauma, which have increasingly emerged (Brown, C., 2017; Brown, C., Johnstone, Ross, & Doll, 2022; Brown, C., Johnstone, & Ross, 2021; Doll, Brown, Johnstone & Ross, 2023; Ross, Brown, C., & Johnstone, 2022, 2023). One approach after another promises overly simplified strategies to address the impact of trauma on people's lives. While therapeutic approaches are not the only relevant responses to violence, where they are used, they need to address the context of the trauma, and often the complex relationship between trauma, mental health and substance-use issues through the development of strong, collaborative therapeutic relationships. Together, through these relationships, the meanings that people attach to their experiences and the coping strategies they have adopted to deal with trauma can be explored. In addition, we advocate for the expansion of state funding for community-based and survivor-led programing, the need for training, resources to support the material needs of survivors, and the intentional intersection of theory and practice across diverse populations. Welfare state policy and legal practices need to explore systematically the ways that violence and trauma are socially situated and how to change this (e.g., violence against Indigenous women, police violence against Black men).

In this chapter, we begin with a review of the historical contribution of feminist trauma work. We then explore the current dominant trauma discourse and practice in the context of postfeminism, neoliberalism, and biomedicalism, which are reflected in the plethora of emerging and ongoing therapeutic strategies (e.g., Dialectical Behavioral Therapy, Trauma-focused Cognitive Behavioral Therapy, Acceptance and Commitment Therapy, Accelerated Resolution Therapy, Eye Movement Desensitization and Reprocessing, and hallucinogenic drugs), which focus on the individual, the body and the brain. We explore the current preoccupation with neuroscience in trauma work and examine its potential hazards. The focus on epi-genetics, while intending to acknowledge intergenerational trauma, also situates and entrenches ongoing experiences of trauma and oppression within genetics rather than the sociopolitical arena. This position locks people genetically into a position with little hope or possibility for escape, and centers the ongoing oppressive life conditions as problems of the body.

We argue that the dominant discursive approach to violence and trauma alongside the lack of adequate programming for social justice-oriented approaches continue to leave women's voices unheard and their despair inadequately addressed. It has been well established that the co-existence of escalating social inequities under neoliberalism, fiscal constraint and lack of adequate mental health programing have produced a mental health care crisis (Baines, Brown, C., & Cabahug, 2024; Brown, C., 2021; Brown, C., Johnstone, & Ross, 2021; Brown, C., Johnstone, Ross, & Doll, 2022; Brown, C., Johnstone, & Ross, 2021; Carney, 2008; Doll, Brown, C., Johnstone, & Ross, 2023; Johnstone, Brown, C., & Ross, 2022; Morrow & Weisser, 2012; Stark, 2018; Yip, 2004). While greater funding and programming are needed, we are not advocating for more of the same funding of biomedical or pathologizing responses. Rather, we advocate for the ongoing importance of a feminist politicized violence and trauma lens while acknowledging unique individual experiences in the aftermath of trauma experiences.

We explore how self-management discourse and subjective disciplinary practices of power reflects the late-capitalist political economy of neoliberalism and how this is translated in the idealized well-regulated neoliberal subject (Baines, Brown, C., Cabahug, & Doll, 2024; Barker, 2013; Braedley & Luxton, 2010; Brown, C., 2007c, 2007d, 2007e, 2014, 2017, 2021, 2022). We then explore the how politics of emotion are intertwined with contemporary individualizing and pathologizing trauma discourse and practice. We acknowledge it is often dangerous and difficult to tell one's trauma story within the context of dominant trauma discourse. Building on feminist approaches to working with women who have experienced violence and trauma, we counterview coping behavior, which is often pathologized, as making sense and as an effort to take care of oneself (Brown, C., 2022). We explore the importance of practitioners listening beyond the words when people speak through their coping efforts. From here, we suggest the need for a counterstorying approach that resists current dominant violence and trauma discourses and enables social justice-based approaches that allow women's voices to be heard (McKenzie-Mohr & Lafrance, 2014; Morrow & Malcoe, 2017; Morrow & Weisser, 2012).

## History of Feminist Trauma Work

Today we talk about "trauma-informed" work as if this were a new discovery. The mainstreaming of trauma talk is detached from the important historical work of the women's movement. and reflects the current more conservative sociopolitical and economic climate. Indeed, in our view, trauma-informed discourse seems a poor imitation, a mere shadow of earlier robustly theorized and politicized discourse and practice. Reflecting the mainstreaming of trauma-informed discourse, the Canadian government for instance advises that the goal of trauma-informed work is to minimize harm, not to treat trauma (Government of Canada, 2018, 2020; Poole, 2013). Minimizing the harm of trauma and alleviating the distress and oppressive effects of trauma through the provision of adequate resources and services are both needed. When adequate resources are not available, and organizations and staff are inadequately trained, receiving services can be both revictimizing and retraumatizing (Brown, C., Johnstone, & Ross, 2021; Ross, Brown, C., & Johnstone, 2023). Feminist work continues to lead the way for women to tell their trauma stories and for them to be heard. Women's struggles to articulate their experiences and be heard has been an ongoing focus within feminism. Despite all this groundbreaking feminist work, women still find themselves struggling to tell their stories, to find a framework for their stories in the context of master narratives that often prevail and to find adequate supports. As talking of trauma is often experienced as dangerous (Brown, C., 2013, 2019), feminist narrative practice makes space for women's trauma stories and appreciates the constraints which often limit their speech (Brown, C., 2014, 2018, 2020a, 2022; Butler, J., 1997; deVault, 1990; Johnstone, 2021; McKenzie-Mohr & Lafrance, 2011; Tseris, 2019e).

Beginning in the 1970s, feminists forged the way to making it known how common violence is toward women and children in patriarchal society, and how significantly violence impacts upon their lives. The *"personal is political"* approach seeks to make sense of rather than pathologize women's responses to trauma and violence by listening to and hearing women's stories and by creating an impact on policy and law. More recently, an intersectional feminist lens allows for a gender analysis of why most perpetrators are male and most victims are female, while also acknowledging non-binary and trans experiences of violence (Ghafournia, 2019; Marecek, 2016; McCall, 2005; McCann & Sharp, 2023; Mehrotra, 2010; Mehrotra, Kimball, & Wahab, 2016). A feminist analysis that acknowledges power and subjugation related to class, race, culture, disability and gender is essential to understanding the trauma of sexual abuse, female sexual victimization and physical abuse (Baines, Bennett, Goodwin, & Rawsthorne 2019; Baines & Waugh, 2019; Brown, L. & Root, 1990).

Judith Herman is one of the most influential feminist thinkers on trauma, beginning with her book *Father-Daughter Incest (1981)* and followed by *Trauma and Recovery* (1992, 1997, 2015), which sought to make sense of the complex ways in which people often cope with trauma. In her 1997 version *of Trauma and Recovery* she forewarned:

> The very strength of recent biological findings in PTSD may foster a narrowed, predominantly biological focus of research. As the field of traumatic stress studies matures, a new generation of researchers will need to rediscover the essential interconnection of biological, psychological, social, and political dimensions of trauma.
>
> *(p. 240)*

In her most recent work, *Truth and repair: How trauma survivors envision justice* (Herman, 2023) we see the interconnection between theory, practice and activism.

While feminists influenced the current "trauma-informed" thinking they differed in that they remained fully political, doing trauma work consistent with feminist politics. To some extent, the political seems to have become more and more personal. Rather than simply recognizing common signs of trauma, early feminist trauma work addressed issues of power and social context in collaboratively based supports (e.g., see Armstrong, 1978; Bass & Davis, 1988, 1990; Brown, L., 1988, 1992, 2004; Brown, L. & Root, 1990; Brownmiller, 1975; Butler, S., 1978; Courtois, 1988, 2004; Forward & Buck, 1988; Herman 1981, 1992, 2015; Pizzey, 1974; Russell, 1986; Shaffer, 1987; Terr, 1990). Correspondingly, feminist therapy approaches reflected the "personal is political" understanding that women's experiences of trauma were political, and they developed an ethical approach to practice centered on not revictimizing or retraumatizing women. This was reflected in a collaborative and empowerment- based way or working that centered on establishing safety and control and addressing relational injury in part through the strength of the therapeutic alliance. Overall, this "personal is political" approach acknowledged the social contexts of trauma and violence rather than centering trauma in individual's bodies and brains.

## Trauma Without Feminism?

Feminist trauma therapy encourages us to understand women's mental health "symptoms" within the context of such experiences as child abuse and sexual violence that disproportionately affect women (Tseris, 2013). For Burstow (2003), "[t]rauma is not a disorder, but a reaction to a kind of wound" (p. 1302). In feminist-based trauma therapy the focus is extended beyond the individual level of the "client in treatment", instead emphasizing the sociopolitical context of women's lives, especially high levels of trauma experienced by women, such as child abuse and sexual violence, and the impact of these experiences on women's mental health. However, mainstream trauma theory is no longer centered on feminist values and intentions (Tseris, 2013). It has become preoccupied with medically oriented issues concerning diagnosis and standardized treatment.

We need a "critical dialogue about this reliance on biological knowledge to promote a social justice framework in mental health services … since it potentially reinforces the privileged status of biology and medical knowledge over social science and women's own narratives" (Tseris, 2013, p. 157). How we make meanings in our lives, interpret life events, our complex and irreducible emotional experiences, the cultures that we live in and the subsequent stories we tell, shapes how we see ourselves and our identities (Brown, C., 2022, Brown, C. & Augusta-Scott, 2007, 2018; Bruner, 1991; Madigan, 2003; White, 2001, 2007).

Trauma is often an overlapping story with many potential mental health and substance-use stories. Sexual assault, domestic violence, incest and sexual abuse have been associated with significant mental health difficulties and co-occurring issues, including depression, anxiety, eating disorders, "borderline" personality disorders, post-traumatic stress and a range of substance-use problems (Anda et al., 2006; Brown, C., 2007c, 2007e, 2011, 2014, 2019, 2020a; Brown, C. & Stewart, 2021; Brown, L., 1992; Cambron, Gringeri, & Vogel-Ferguson, 2015; Chapman et al., 2004; Herman, 1992, 2015; Herman, Perry, & van der Kolk, 1989; Kagi & Regala, 2012; Perry & van der Kolk, 1989; Plant, 2008; Ross, Brown, C., & Johnstone, 2023; Stewart & Israeli, 2003). Herman notes that "[p]rotracted depression is the most common finding in virtually all clinical studies of chronically traumatized people" (1992, p. 94). It is not uncommon for people to seek ways of coping with the effects of trauma including depression/suicidality, anxiety, fear, panic or profound despair with, for instance, self-harm, cutting, binge-eating, self-starvation and substance use. We do not question the immense suffering that can accompany violence and abuse, but how we understand it, name it and respond to it is open to question. Psychiatric language and responses offer only one narrow avenue.

Beginning with feminist advocacy, practice and research on violence and trauma in the 1970s, and supported by more recent research findings, it is clear we need to significantly enhance direct service programs that acknowledge how trauma is often at the roots of people's mental health struggles. Further, specific attention to gender, race and poverty is needed, and this response must be extended to the larger society (Crenshaw, 1989; Collins, 2000a, 2000b; hooks, 1990; Lorde, 1984).

While rejecting the medicalization of women's pain and suffering, we must also be conscious of not simply psychologizing the effects of trauma on women. Instead:

> [a] de-therapising agenda can challenge psychocentric thinking about violence and its effects – while also keeping in mind the pitfalls of neoliberal thinking about the triviality of women's despair, and an individualized resilience agenda that places the burden squarely upon women to manage the effects of violence as isolated individuals.
>
> *(Tseris, 2019b, p. 113)*

Burstow suggests that standard cognitive behavioral therapy strategies, such as interventions for "maladaptive" thoughts and relaxation/mindfulness/self-soothing strategies, can be useful treatments but are likely to be superficial and inadequate to support women who have experienced complex trauma, and they could even be harmful. Alternatively, Burstow suggests that we need to address themes of power, betrayal, self-blame, and stigma as critical components of complex trauma work. These are often overlooked in mental health contexts that emphasize short-term interventions and that require interventions to fit neatly within "evidence-based practice" paradigms. The complexity of strengths and problems disrupts simplistic understandings of resilience as being merely the absence of symptomatology. As practitioners, we have often pathologized the very behaviors that have helped people to survive (Burstow, 2003, p. 1306):

Just as trauma is properly understood as a series of responses to a concrete situation—not as symptoms or free-floating feelings or orientations—traumatic events and situations must be seen as concrete events within contexts. Specific traumatic events happen to specific people in specific locations and within specific contexts, and they inevitably involve other human beings. As such, trauma is inherently political.

## Critically Engaging with Neurocentric Perspectives on Trauma

It is impossible to ignore the turn to neuroscience as a key source of knowledge for shaping understandings of trauma within the contemporary context. Despite the now-pervasive influence of neuroscientific discourses on understandings of trauma, both critical scholars and neuroscientists themselves have challenged the attention and resources that have been allocated to a neurocentric approach within human service policy, research and practice. Neuroscientific knowledge is at an early and provisional stage, and yet often is granted powerful, totalizing status in developing "truths" about trauma and social disadvantage (Wastell & White, 2012). As such it is regarded as uncontestable truth, which most people do not feel qualified to question or challenge.

The notion that the brain is wholly constitutive of the "self" in contemporary Western societies is a captivating and yet problematic claim (Thompson, 2021). While we do not wish to deny the role that the brain, or the body, play in our lives and experiences, we are curious about the over-emphasis on the brain as an explanatory framework for trauma. This represents a "biologically privileged worldview" (Wastell & White, 2012, p. 399) that reduces our ability to engage with multiple knowledges and diverse ways of engaging with trauma. Further to this we do not wish to focus on the brain and negate the importance of mind, culture and the meaning making so often attached to struggles associated with trauma.

Social workers and other professionals may draw upon the authority of neuroscientific understandings with good intentions and as a strategy to add weight to the voices of survivors of violence through invoking a high-status discourse. It is important, however, to note the costs of such an approach to advocacy, and the bolstering of positivist assumptions about trauma, which are quite incongruent with feminist understandings of the role of culture, language and discourse in mediating individual experiences and producing multiple realities (Johnson & Flynn, 2021). Through viewing trauma as a mainly biological process, a sociopolitical explanation of violence is concealed (Thompson, 2021). This reduces our ability to take actions to address and prevent social injustices by maintaining a focus on "unwell" individuals.

As the majority of trauma survivors do not have specialized training in neuroscience, the continued emphasis on neuroscience knowledge justifies professional expertise as a core response to trauma (Thompson, 2021). The enthusiastic pursuit of neuroscience today rests on these authoritative professional knowledge claims, presented as objective, scientific and evidence-based, Mirroring the ways in which women's experiences of abuse and oppression have been silenced throughout history, neurocentric approaches to trauma may mean that women's own understandings of violence and its impacts on their lives are subjugated and viewed as less valid or reliable sources of knowledge. Through ignoring the individual and collective knowledges of survivors, and sidelining community-led and grassroots responses to violence in favour of professional expertise, neurocentric understandings of trauma participate in epistemic injustice, whereby survivors experience discrimination and exclusion in knowledge generation (Sweeney et al., 2019, drawing on Fricker, 2007). In addition, the contributions of other sources of knowledge, including social sciences, intersectional feminism and First Nations' perspectives, are minimized, ignored or elevated only when they are positioned alongside neuroscientific expertise. Indeed, any approach to knowledge-building in trauma that adopts Western perspectives and ignores First Nations' knowledges is very likely to cause further harm and undermine justice (Tudor, 2023).

Women are often told that neuroscientific approaches enable the broader community to take gendered violence more seriously, as the impacts of violence are made more visible through the authority of biological discourses, however this comes at the cost of conceptualizing women's responses to violence in deficit-laden and medicalized language. Here, we see the focus on "fixing" individual women and children, at the expense of collective and politicized perspectives on domestic and family violence, child abuse and sexual assault. Neuroscience informs an approach to working with people that is focused on standardized, "evidence-based" interventions and programs, precluding other forms of support and practical help, which are approaches that do not hold as much status because they are not so easily measured (Wastell & White, 2012). Standardized interventions often cement the status quo, by concealing power relations such as patriarchy, positioning individuals who have survived violence as problematic, and focusing on the development of therapeutic "techniques" and clinical competencies (Birnbaum, 2019). While we recognize that knowledge of brain-based processes is not irrelevant to developing a comprehensive approach to trauma, the current preoccupation with a neurocentric perspective on trauma reinforces a hierarchical approach to knowledge production, whereby certain forms of knowledge are privileged much more than others. This encourages a reliance upon highly reductionist explanations of trauma. Ultimately, our concern lies in the potential for neurocentric and biomedical knowledge production to lead us away from the social conditions that give rise to despair and suffering. In her work on depression among women, Lafrance (2014) argued that the "hegemony of the biomedical model can be understood as less a matter of 'truth' than of power" (p. 141). Just as we argue here about authoritative biomedical truth claims about trauma, she notes biomedical explanations are rarely enough.

*The Body Keeps the Score*, van der Kolk's often-cited book, emphasizes the body's responses to trauma (2014). Along with Herman, his work may be among the more nuanced efforts, acknowledging the complex relationship between the mind, body, emotion, lived experience and social life. While van der Kolk is unabashedly critical of the efforts of the *Diagnostic and Statistical Manual of Mental Disorders* (DSM) to produce endless diagnoses of responses to trauma, most specifically "Borderline Personality Disorder" (Herman, Perry, & van der Kolk, 1989; van der Kolk, 2014), he nonetheless proposes his own preferred diagnosis – Developmental Trauma Disorder (DTD), which the DSM rejected.

Even when the approach seeks to acknowledge nuanced interconnections between the body, the individual and social life, the narrowing process of science that Herman (1997) refers to seems inescapable in the current sociopolitical landscape. The body as a separate and distinct entity is too often the common takeaway from van der Kolk's work. He asserts the significance of polyvagal theory for trauma work and the popular uptake of his work overdetermines its importance. While emotion has corresponding biochemical responses, like the body, emotion is always in the grip of culture and thus so is experience. The meaning-making process of safety and connection in relation to trauma cannot be reduced to polyvagal theory.

In fairness to van der Kolk, he is saying much more, but his ideas about polyvagal theory are compelling to those who find neuroscience and biomedical frameworks both convincing and conclusive. Popular writing, such as *The Grieving Brain* (O'Connor, 2022), draws on MRI brain imaging as neuroscientific evidence of how grief works. Others argue polyvagal theory oversimplifies complex issues, and that it does not have significant research support. Martin (2023) notes that polyvagal theory "offers uncertain science in the name of self-help" and that these contemporary neuroscience books "oversimplify and overstate" the importance of neuroscience. She reports that many researchers now claim the vagal nerve theory itself holds little merit.

It seems the material discursive approach that has been advanced by feminists critiquing "madness" and the "medicalization of misery" is useful here (Ussher, 2010, 2011b). A material discourse approach has been offered as an alternative to the two culturally competing discourses of either the dominant biochemical or women's live approach (Lafrance, 2007; Lafrance & Stoppard, 2007; Stoppard, 2000). This alternative avoids the body/mind or individual/society binaries, suggesting that all human experience is a complex biopsychosocial phenomenon that "involves experiences grounded in the materiality of the body which continually, and reciprocally, feed back into people's experiences in the social context of their everyday lives" (Stoppard, 2000, p. 21). From this perspective the discursive construction of meaning and women's embodied experiences are taken as inseparable from the circumstances of their lives.

It is our view that the body indeed speaks, but its stories are messy, and involve pain and suffering as people seek to make meaning from experiences that often feel incomprehensible and sometimes unmanageable. We cannot overlook the co-existence of normalizing social practices, which demand a heightened self-surveillance and compliance to a regulated, controlled, managed self. Gaining regulatory control over the body is tied to gaining control over the self. Arguably gaining regulatory control over the body has taken over the therapeutic milieu. The lure of science, like that of diagnoses, is rooted in unquestioned epistemic privilege, detached from the context of people's lives (Lafrance & McKenzie-Mohr, 2013; Strong, 2012; Szasz, 1970).

## Dominant Trauma Discourse: The Influence of Postfeminism, Neoliberalism and Biomedicalism

Postfeminism is not simply a backlash. It is *"a sensibility* characterized by a set of entangled and contradictory feminist and anti-feminist discourses about feminism and femininity" (Adamson, 2017, p. 315). Together, these discourses shape who women want to be and who they are expected to be. "What makes a postfeminist sensibility quite different from both prefeminist constructions of gender or feminist ones is that it is clearly a response to feminism" (Gill, 2008, p. 442). Feminist ideas are not used to advance the feminist cause, but to celebrate a rhetoric of individuality, individual choice and freedom (Chen, 2013; McRobbie, 2007) without attention to issues of power or oppression. Within a postfeminist, neoliberal era, we need to resist this discourse. This is particularly important when we think about how to best understand the political construction of gendered violence and trauma and its effects. Additionally, this discursive resistance is critically central to trauma-based work if we wish to disrupt the medicalization of women's misery and suffering (Francis 2012a, 2012b; Francis & Widiger, 2012; Gavey & Schmidt, 2011; Lafrance & McKenzie-Mohr, 2013; Marecek & Gavey, 2013; McKenzie-Mohr & Lafrance, 2011; Moulding, 2015; Penfold & Walker, 1983; Ross, Brown, C., & Johnstone, 2023; Teghtsoonian, 2009; Tseris, 2019c, 2019d, 2019e; Ussher, 1991, 2005, 2010, 2011a, 2011b; Webster & Dunn, 2005; Wunke, 2016). Many have rejected the use of diagnosis, pathologization, psychiatrization and the authorative use of the DSM (Becker & Lamb, 1994; Brown, C., 2020b; Brown, C., Johnstone, & Ross, 2021; Brown, P., 1995; Burstow, 1992, 2003; Burstow & Weitz, 1988; Caplan, 1987, 1995; Capponi, 1992; Cermele, Daniels, & Anderson, 2001; Chesler, 1972; Foucault, 1964; LeFrancois, Menzies, & Reaume, 2013; Penfold & Walker,1983; Smith & David, 1975; Strong, 2012; Szasz, 1961, 1970).

Feminist approaches view the self as influenced by the social world, whereas postfeminist approaches center on the success and ability of individual women, while applauding "individuality". Postfeminist sensibility and neoliberalism stress discourses of freedom, choice, agency and feeling good about oneself. The ideal image of women is of the empowered, assertive, pleasure-seeking, "have-it-all", "can do", "never stopping", "bounce-backable" women with sexual and financial agency (Chen 2013, p. 441; Gill, 2008).

Despite a growth of trauma-awareness, trauma-based services and programming are inadequately resourced and the system is increasingly minimized and individualized. Taken in tandem, in the context of neoliberalism, there has been a dissolution of the welfare state and corresponding intensification of fiscal constraints and limited community resources (Brown, C., Johnstone, Ross, & Doll, 2022; Ferguson & Lavalette, 2013). "Feminism is under siege" according to Carrington (2016), who explores the impact of neoliberalism and managerialism on feminist practice. A focus on biomedical discourse and the lack of focus on the sociopolitical context of women's lives, produce a decontextualized and depoliticized focus on the individual. While those experiencing trauma often feel hopeless, vulnerable and out of control, those who work with trauma feel increasingly desperate as they struggle to find the time and resources they need to do this work. Morley and Dunstan (2016) note that neoconservative or neoliberal governments have degendered and depoliticized domestic violence in Australia, often defunding feminist services and viewing this as a privatized relationship problem rather than a broad sociopolitical patriarchal issue. They argue that practitioners need to adopt a "personal is political" approach, which includes a feminist structural analysis and reflection on how to create broader social change through education and policy development.

The constrained welfare state and its associated managerialized and rationalized service provision often produces a sense of moral distress (Brown, C., Johnstone, & Ross, 2021; Spolander et al., 2014; Yip, 2004). Managerialism refers to a type of management where labor is reduced and simplified to enable ongoing control over labor costs with an emphasis on cost and time efficiency in the delivery of work/services (Johnstone, Brown, C., & Ross, 2022). Management controls the work process, reducing the power and responsibility of workers, resulting in the deskilling of workers and the reconceptualization of their work (Arnfjord & Hiybsgiidm, 2015; Baines, Clarke, & Bennett, 2022; Brown, C., Johnstone, Ross, & Doll, 2022; Brown, C., Doll, Baines, & Johnstone, 2024, under review; Baines, Brown, C., & Cabahug, 2024; Johnstone, Brown, C., & Ross, 2022).

Neoliberal capitalist economic policy is reflected in the ongoing dismantling of the welfare state in the current managerialist mental health service provision whereby individuals can no longer expect that the state will provide for their mental health needs. The entrenched policy of fiscal constraint is evidenced by rationalized health care costs and skeletal mental health service provision, now based primarily in surveillance and coercion, with little understanding of the complexity of mental health issues (Spark, 2020). The hegemony of the biomedical perspective reinforces the dominance of medical professionals in team-based care and the concomitant medical model (Brown, C., 2022; Brown, C., Johnstone, Ross, & Doll, 2022; Mahboube, Talebi, Porouhan, Orak, & Farahani, 2019; Migotto et al., 2019; Nathan & Webber, 2010). The convergence of the twin prevailing discourses of neoliberalism and biomedicalism represent an epistemic injustice through their invisibilizing of the social influences on mental health. Fricker (2003, 2007) identifies unquestioned hegemonic views as a form of epistemic injustice that obscures and delegitimizes alternative interpretations. Alternative interpretations that center of social context and meaning, and on significant critiques of the psychiatrization and medicalization of social life through the emphasis on diagnosis, pathologization and labeling have significantly less power and authority. Alongside the dominance of the biomedical model is the mutually reinforcing claim of objectivity and emphasis on evidence-based practice (Bullen, Deane, Meissel, & Bhatnager, 2020; Webb, 2001). Yet, the argument that biomedical models are objective and evidence-based obscures the political positions they support, and reinforces and renders invisible alternative views.

## Self-management and Disciplinary Practices of Power

The cultural imperative of self-management reflects a normative cultural expectation that individuals discipline and control themselves. The discursive shift of postfeminist neoliberalism "call[s] into being a subject who is compelled and encouraged to conform to the norms of the market while assuming responsibility for her own well-being" (Rottenberg, 2014, p. 426). The recovery movement was once a progressive reflection of the mental health consumer/survivor movement. Today the notion of recovery has been co-opted and reconfigured by the new focus on self-management and the alignment of self-help with positive psychology, the celebration of the individual and neoliberalism (McWade, 2016; Rose, 2014). Not surprisingly, the popularity of positive psychology today corresponds with the legitimation of individualism (Cabanas, 2018).

Recovery is associated with the responsibilization of the individual through successful self-management (Scott & Wilson, 2011). This focus on *responsibilization* is characteristic of the psychological project of neoliberalism: the self-sufficient individual without much need for external social support or resources in a diminished welfare state (Brown, C., 2019; Pyysiinen, Halpin, & Guilfoyle, 2017; Shamir, 2008). Resilience is part of the current gendered, classed and racialized regulatory ideal and is demanded and promoted by public policy in the context of austerity and worsening inequality (Morrow & Weisser, 2012). The resilient individual is encouraged to reveal their psychological efforts as evidence of their resilience or that they are "bounce-backable" subjects (Gill & Orgad, 2018). Garrett (2016) questions the neoliberal reasoning that constructs resilience as "ordinary magic" and a lack of resilience as individual failure, rather than social inequity, social injustice and the need for social transformation (Gill & Orgad, 2018; Morrow & Weisser, 2012; Schraff, 2016). In this process the sociocultural and political contexts of individuals lives are invisibilized.

Not only does neoliberalism emphasize market rationality located in regulatory and state structures, it also emphasizes a corresponding ideal citizen (Braedley & Luxton, 2010; Lemke, 2001). This mechanism of power works by encouraging individual participation and belief in their responsibility by focusing on disciplinary practices which emphasize self-care, self-improvement and misleading notions of choice and resilience (Brown, C., 2007b, 2014, 2022). The social message widely circulated is that practices of self are freely chosen individual preferences, without questioning the sociopolitical regulation that shapes self-surveillance, self-monitoring and self-discipline (Chen, 2013). "Indeed it is not simply that subjects are governed, disciplined or regulated in ever more intimate ways, but even more fundamental that notions of choice, agency and autonomy have become central to the regulatory project" (Gill, 2008, p. 444).

Foucault (1980b) refers to the docile body, or social practices in which "individuals participate in normalizing and disciplinary practices of self, wherein we turn ourselves into subjects, absorbed by improvement, management and performance of self" (Brown, 2014, p. 176). People are then active in the creation of themselves, but not always in a way that benefits them – believing this is choice, not regulation. But our stories of self are creations that can encourage or limit self-agency, and thus these stories may be helpful, hurtful or both. A critical approach to understanding violence and trauma must ensure that we are not reinforcing these social mechanisms of power through essentialist notions of the self.

In the analysis of the influence of dominant social discourses of neoliberalism and biomedicalism we can see how humans govern and regulate themselves and others through the production of truth. According to Foucault, "We are subjected to the production of truth through power and we cannot exercise power except through the production of truth" (Foucault, 1980a, p. 93). Following Foucault, White and Epston (1990, p. 19) argue that "We are subject to power through the normalizing 'truths' that shape our lives and relationships". For Foucault (1972), knowledge and power are joined through discourses, which are social "practices that systematically form the objects of which they speak" (p. 49). Knowledge and power are viewed as inseparable whereby "a domain of knowledge is a domain of power, and a domain of power is a domain of knowledge" (White & Epston, 1990, p. 22).

Importantly, while power and knowledge imply each other they cannot be reduced to each other, as knowledge is not simply an instrument of power. As such, challenge and resistance to dominant discourse can be created (Butler, J., 1997). Judith Butler suggests that while choices are constrained, resistance is always possible (1997). The reflexivity necessary for social justice-based theory and practice challenges both what we think we know and how we practice (Chambon, 1999; Fook, 2016). The production of transformative critical knowledge disturbs or disrupts normalizing truths, as does the narrative process of unpacking and resisting the influence of dominant discourse on people's lives. Feminist narrative therapy is then a social justice-rooted political activity that challenges the normalizing truths constituting people's lives and critically uncovers techniques of power that subjugate people to a dominant ideology (Brown, C., 2007a; Foucault, 1980b; White 2001, 2007).

## Normalizing Processes of Self and the Regulating Project

Socially constructed notions of emotion are connected to these practices of self. The "self is a vehicle of power in which individuals enact and reify culturally encoded normative practices of self" (Brown, C., 2014, p. 176). The emotional expressions of self are seen to be individual and freely chosen and, yet, co-exist with self-surveillance, self-monitoring and self-discipline (Chen, 2013). "Indeed, it is not simply that subjects are governed, disciplined or regulated in ever more intimate ways, but even more fundamental that notions of choice, agency and autonomy have become central to the regulatory project" (Gill, 2008, p. 444).

The emotional experience within stories is not separate from the psychological or social world. Emotional experiences deepen the sense of meaning, possibility and danger in stories and how we live them. The social construction of emotion is a central ingredient to individual participation in self-discipline and self-regulation. Engaging in these self-management practices requires ongoing self-surveillance and is often motivated by how one expects to benefit from doing so. Participation in self-management reifies the sense the that one has choice, agency and autonomy and produces a sense of satisfaction with perceiving oneself to be in control of oneself and one's life. This sense of mastery is reflected in a series of symbolic metaphors. One is valued, for instance, for being attractive, fit and professionally successful. Intersubjectively shared meaning circulating the message that mastery and self-regulation represent individual choice, capacity, power and freedom is a powerfully effective way of encouraging individuals' participation in capitalist and patriarchal norms. The power of social control is strengthened and reinforced through collective participation that, taken together, uphold the values, assumptions and regulatory discourse, practices and policies.

## Self-management Discourse, Emotional Regulation and Neoliberalism

Dominant discourse renders invisible the social and political context of emotion as the focus remains on the individual. As "emotional life is in the grip of cultural practice" (Brown, C., 2019, p. 158), it "is not subjectively innocent" (Brown, C., 2022, p. 7). There is a need to both recognize and understand how we are simultaneously emotionally embodied cognitive subjects and that emotions are always social things. As such, emotions are socially constituted (Ahmed, 2004a, 2004b; Turner, 2009).

The dominant culture of self-management shapes the expectations and performance of emotion management. Emotions are expected to be tightly controlled within neoliberal emotional regimes. Ahmed's (2004a, 2004b) view that emotions are cultural practices leads her to ask: "what do emotions do?" (p. 4). The emotional threads of trauma are inseparable from the meaning we associate with lived events. According to Ahmed (2004a), "emotions 'matter' for politics; emotions show us how power shapes the very surface of bodies as well as worlds. So in a way, we do 'feel our way'" (p. 12). Once we enter the realm of meaning-making, we are in the social realm, and, thereby, the political. As we seek to make sense or meaning of our life experiences, we necessarily move beyond a one-dimensional notion of emotional embodiment that results in the essentialism of emotion, and enter the cultural politics of emotion experienced in daily life. We need to be aware of the co-existing impact of social regulatory influence and individual agency in how people make meaning of their trauma stories (Foucault, 1980a, 1980b, 1991, 1995). In trauma stories we need to be conscious of disrupting the unhelpful influence of individual choice, self-management and responsibilization, which currently fail to situate trauma stories within a social and political context, and which devalue messiness, complexity and sitting with distress, in favor of technical, "fixing" approaches.

## Counterviewing Dominant Discourse

Dominant social discourses often shape people's stories of experience and can contribute to unhelpful and oppressive identity conclusions. Feminist narrative approaches see people's stories as socially constructed within existing social relations and available social discourses.

There is little doubt that women's trauma stories are constrained by the limited discourses available to them that fit well with their experiences. According to Judith Butler (1997), the coercive effect of dominant discourse produces injurious speech as it constrains not only what can be said, but by whom and to whom. Dominant discursive frameworks often represent *epistemic gaps which produce epistemic injustice* (Fricker, 2003, 2007). Where there is power, however, there is often resistance (Foucault, 1980a, 1980b). Resisting the dominant discursive constructions on violence and trauma simultaneously resists neoliberal mechanism of power. It is important, then, that we engage in discursive resistance in the mainstreaming of trauma-informed discourse (Brown, C., 2022).

## Counterstorying the Impact of Trauma –
## Social Justice Trauma-based Care

We need to challenge an individual and medicalizing approach to violence and trauma and recognize that trauma is political (Brown, C., Johnstone, Ross, & Doll, 2022; Burstow, 2003). Narrative therapeutic conversations focus on meaning-making which is viewed as both social and political. "Counterviewing solicits counterstories that disrupt and challenge unhelpful dominant social discourses which reinforce social inequity and oppression. Counternarratives resist the discursive power mechanisms within stories and disrupt their hegemony" (Brown, C., 2022, p. 3). Through double listening, listening beyond the words, we can unpack injurious speech and the political and social context in which they emerge (Brown, C., 2019, Madigan 2003; White, 2000, 2001, 2004, 2007). Counterviewing questions about trauma offer potentially new entry points in therapeutic conversations (Brown, C., 2019; Madigan 2003) that shift stories away from individual blame and pathology to understanding people's coping responses and how they make sense. Counterviewing questions can facilitate greater depth and specificity to the meaning, experience and context of trauma and coping. Trauma work necessarily appreciates how dangerous it often is to tell unspeakable trauma stories in a social context that minimizes, blames and encourages silence. A strong, collaborative, therapeutic alliance can support the process of storying and counterstorying experiences of trauma (Brown, C., 2022).

We need to change how people who experience the burden of trauma are too often held responsible for not just the trauma but for the expectation they "recover" with inadequate available resources. Resistance to gender expectation and counterstorying co-occurring trauma, depression and anxiety appears to be central in reducing and managing traumatic aftermath. While the idea of resilience appears on the surface to emphasize choice, strengths and empowerment, a deeper reading of its neoliberal cultural uptake suggests that it obscures inequalities, violence, injuries and injustice.

To reduce trauma and stress experienced in childhood and throughout the lifespan, cultural and structural changes are necessary to challenge the dominant discourses that "normalize" violence, provide education and build the capacity of communities to define and solve problems (Gavey & Schmidt, 2011; Wunke, 2016). Research on trauma and violence points to the need for awareness of intergenerational trauma (Matz, Vogel, Mattar, & Montenegro, 2015; Wiesel, 2006) and intergenerational healing within families and communities and recommends engaging with communities to learn what is most relevant to them to generate new cultural norms that mirror the values and aspirations that community members have for their children (Porter, Martin, & Anda, 2017; Sheppard, 2016). Violence, trauma and intergenerational trauma, in particular among First Nations and African Canadians, must also be addressed (Bombay, Matheson, & Anisman, 2009; Brownridge, 2003; Culhane, 2003; Denham, 2008; Menzies, 2008; Waldron, 2021). We need to resist the neoliberal psychological and biomedical turn if we wish to advance a social justice approach to mental health and trauma.

We know that many experience complex trauma in their lives, face extreme social and economic disadvantage, and/or struggle with co-occurring mental health and substance-use issues, which often require more extensive supports and the building of a trusting therapeutic relationship or community development approaches (Brown, V., Huba, & Melchior, 1995). We need to provide mental health care that addresses struggles that often arise in tandem from the combination of adverse life experiences, such as trauma and relational injury, alongside marginalization, oppression and inequity (Brown, C. & MacDonald, 2022; Sangalang & Vang, 2017). The critical thought of Black feminists (Collins, 2000a, 2000b, 2007, 2015; Crenshaw, 1989; hooks, 1990, 2000; Jordan-Zachery, 2007; Lorde, 1984; Waldron, 2021), Indigenous (Baskin & Davey, 2017; Bombay, Matheson, & Anisman 2014; Baikie, 2020), lesbian (Brown, L., 1988; Brown, L. & Root, 1990; Butler, J., 1997, 2010, 2011; Kopelson, 2002) and (dis)Ability activists and writers have provided an important foundation for intersectional critical analysis (Brown, C. & MacDonald, 2022; Carter, Hanes, & MacDonald, 2017; Chapman,

2022; Garland-Thompson, 2005; Hanes, Carter, & MacDonald, 2022; MacDonald, 2020; MacDonald, Brown, & Jones, 2022; Meyer, 2002; Tseris, 2019a).

## Conclusion

We have argued that the current rationalized approach to mental health service delivery is often based on an individualized approach that is too narrowly focused and time-limited to allow for the development of the strong therapeutic alliance or community development approaches needed to adequately address the level of distress and suffering, material needs and social justice needs that arise within the conditions of violence and mental health inequity.

With growing social inequities and injustices in society, there is now an even greater need to intentionally advocate for and adopt critical social justice practices (Brown, C., 2020a; Brown, C., Johnstone, & Ross, 2021; Brown, C. & Macdonald, 2020; Pease, Goldingay, Hosken, & Nipperess, 2016; Morrow & Weisser, 2012; Weisser, Morrow, & Jamer, 2011). Moving forward we need to resist co-optation into neoliberal constructions of service provision (e.g., biomedicalization, pathologization, individualization, responsibilization, privatization) (Brown, C., Johnstone, Ross, & Doll, 2022; Johnstone, Brown & Ross, 2022; Ross, Brown, C., & Johnstone, 2022; Nathan & Webber, 2010; Wallace & Pease, 2011). On the whole, dominant postfeminist neoliberal discourse is at odds with a social justice approach to trauma and its effects on mental health and substance use (Brown, C., Johnstone, & Ross, 2021; Johnstone, 2021).

## References

Adamson, M. (2017). Postfeminism, neoliberalism, and a "successfully" balanced femininity in celebrity CEO autobiographies. *Gender, Work and Organization*, 24(3), 314–327.

Ahmed, S. (2004a). *The cultural politics of emotion*. Edinburgh University Press.

Ahmed, S. (2004b) Affective economies. *Social Text*, 79, 22(2), 117–139.

Anda, R., Felitti, V., Bremner, J., Walker, J., Whitfield, C., Perry, B., et al. (2006).The enduring effects of abuse and related adverse experiences in childhood. A convergence of evidence from neurobiology and epidemiology. *European Archives of Psychiatry and Clinical Neuroscience*, 256(3), 174–186. https://doi.org/10.1007/s00406-005 -0624-4 PMID:16311898.

Armstrong, L. (1978). *Kiss daddy goodnight*. Hawthorn.

Arnfjord, S. & Hiybsgiidm, L. (2015). Problems of professional disempowerment: An initial study of social work conditions in Greenland. *Intersectionalities: A Global Journal of Social Work Analysis, Research, Polity, and Practice*, (4)1, 40–58.

Baikie, G. (2020). (De)Colonizing Indigenous social work within the borderlands. In C. Brown & J. Macdonald (Eds.), *Critical clinical social work. Counterstorying for social justice* (pp. 328–340). Canadian Scholars Press.

Baines, D., Bennett, B., Goodwin, S., & Rawsthorne, M. (Eds.) (2019). *Working across difference. Social work, social policy, and social justice* (pp. 247–260). Red Globe Press.

Baines, D., Brown, C., & Cabahug, F. (2024). The shifting labour process in professional care: Recreating dominance and the managerialised mental health social worker. *The British Journal of Social Work.* 1(54), 475–493. https://doi.org/10.1093/bjsw/bcad210.

Baines, D., Clarke, N., & Bennett, B. (Eds.) (2022). *Doing anti-oppressive social work. Rethinking theory and practice* (4th ed.). Fernwood.

Baines, D., & Waugh, F. (2019). Afterword: Resistance, white fragility and late neo-liberalism. In D. Baines, B. Bennett, S. Goodwin, & M. Rawsthorne (Eds.), *Working across difference. Social work, social policy, and social justice* (pp. 247–260). Red Globe Press.

Barker, M. (2013) New femininities: Postfeminism, neoliberalism and subjectivity. *Psychology & Sexuality,* 4(3), 323–325.

Baskin, C., & Davey, C. (2017). Parallel pathways to decolonization: Critical and Indigenous social work. In S. Wehbi & H. Parada (Eds.), *Reimagining anti-oppression social work practice* (pp. 3–16). Canadian Scholars Press.

Bass, E., & Davis, L. (1988). *The courage to heal. A guide for women survivors of child sexual abuse.* Harper and Row.

Bass, E., & Davis, L. (1990). *Beginning to heal. First book for survivors of child sexual abuse.* Harper Perennial.

Becker, D., & Lamb, S. (1994). Sex bias in the diagnosis of borderline personality disorder and posttraumatic stress disorder. *Professional Psychology: Research and Practice,* 25(1), 55–61.

Birnbaum, S. (2019). Confronting the social determinants of health: Has the language of trauma informed care become a defense mechanism? *Issues in Mental Health Nursing,* 40(6), 476–481.

Bombay, A., Matheson, K., & Anisman, H. (2009). Intergenerational trauma: Convergence of multiple processes among First Nations peoples in Canada. *International Journal of Indigenous Health,* 5(3), 6–47.

Bombay, A., Matheson, K., & Anisman, H. (2014). The intergenerational effects of Indian Residential Schools: Implications for the concept of historical trauma. *Transcultural Psychiatry,* 51(3), 320–338. https://journals.sagepub.com/doi/abs/10.1177/1363461513503380.

Braedley, S., & Luxton, M. (2010). Competing philosophies. Neo-liberalism and challenges of everyday life. In S. Braedley & M. Luxton (Eds.), *Neo-liberalism and everyday life* (pp. 3–21). McGill-Queen's University Press.

Brown, C. (2007a). Dethroning the suppressed voice: Unpacking experience as story. In C. Brown & T. Augusta-Scott (Eds.), *Narrative therapy. Making meaning, making lives* (pp.177–196). Sage.

Brown, C. (2007b). Discipline and desire: Regulating the body/self. In C. Brown & T. Augusta-Scott (Eds.), *Narrative therapy. Making meaning, making lives* (pp. 105–131). Sage.

Brown, C. (2007c). Feminist therapy, violence, problem drinking and re-storying women's lives: Reconceptualizing anti-oppressive feminist therapy. In D. Baines (Ed.). *Doing anti-oppressive practice: Building transformative, politicized social work* (pp.128–144). Fernwood Press.

Brown, C. (2007d). Situating knowledge and power in the therapeutic alliance. In C. Brown & T. Augusta-Scott (Eds.), *Narrative therapy. Making meaning, making lives* (pp. 3–22). Sage.

Brown, C. (2007e). Talking body talk: Blending feminist and narrative approaches to practice. In C. Brown & T. Augusta-Scott (Eds.), *Narrative therapy. Making meaning, making lives* (pp. 269–302). Sage.

Brown, C. (2011). Reconceptualizing feminist therapy: Violence, problem drinking and re-storying women's lives. In D. Baines (Ed.). *Doing anti-oppressive practice: Building transformative, politicized social work* (2nd ed.) (pp. 95–115). Fernwood Press.

Brown, C. (2012). Anti-oppression through a postmodern lens: Dismantling the master's tools. *Critical Social Work*, 3(1), 34–65.

Brown, C. (2013). Women's narratives of trauma: (Re)storying uncertainty, minimization and self-blame. *Narrative Works: Issues, Investigations & Interventions*, 3(1), 1–30.

Brown, C. (2014). Untangling emotional threads, self-management discourse and women's body talk. In M. LaFrance & S. McKenzie-Mohr (Eds.), *Women voicing resistance. Discursive and narrative explorations* (pp. 174–190). Routledge.

Brown, C. (2017). Creating counterstories: Critical clinical practice and feminist narrative therapy. In D. Baines (Ed.), *Doing anti-oppressive practice: Building transformative, politicized social work* (3rd ed.) (pp. 212–232). Fernwood Press.

Brown, C. (2018). The dangers of trauma talk: Counterstorying co-occurring strategies for coping with trauma. *Journal of Systemic Therapies*, 37(3), 38–55.

Brown, C. (2019). Speaking of women's depression and the politics of emotion. *Affilia: Journal of Women and Social Work*, 34(2), 151–169.

Brown, C. (2020a). Critical clinical social work: Theoretical and practical considerations. In C. Brown & J. MacDonald (Eds.), *Critical clinical social work: Counterstorying for social justice* (pp. 16–58). Canadian Scholars Press.

Brown, C. (2020b). Feminist narrative therapy and complex trauma: Critical clinical work with women diagnosed as "borderline". In C. Brown & J. MacDonald (Eds.), *Critical clinical social work: Counterstorying for social justice* (pp. 82–109). Canadian Scholars Press.

Brown, C. (2021). Critical clinical social work and the neoliberal constraints on social justice in mental health. Special Issue on Social Justice. *Research on Social Work Practice*, 1–9. doi: 0.1177/1049731520984531.

Brown, C. (2022). Postmodern theory: The case of narrative theory in social work. In R. Hugman, D. Holscher, & D. McAuliffe (Eds.), *Social work theory and ethics* (pp. 79–100). Springer.

Brown, C., & Augusta-Scott, T. (Eds.) (2007). *Narrative therapy. Making meaning, making lives*. Sage.

Brown, C., & Augusta-Scott, T. (2018). Reimagining the intersection of gender, knowledge and power in collaborative therapeutic conversations with women and eating disorders and men who use violence. In D. Pare & C. Audet (Eds.), *Social justice and narrative therapy* (pp.143–158). Routledge.

Brown, C., Doll, K., Baines, D., & Johnstone, M. (2024). All dressed up and nowhere to go: The impact of neoliberalism on social justice-based scope of practice with mental health and substance use. *Canadian Review of Social Work*.

Brown, C., Johnstone, M., & Ross, N. (2021). Repositioning social work practice in mental health in Nova Scotia. Report. Nova Scotia College of Social Workers. https://nscsw.org/wp-content/uploads/2021/01/NSCSW-Repositioning-Social-Work-Practice-in-Mental-Health-in-Nova-Scotia-Report-2021.pdf.

Brown, C., Johnstone, M., Ross, N., & Doll, K. (2022). Challenging the constraints of neoliberalism and biomedicalism: Repositioning social work in mental health. *Qualitative Health Research*, 32(5), 771–787. https://doi.org/10.1177/10497323211069681.

Brown, C., & Macdonald, J. (Eds.) (2020). *Critical clinical social work: Counterstorying for social justice.* Canadian Scholars Press.

Brown, C., & Macdonald, J. (2022). Critical clinical social work. Working in the context of trauma and (dis)Ability. In D. Baines (Ed.), *Doing anti-oppressive practice: Building transformative, politicized social work* (4th ed.). Fernwood Press.

Brown, C., & Stewart, S. (2021). Harm reduction for women in treatment for alcohol use problems: Exploring the impact of dominant addiction discourse on policy and practice. *Qualitative Health Research*, 31(1), 54–69.

Brown, L. (1988). From perplexity to complexity: Thinking about ethics in the lesbian therapy community. *Women & Therapy*, 8, 13–26.

Brown, L. (1992). A feminist critique of personality disorders. In L.S. Brown & M. Ballou (Eds.), *Personality and psychopathology: Feminist reappraisals* (pp. 206–228). Guilford Press.

Brown, L. (2004). Feminist paradigms of trauma treatment. *Psychotherapy: Theory, Research, Practice, Training*, 41(4), 464–471.

Brown, L., & Root, M. (Eds.) (1990). *Diversity and complexity in feminist therapy.* Routledge.

Brown, P. (1995). Naming and framing: The social construction of diagnosis and illness. *Journal of Health and Social Behavior, Suppl. Extra Issue: Forty Years of Bio-medical Sociology*, 34–52.

Brown, V., Huba, G., & Melchior, L. (1995). Level of burden: Women with more than one co-occurring disorder. *Journal of Psychoactive Drugs*, 27, 339–346.

Brownmiller, S. (1975). *Against our will: Men, women, and rape.* Simon and Schuster.

Brownridge, D. (2003). Male partner violence against aboriginal women in Canada. An empirical analysis. *Journal of Interpersonal Violence*, 18(1), 65–83.

Bruner, J. (1991). The narrative construction of reality. *Critical Inquiry*, (Fall), 1–21.

Bullen, P., Deane, K., Meissel, K., & Bhatnager, S. (2020). What constitutes lobalized evidence? Cultural tensions and critical reflections of the evidence-based movement in New Zealand. *International Journal of Psychology*, 55(1), 16–25.

Burstow, B. (1992). *Radical feminist therapy: Working in the context of violence.* Sage.

Burstow, B. (2003). Toward a radical understanding of trauma and trauma work. *Violence Against Women*, 9(11), 1293–1317.

Burstow, B., & Weitz, D. (1988). *Shrink resistant. The struggle against psychiatry in Canada.* New Star Books.

Butler, J. (1997). *Excitable speech: A politics of the performative.* Routledge.

Butler, J. (2010). Performative agency. *Journal of Cultural Economy*, 3(2), 147–161. doi: 10.1080/17530350.2010.494117.

Butler, J. (2011). *Bodies that matter: On the discursive limits of sex.* Taylor & Francis.

Butler, S. (1978). *The conspiracy of silence. The trauma of incest.* Volcano Press.

Cabanas, E. (2018). Positive psychology and the legitimation of individualism. *Theory & Psychology*, 28(1) 3–19. https://doi.org/10.1177/0959354317747988.

Cambron, C., Gringeri, C., & Vogel-Ferguson, M.B. (2015). Adverse childhood experiences, depression and mental health barriers to work among low-income women. *Social Work in Public Health*, 30(6), 504–515. https://www.tandfonline.com/doi/abs/10.1080/19371918.2015.1073645.

Caplan, P. (1987). The psychiatric association's failure to meet its own standards: The dangers of self-defeating personality disorder as a category. *Journal of Personality Disorders*, 1(2), 178–182.

Caplan, P. (1995). How do they decide who is normal? In *They say you're crazy. How the world's most powerful psychiatrists decide who's normal* (pp. 1–32). Addison-Wesley.

Capponi, P. (1992). *Upstairs in the crazy house. The life of a psychiatric survivor.* Viking.

Carney, T. (2008). The mental health service crisis of neoliberalism – An Antipodean perspective. *International Journal of Law and Psychiatry,* 31, 101–115.

Carrington, A. (2016). Feminism under siege: Critical reflections on the impact of neoliberalism and managerialism for feminist practice. In B. Pease, S. Goldingay, N. Hosken, & S. Nipperess (Eds.), *Doing critical social work. Transformative practices for social justice* (pp. 226–240). Allen and Unwin.

Carter, I., Hanes, R., & MacDonald, J.E. (2017). Beyond the social model of disability: Engaging in anti-oppressive social work practice. In D. Baines (Ed.), *Doing anti-oppressive practice: Social justice social work* (3rd ed.) (pp. 153–171). Canadian Scholars Press.

Cermele, J., Daniels, S., & Anderson, K. (2001). Defining normal: Constructions of race and gender in the DSM-IV Casebook. *Feminism & Psychology,* 11(2), 229–247.

Chambon, A. (1999). Foucault's approach: Making the familiar visible. In A. Chambon, A. Irving, and L. Epstein (Eds.), *Reading Foucault for social work.* Columbia University Press.

Chapman, C. (2022). Disability studies insights for critical social work. In S.S. Shaikh, B. LeFrançois, & T. Macías (Eds.), *Critical social work praxis* (pp. 432–442). Fernwood.

Chapman, D.P., Whitfield, C.L., Felitti, V.J., Dube, S.R., Edwards, V.J., & Anda, R.F. (2004). Adverse childhood experiences and the risk of depressive disorders in adulthood. *Journal of Affective Disorders,* 82(2), 217–225. https://www.sciencedirect.com/science/article/pii/S016503270400028X.

Chen, E. (2013). Neoliberalism and popular women's culture: Rethinking choice, freedom and agency. *European Journal of Cultural Studies,* 16(4), 440–452.

Chesler, P. (1972). *Women & madness.* Avon.

Collins, P.H. (2000a). *Black feminist thought: Knowledge, consciousness and the politics of empowerment* (2nd ed.). Routledge.

Collins, P.H. (2000b). Gender, Black feminism, and Black political economy. *The Annals of the American Academy of Political and Social Science,* 568(4), 41–53.

Collins, P.H. (2007). Black feminist epistemology [1990]. In C.J. Calhoun (Ed.), Contemporary *sociological theory* (p. 327). Blackwell.

Collins, P.H. (2015). Intersectionality's definitional dilemmas. *Annual Review of Sociology,* 41, 1–20. https://www.annualreviews.org/doi/abs/10.1146/annurev-soc-073014-112142.

Courtois, C. (1988). Philosophy, process, and goals of incest therapy. In *Healing the incest wound* (pp. 165–182). W.W. Norton.

Courtois, C. (2004). Complex trauma, complex reactions: Assessment and treatment. *Psychotherapy: Theory, Research, Practice, Training,* 41(4), 412–425.

Crenshaw, K. (1989). Demarginalizing the intersection of race and sex: A Black feminist critique of antidiscrimination doctrine, feminist theory and antiracist politics. *University of Chicago Legal Forum,* 1(8), 139–167.

Culhane, D. (2003). Their spirits live within us. Aboriginal women in downtown Eastside Vancouver emerging into visibility. *American Indian Quarterly,* 27, 593–606.

Denham, A. (2008). Rethinking historical trauma: Narratives of resilience. *Transcultural Psychiatry,* 45(3), 391–414. https://doi.org/10.1177%2F1363461508094673.

DeVault, M.L. (1990). Talking and listening from women's standpoint: Feminist strategies for interviewing and analysis. *Social problems,* 37(1), 96–116. https://academic.oup.com/socpro/article-abstract/37/1/96/1654874.

Doll, K., Brown, C., Johnstone, M., & Ross, N. (2023). Neoliberalism, control of trans and gender diverse bodies and social work. *Journal of Evidence-Focused Social Work*, 20(4), 568–594. doi: 10.1080/26408066.2023.2192707.

Ferguson, I., & Lavalette, M. (2013). Crisis, austerity and the future(s) of social work in the UK. *Critical and Radical Social Work*, 1(1), 95–110.

Fook, J. (2016). *Social work: A critical approach to practice* (3rd ed.). Sage.

Forward, S., & Buck, C. (1988). *Betrayal of innocence: Incest and its devastation*. Penguin Books.

Foucault, M. (1964). *Madness and civilization*. Vintage Books.

Foucault, M. (1972). *The archeology of knowledge and the discourse on language*. Pantheon Books.

Foucault, M. (1980a). *Power/knowledge: Selected interviews and other writings 1972–1977*. Pantheon.

Foucault, M. (1980b). *The history of sexuality. Vol 1. An introduction*. Vintage.

Foucault, M. (1991). Politics and the study of discourse. In G. Burchell, C. Gorden, & P. Miller (Eds.), *The Foucault effect, studies in governmentality* (pp. 53–72). Harvester.

Foucault, M. (1995). Strategies of power. In W. Anderson (Ed.), *The truth about the truth: De- and re-confusing the postmodern world* (pp. 40–45). Tarcher/Putnam.

Francis, A. (2012a). DSM 5 is guide not bible – ignore ten worst changes. APA approval of DSM-5 is a sad day for psychiatry. https://www.psychologytoday.com/blog/dsm5-in-distress/201212/dsm-5-is-guide-not-bible-ignoreits-ten-worst-changes.

Francis, A. (2012b). Two fallacies invalidate the DSM-5 field trials. *Psychology Today*. http://www.psychologytoday.com/blog/dsm5-in-distress/201201/two-fallacies-invalidate-the-dsm-5-field-trials.

Francis, A., & Widiger, T. (2012). Psychiatric diagnosis: Lessons from the DSM-IV past and cautions for the DSM-5 Future. *Annual Review of Clinical Psychology*, 8, 109–130.

Fricker, M. (2003). Epistemic injustice and a role for virtue in the politics of knowing. *Metaphilosophy*, 34, 154–173.

Fricker, M. (2007). *Epistemic justice. Power and the ethics of knowing*. Oxford University Press.

Garland-Thompson, R. (2005). Feminist disability studies. *Signs: Journal of Women in Culture and Society*, 30(2), 1557–1587. http://ezproxy.library.dal.ca/login?url=http://www.jstor.org/stable/10.1086/423352.

Garrett, P.M. (2016). Questioning tales of "ordinary magic": "Resilience" and neo-liberal reasoning. *British Journal of Social Work*, 46, 1909–1925.

Gavey, N., & Schmidt, J. (2011)."Trauma of rape" discourse: A double-edged template for everyday understandings of the impact of rape? *Violence Against Women*, 17(4) 433–456. doi: 10.1177/1077801211404194.

Ghafournia, N. (2019). Pushing back against stereotypes: Muslim immigrant women's experiences of domestic violence. In D. Baines, B. Bennett, S. Goodwin, & M. Rawsthorne (Eds.), *Working across difference. Social work, social policy and social justice* (pp. 71–84). Red Globe Press.

Gill, R. (2008). Culture and subjectivity in neoliberal and postfeminist times. *Subjectivity*, 25, 432–445.

Gill, R., & Orgad, S. (2018). The amazing bounce-backable woman: Resilience and the psychological turn in neoliberalism. *Sociological Research Online*, 23(2), 477–495. https://journals.sagepub.com/doi/abs/10.1177/1360780418769673.

Government of Canada. (2018). Trauma and violence-informed approaches to policy and practice. Ottawa. https://www.canada.ca/en/public-health/services/publications/health -risks-safety/trauma-violence-informed-approaches-policy-practice.html.

Government of Canada. (2020). Federal framework on posttraumatic stress disorder: Recognition, collaboration and support. Ottawa. https://www.canada.ca/en/public -health/services/publications/healthy-living/federal-framework-post-traumatic-stress -disorder.html.

Hanes, R., Carter, I., & MacDonald, J.E. (2022). Getting to the heart of the matter: A social-oppression model of disability. In D. Baines, N. Clark, & B. Bennett (Eds.), *Doing anti-oppressive social work: Rethinking theory and practice* (4th ed.) (pp. 244– 266). Fernwood.

Herman, J. (1981). *Father-daughter incest*. Harvard University Press.

Herman, J. (1992). *Trauma and recovery: The aftermath of violence – From domestic abuse to political terror* (1st ed.). Basic Books.

Herman, J. (1997). *Trauma and recovery: The aftermath of violence – From domestic abuse to political terror* (2nd ed.). Basic Books.

Herman, J. (2015). *Trauma and recovery: The aftermath of violence – From domestic abuse to political terror* (3rd ed.). Basic Books.

Herman, J. (2023). *Truth and repair: How trauma survivors envision justice*. Basic Books.

Herman, J., Perry, C., & van der Kolk, B. (1989). Childhood trauma in borderline personality disorder. *American Journal of Psychiatry*, 146, 490–495.

hooks, b. (1990). Postmodern Blackness. *Postmodern Culture*, 1(1), Johns Hopkins University Press. 10.1353/pmc.1990.0004.

hooks, b. (2000). *Feminist theory: From margin to center*. Pluto Press.

James, W. (1890). *The Principles Of Psychology Volume II By William James (1890)*.

Johnson, H., & Flynn, C. (2021). Collaboration for improving social work practice: The promise of feminist participatory action research. *Affilia*, 36(3), 441–459.

Johnstone, M. (2021). Centering social justice in mental health practice: Epistemic justice, narrative social work and the hermeneutic gap. Special edition in *Research in Social Work Practice*, 31(6), 634–643. https://doi.org/10.1177/10497315211010957.

Johnstone, M., Brown, C., & Ross, N. (2022). The Macdonaldization of social work: A critical analysis of mental health care services using the choice and partnership approach (CAPA) in Canada. *Journal of Progressive Social Services*, 33(3), 223–243. DOI: 10.1080/10428232.2022.2050117.

Jordan-Zachery, J.S. (2007). Am I a Black woman or a woman who is Black? A few thoughts on the meaning of intersectionality. *Politics & Gender*, 3(2), 254–263.

Kagi, R., & Regala, R. (2012). Translating the adverse childhood experiences (ACE) study into public policy: Progress and possibility in Washington State. *Journal of Prevention & Intervention in the Community*, 40(4), 271–277. doi: 10.1080/10852352.2012.707442.

Kopelson, K. (2002). Dis/integrating the gay/queer binary: "Reconstructing identity politics" for a performative pedagogy. *College English*, 65(1), 17–35. http://ezproxy .library.dal.ca/login?url=http://www.jstor.org/stable/3250728.

Lafrance, M. (2007). A bitter pill. A discursive analysis of women's medicalized accounts of depression. *Journal of Health Psychology*, 12, 127–140.

Lafrance, M. (2014). Depression as oppression: Disrupting the biomedical discourse in women's stories of sadness. In S. McKenzie-Mohr & M. Lafrance (Eds.), *Creating counterstories: Women resisting dominant discourses in speaking their lives* (pp. 141– 158). Routledge.

Lafrance, M., & McKenzie-Mohr, S. (2013). The DSM and its lure of legitimacy. *Feminism and Psychology*, 23(1), 119–140.

Lafrance, M., & Stoppard, J. (2007). Re-storying women's depression: A material-discursive approach. In C. Brown & T. Augusta-Scott (Eds.), *Narrative therapy. Making meaning, making lives* (pp. 23–38). Sage.

LeFrancois, B., Menzies, R., & Reaume, G. (Eds.) (2013), *Mad matters. A critical reader in Canadian mad studies*. Canadian Scholars Press.

Lemke, T. (2001). The "birth of bio-politics": Michel Foucault's lecture at the College de France on neo-liberal governmentality. *Economy and Society*, 30(2), 190–207.

Lorde, A. (1984). Age, race, class, and sex: Women redefining difference. In *Sister outside. Essays and speeches* (pp. 114–123). The Crossing Press.

McCall, L. (2005). The complexity of intersectionality. *Signs: Journal of Women in Culture and Society*, 30(3), 1771–1800.

McCann, H., & Sharp, M. (2023). #MeToo, cisheteropatriarchy and LGBTQ+ sexual violence on campus. *Sexualities*. https://doi.org/10.1177/13634607231170770.

MacDonald, J.E., Brown, M., & Jones, S. (2022). Social policy across social identities. In B. MacKenzie & B. Wharf (Eds.), *Connecting policy to practice in the human services* (5th ed.) (pp. 272–290). Oxford University Press.

McKenzie-Mohr, S., & Lafrance, M. (2011). Telling stories without the words: Tightrope talk in women's accounts of coming to live well after rape or depression. *Feminism and Psychology*, 21(1), 49–73.

McKenzie-Mohr, S., & Lafrance, M. (2014). Women's discursive resistance: Attuning to counter-stories and collectivizing for change. In S. McKenzie-Mohr & M. Lafrance (Eds.), *Creating counterstories: Women resisting dominant discourses in speaking their lives* (pp. 191–205). Routledge.

McRobbie, A. (2007). Top girls? *Cultural Studies*, 21(4–5), 718–737.

McWade, B. (2016). Recovery-as-policy as a form of neoliberal state making. *Intersectionalities: A Global Journal of Social Work Analysis, Research, Polity, and Practice*, 5(3) 62–81.

Madigan, S. (2003). Counterviewing injurious speech acts: Destabilizing eight conversational habits of highly effective problems. *International Journal of Narrative Therapy and Community Work*, 1, 43–59.

Mahboube, L., Talebi, E., Porouhan, P., Orak, R.J., & Farahani, M.A. (2019). Comparing the attitude of doctors and nurses toward factor of collaborative relationships. *Journal of Family Medicine and Primary Care*, 8(10), 3263. doi: 10.4103/jfmpc.jfmpc_596_19.

Marecek, J. (2016). Invited reflection: Intersectionality theory and feminist psychology. *Psychology of Women Quarterly*, 40(2), 177–181.

Marecek, J., & Gavey, N. (2013). DSM-5 and beyond: A critical feminist engagement with psychodiagnosis. *Feminism & Psychology*, 23(1), 3–9.

Martin, K. (August 2, 2023). "The body keeps the score". Offers uncertain science in the name of self-help. It's not alone. *Washington Post*.

Matz, D., Vogel, E.B., Mattar, S., &. Montenegro, H. (2015). Interrupting intergenerational trauma: Children of Holocaust survivors and the Third Reich. *Journal of Phenomenological Psychology*, 46, 185–205.

Mehrotra, G. (2010). Toward a continuum of intersectionality theorizing for feminist social work scholarship. *Affilia: Journal of Women and Social Work*, 25(4), 417–430.

Mehrotra, G., Kimball, E., & Wahab, S. (2016). The braid that binds us: The impact of neoliberalism, criminalization, and professionalization on domestic violence work. *Affilia*, 31(2), 153–163. doi: https://doi-org.ezproxy.library.dal.ca/10.1177 /088610991664387.

Menzies, P. (2008). Developing an Aboriginal healing model for intergenerational trauma. *International Journal of Health Promotion and Education*, 46(2), 41–48. https://doi.org /10.1080/14635240.2008.10708128.

Meyer, B. (2002). Extraordinary stories: Disability, queerness and feminism. *NORA-Nordic Journal of Feminist and Gender Research*, 10(3), 168–173. http://ezproxy.library .dal.ca/login?url=http://www.tandfonline.com/doi/abs/10.1080/0803874023 21012199.

Migotto, S., Garlatti Costa, G., Ambrosi, E., Pittino, D., Bortoluzzi, G., & Palese, A. (2019). Gender issues in physician–nurse collaboration in healthcare teams: Findings from a cross-sectional study. *Journal of Nursing Management*, 27(8), 1773–1783. https://doi .org/10.1111/jonm.12872.

Morley, C., & Dunstan, J. (2016). Putting gender back on the agenda in domestic and family violence policy and service responses: Using critical reflection to create cultural change. *Social Alternatives*, 35(4), 43–48.

Morrow, M.H., Jamer, B., & Weisser, J. (2011). *The recovery dialogues: A critical exploration of social inequities in mental health recovery*. Centre for the Study of Gender, Social Inequalities and Mental Health, Simon Fraser University. https://www.researchgate .net/profile/Marina-Morrow/publication/264877917_The_Recovery_Dialogues_A _Critical_Exploration_of_Social_Inequities_in_Mental_Health_Recovery/links/5a2 d66e6aca2728e05e2e06e/The-Recovery-Dialogues-A-Critical-Exploration-of-Social -Inequities-in-Mental-Health-Recovery.pdf.

Morrow, M., & Malcoe, L. (2017). Critical inquiries for social justice in mental health. University of Toronto Press.

Morrow, M., & Weisser, J. (2012). Towards a social justice framework for mental health recovery. *Studies in Social Justice*, 6(1), 27–43.

Moulding, N. (2015). *Gendered violence, abuse and mental health in everyday lives: Beyond trauma*. Routledge.

Nathan, J., & Webber, M. (2010). Mental health social work and the bureau medicalisation of mental health care: Identity in a changing world. *Journal of Social Work Practice*, 24(1), 15–28.

O'Connor, M. (2022). *The grieving brain: The surprising science of how we learn from love and loss*. Harper.

Pease, B., Goldingay, S., Hosken, N., & Nipperess, S. (Eds.) (2016). *Doing critical social work. Transformative practices for social justice*. Allen and Unwin.

Penfold, S., & Walker, G. (1983). *Women and the psychiatric paradox*. Eden Press.

Pizzey, E. (1974). *Scream quietly or the neighbours will hear*. Penguin Books.

Plant, M. (2008). The role of alcohol in women's lives: A review of issues and responses. *Journal of Substance Use*, 13(3), 155–191.

Poole, N. (2013). Trauma informed practice. [PDF document.]. Retrieved from http:// pacificaidsnetwork.org/wp-content/uploads/2013/02/PAN-presentation-on-TIP.pdf.

Porter, L., Martin, K., & Anda, R. (2017). Culture matters: Direct service programs cannot solve widespread, complex, intergenerational social problems. Culture change can. *Academic Pediatrics*, 17(7), S22–S23. https://www.academicpedsjnl.net/article/S1876 -2859(16)30496-X/abstract.

Pyysiinen, J., Halpin, D., & Guilfoyle, A. (2017). Neoliberal governance and "responsibilization" of agents: Reassessing the mechanisms of responsibility-shift in neoliberal discursive environments. *DISTINKTION: Journal of Social Theory*, 18(2), 215–235.

Rose, D. (2014). The mainstreaming of recovery. *Journal of Mental Health*, 23(5), 217–218.

Ross, N., Brown, C., & Johnstone, M. (2022). Dismantling addiction services: Neoliberal, biomedical and degendered constraints on social work practice. *International Journal of Mental Health and Addiction*, 1–14. https://doi.org/10.1007/s11469-022-00779-0.

Ross, N., Brown, C., & Johnstone, M. (2023). Beyond medicalised approaches to violence and trauma: Empowering social work practice. *Journal of Social Work*, 1–19.

Rottenberg, C. (2014). The rise of neoliberal feminism. *Cultural studies*, 28(3), 418–437. https://www.tandfonline.com/doi/abs/10.1080/09502386.2013.857361

Russell, D. (1986). *The secret trauma: Incest in the lives of girls and women*. Basic Books.

Sangalang, C.C., & Vang, C. (2017). International trauma in refugee families. A systematic review. *Journal of Immigrant Minority Health*, 19, 745–754. doi: 10.1007/s10903-016-0499-7.

Scharff, C. (2016). The psychic life of neoliberalism: Mapping the contours of entrepreneurial subjectivity. *Theory, Culture and Society*, 33(6), 107–122. https://journals.sagepub.com/doi/abs/10.1177/0263276415590164.

Scott, A., & Wilson, L. (2011). Valued identities and deficit identities. Wellness recovery action planning and self-management in mental health. *Nursing Inquiry*, 18(1), 40–49. doi: 10.1111/j.1440-1800.2011.00529.x.PMID:21281394.

Shaffer, B. (1987). Film. *To a safer place*. National Film Board, Canada.

Shamir, R. (2008). The age of responsibilization: On market-embedded morality. *Economy and Society*, 37(1), 1–19.

Sheppard, R. (2016). *Mental illness and African Nova Scotian communities. Understanding heritage and ethnicity is the difference between healing and isolation*. The Coast. Available online: https://www.thecoast.ca/halifax/mental-illness-and-african-nova-scotian-communities/Content?oid=5249498.

Smith, D., & David, S. (Eds.) (1975). *Women look at psychiatry: I'm not mad, I'm angry*. Press Gang Publishing.

Spark, M. (2020). Neoliberal regime change and the remaking of global health: From rollback disinvestment to rollout reinvestment and reterritorialization. *Review of International Political Economy*, 27(1), 48–74. https://doi.org/10.1080/09692290.2019.1624382.

Spolander G., Engelbrecht, L., Martin, L., Strydom, M., Pervova, I., Marjanen, P., Tani, P., Sicora, A., & Adaikalam, F. (2014). The implications of neoliberalism for social work: Reflections from a six-country international research collaboration. *International Social Work*, 57(4), 301–312.

Stark, C. (2018). The neoliberal ideology, its contradictions, the consequences and challenges for social work. *Ljetopis socijahnog rada*, 25(1), 39–63.

Stewart, S., & Israeli, A. (2003). Substance abuse and co-occurring psychiatric disorders in victims of intimate violence. In C. Wekerle & A.M. Wall (Eds.), *The violence and addiction equation: Theoretical and clinical issues in substance abuse and relationship violence* (pp. 98–122). Brunner-Mazel.

Stoppard, J. (2000). *Understanding depression: Feminist social constructionist approaches*. Routledge.

Strong, T. (2012). Talking about the DSM-V. *International Journal of Narrative Therapy & Community Work*, 2, 54–64.

Sweeney, A., Perôt, C., Callard, F., Adenden, V., Mantovani, N., & Goldsmith, L. (2019). Out of the silence: towards grassroots and trauma-informed support for people who have experienced sexual violence and abuse. *Epidemiology and Psychiatric Sciences*, 28(6), 598–602.

Szasz, T. (1961). The myth of mental illness. *The American Psychologist*, 15(2), 59–65.

Szasz, T. (1970). *Ideology and insanity. Essays on the psychiatric dehumanization of man.* Anchor.

Teghtsoonian, K. (2009). Depression and mental health in neoliberal times: A critical analysis of policy and discourse. *Social Science & Medicine*, 69(1), 28–35.

Terr, L. (1990). *Too scared to cry: Psychic trauma in childhood.* Harper & Row.

Thompson, L. (2021). Toward a feminist psychological theory of "institutional trauma". *Feminism & Psychology*, 31(1), 99–118.

Tseris, E. (2013). Trauma theory without feminism? Evaluating contemporary understandings of traumatized women. *Affilia: Journal of Women and Social Work*, 28(2), 153–164.

Tseris, E. (2019a). Accepting my illness? Problematising the claims of mental health anti-stigma efforts. In D. Baines, B. Bennett, S. Goodwin, & M. Rawsthorne (Eds.), *Working across difference. Social work, social policy and social justice* (pp. 155–170). Red Globe Press.

Tseris, E. (2019b). De-therapizing trauma: Negotiating the contested trauma concept. In *Trauma, women and mental health and social justice. Possibilities and pitfalls* (pp. 105–123). Routledge.

Tseris, E. (2019c). Interrogating biomedical dominance: Critical and feminist perspectives on mental health. In *Trauma, women and mental health and social justice. Possibilities and pitfalls* (pp. 14–31). Routledge.

Tseris, E. (2019d). The mainstreaming of trauma in mental health: Radical critique or business as usual? In *Trauma, women and mental health and social justice. Possibilities and pitfalls* (pp. 32–58). Routledge.

Tseris, E. (2019e). *Trauma, women and mental health and social justice. Possibilities and pitfalls.* Routledge.

Tudor, R. (2023). "Making cuts that matter" in social work: A diffractive experiment with trauma-informed practice. *Ethics and Social Welfare*, online first: https://doi.org/10.1080/17496535.2023.2198774.

Turner, J. (2009). The sociology of emotions. Basic theoretical arguments. *Emotion Review*, 1(4), 340–354.

Ussher, J. (1991). *Women's madness: Misogyny or mental illness?* Harvester Wheatsheaf.

Ussher, J. (2005). Unravelling women's madness. Beyond positivism and constructivism and towards a material discursive – intrapsychic approach. In R. Menzies, D. Chunn, & W. Chan (Eds.), *Women, madness and the law: A feminist reader* (pp. 19–41). Glasshouse.

Ussher, J. (2010). Are we bio-medicalizing women's misery? A critical review of women's higher rates of reported depression. *Feminism & Psychology*, 20(1), 9–35.

Ussher, J. (2011a). Gender matters: Differences in depression between women and men. In D. Pilgrim, A. Rogers, & B. Pescosolido (Eds.), *The Sage handbook of mental health and illness* (pp. 103–126). Sage.

Ussher, J. (2011b). *The madness of women. Myth and experience.* Routledge.

van der Kolk, B. (2014). *The body keeps the score: Brain, mind, and body in the healing of trauma.* Penguin Books.

Waldron, I.R. (2021). The wounds that do not heal: Black expendability and the traumatizing aftereffects of anti-Black police violence. *Equality, Diversity and Inclusion: An International Journal*, 40(1), 29–40. https://www.emerald.com/insight/content/doi/10.1108/EDI-06-2020-0175/full/html.

Wallace, J., & Pease, B. (2011) Neoliberalism and Australian social work: Accommodation or resistance? *Journal of Social Work*, 11(2), 132–142.

Wastell, D., & White, S. (2012). Blinded by neuroscience: Social policy, the family and the infant brain. *Families, Relationships and Societies*, 1(3), 397–414.

Webb, A. (2001). Some considerations on the validity of evidence-based practice in social work. *British Journal of Social Work*, 31(1), 57–79.

Webster, D., & Dunn, E. (2005). Feminist perspectives on trauma. *Women & Therapy*, 28(3–4), 111–142.

White, M. (2000). Re-engaging with history: The absent but implicit. In M. White, *Reflections on narrative practice: Essays and interviews* (pp. 35–58). Dulwich Centre Publications.

White, M. (2001). Narrative practice and the unpacking of identity conclusions. *Gecko: A Journal of Deconstruction and Narrative Ideas in Therapeutic Practice*, 1, 28–55.

White, M. (2004). Working with people who are suffering the consequences of multiple trauma: A narrative perspective. *International Journal of Narrative Therapy and Community Work*, 1, 45–76. https://search.informit.org/doi/abs/10.3316/informit.228819554854851.

White, M. (2007). *Maps of narrative practice*. Norton.

White, M., & Epston, D. (1990). *Narrative means to therapeutic ends*. Norton.

Wiesel, E. (2006). *Night* (2nd ed.). Farrat, Straus and Giroux. (Originally published 1958: Editions de Minuit.)

Wunke, E. (2016). Notes on rape culture. In *Notes from a feminist killjoy. Essays on everyday* life (pp. 47–108). Book Thug.

Yip, Kam-Shing. (2004). Bio-medicalization of social workers in mental health services in Hong Kong. *British Journal of Social Work*, 34, 413–435.

# 2

# REPOSITIONING OUR UNDERSTANDING OF TRAUMA THROUGH THE LENS OF EPISTEMIC INJUSTICE AND HERMENEUTIC OMISSIONS

*Marjorie Johnstone and Eunjung Lee*

## Introduction

This chapter aims to reframe ways we understand pervasive discourses of trauma in a domain of epistemology and human dignity. We will explore the theoretical framework of epistemic injustice in detail and apply it to examine the diagnosis and conceptualization of trauma. The fundamental premise of epistemic justice is that validation of our lived experience and respect for our testimony is a fundamental part of being human and an essential part of inclusion and membership in our collective humanity. Mainstream psychiatric and psychological approaches to trauma have used a biomedical framework to interpret and diagnose the individual harm resulting from traumatic experiences. However, it is widely understood that trauma is the human imprint of violent occurrences, whether from human engineered or natural/accidental events. The separation of the context and circumstances of the source of the trauma from the human response to these kinds of experiences reflects a scientific approach that examines component parts in depth. We argue that it is important to understand the composition of the whole experience and so we propose a new frame that honors human experience, power and dignity. We will follow the path from diagnosis to treatment in the biomedical model and then contrast this with an approach that begins with a holistic assumption that examination of the total phenomenon, the precipitating events or circumstances and the testimony of the persons who experienced the violence must be considered in their totality. For this purpose, we will discuss Judy Atkinson's work (2002), which theorizes from her work on generational trauma with Australian Indigenous people who have endured centuries of violent dispossession and enforced dependency. Throughout this comparison we will consider the achievement of epistemic justice as a tool to evaluate the effectiveness of these approaches.

DOI: 10.4324/9781003379591-3

## Theoretical Framework of Epistemic Injustice and Epistemic Oppression

The ideas and concepts developed in the philosophical study of epistemic injustice are, in the opinion of the authors, very pertinent to clinical practice in social work. This area of justice-related scholarship is a growing field, with the number of scholars (from a range of other fields) increasing all the time. We will briefly outline some of the key ideas that are central to this discussion.

In a study of epistemic injustice, Miranda Fricker (2010) stated that to not be respected and believed as a credible knower is to be denied your fundamental humanity, as knowing is central to *being* human. Furthermore, she observed, this epistemic form of injustice becomes institutionalized when it is attached to a specific identity and becomes a source of prejudice. This prejudice is disseminated through the circulation of pejorative discourses that not only appear in individual interactions but can *become systemic* when an identity is established that can then track "the subject through different dimensions of social activity – economic, educational, professional, sexual, legal, political, religious" (p. 27). Fricker (2010) distinguished two forms of injustice, testimonial injustice and hermeneutic injustice. She described *testimonial injustice* as that which "occurs when prejudice causes a hearer to give a deflated level of credibility to a speaker's word" (p. 1). Fricker went to some lengths to describe the construction of negative stereotypes that, once disseminated, result in the person becoming the target of prejudicial discrimination, a significant part of which was being given little or no credibility. This lack of credibility positions the person as an object, as less than human, as not worthy of being listened to, and their account of lived experience is silenced. A good example of this is the lack of credibility given to a "known criminal" in the criminal justice system (Johnstone & Lee, E., 2018) or to a person in the mental health system labelled/diagnosed as insane (Johnstone, 2021; Lee, E., Tsang, Bogo, Johnstone, Herschman, & Ryan, 2019; Lee, E., Tsang, Bogo, Johnstone, & Herschman, 2019; Lee, E., Herschman, & Johnstone, 2019).

The other major form of injustice Fricker described is *hermeneutic injustice*, which she stated is "the injustice of having some significant area of one's social experience obscured from collective understanding" (p. 155). This is the epistemic consequences that can occur when testimony is blocked or silenced, or there is an absence of public discussion and debate on certain experiences so that they are not conceptualized, refined and named, thus creating an epistemic gap. This gap intensifies the isolation and oppression of those experiencing this form of epistemic injustice, as their experience is not represented in the collective epistemic resource. A telling example of this is gender violence where, historically, until the work of second wave feminism in the 1970s, the prevalence of sexual abuse and sexual harassment were undertheorized and unacknowledged in the wider public domain. As a result, women were aware that something was uncomfortable or unsettling but were not able to clearly articulate those feelings so there was no language for reporting or complaining. Furthermore, these issues were then not represented legislatively or in governing policies so there were no formal recourse channels available.

Dotson (2012) built on Fricker's ideas of hermeneutic epistemic injustice by introducing what she calls *contributory epistemic injustice*. This expands Fricker's concept of hermeneutic injustice, by introducing the idea that there are hermeneutically marginal resources, i.e., places where marginal groups have created their own collective resource of understanding but because of power relations they are unable to contribute their hermeneutical resources into the governing collective resource. This phenomenon can be seen in grassroots organizing when persons with a common experience of exclusion and disempowerment begin meeting and sharing their experiences. A historical example of this is, at the turn of the twentieth century, when the Western women's suffrage movement began, White women met amongst themselves to discuss their exclusion from public life and their exclusion from voting and participation in governance. Through these meetings and sharing of experiences they built a marginalized hermeneutic resource which then provided a shared epistemic resource for them to organize a social movement to address the contributory epistemic injustice they were experiencing. Similarly, the civil rights movement in the United States in the 1960s began with a grassroots pooling of lived experience and dissatisfaction with the inequitable legal structures of post-Civil War reconstruction America, which then developed into the civil rights movement led by Martin Luther King – which directly challenged epistemic contributory injustice.

A corollary to the concept of contributory injustice is the concept of *willful ignorance* where the perceiver has evidence of the contributory injustice before them but refuses "to acknowledge and acquire the necessary tools for knowing whole parts of the world" (Polhaus, 2011, p. 15). For example, it could be fruitfully argued that the injustices intrinsic to reconstruction America were plain for anyone to see, but the acknowledgement of these injustices would compromise the hegemony of the White ruling class who benefitted from them, thus there was no public discussion or acknowledgement of this injustice. There is usually a collective vested interest in ignoring the voices of those who are oppressed, and this is what Polhaus is describing as willful ignorance.

Dotson (2012, 2014) outlines a theory of *epistemic oppression* in which she seeks to describe and identify the mechanics of contributory injustice. She states that epistemic oppression refers to "epistemic exclusions afforded positions and communities that produce deficiencies in social knowledge" (p. 24). In other words, the epistemic exclusion or oppression that occurs prevents the lived experiences of the excluded members from being part of the collective epistemic resources that the community draws upon. This absence is huge as not only are the excluded community members confronted with silencing mechanisms (such as prejudicial low credibility) that deny their right to speak up, but it also means that if they do have an opportunity to speak, their communication potential is severely limited as their experience is not part of the collective epistemic resource, so it is as though they are speaking a foreign language. The corollary to this injurious exclusion is *epistemic agency*, which is the ability to be a participant in knowledge production. This means that the harms from epistemic oppression include exclusion, isolation and a lack of epistemic agency, which are collectively a denial of the fundamental part of being human and belonging to humanity. We will consider these ideas of epistemic injustice when examining the biomedicalization of trauma diagnosis and some of the ensuing healing approaches to trauma that have been adopted in response to the assessment framing. We will discuss these issues in greater depth with a case example from Aboriginal Australia.

## The Assessment of Trauma and Violence

The biomedical definition of trauma is that it is the individual experiential response to overwhelming experiences, which include relational violence and occurrences such as natural disasters and war (SAMHSA (Substance Abuse and Mental Health Services), 2014). Biomedicalization approaches trauma according to a disease model, where the first task is individual assessment and diagnosis of the designated "patient" and then the treatment and cure follow. The criteria for diagnosis of pathological trauma are described in the DSM-5 (Diagnostic and Statistical Manual of Mental Disorders, 5th ed.) as symptoms within the broader categories of intrusion avoidance symptoms, dissociative cognitive and mood alterations, changes in arousal and reactivity, and interference in intimate relations and workplace function; and it is stated that if these symptoms persist beyond a month of the traumatic event, then this diagnosis of trauma pathology is warranted (American Psychiatric Association, 2013). Post-traumatic stress disorder (PTSD) is an associated trauma diagnosis, and the DSM-5 states that exposure to actual or threatened death, serious injury or sexual violence, either directly or as a witness, or learning of this occurring to a close family member or friend constitutes the grounds for a trauma diagnosis of PTSD (American Psychiatric Association, 2013).

The DSM-5 is a manual to aid and standardize professional diagnosis and there is little space given in this manual to treatment options. The diagnostic process uses a biomedical blueprint where the presence of a series of symptomatic clusters are identified and described in detail and the assumption is that the treatment will then focus on eliminating those symptoms. This is a standard medical approach to physical health disorders that has been applied to mental distress. Mirroring the response to physical disorders, this diagnostic style favors treatment that consists of technical targeting of the various individual "symptoms". This reductive and specialized approach invites a reliance on specific symptom reduction therapies to complement the use of pharmaceutical interventions that target the reduction or elimination of specific "undesirable" symptoms. Not only are the contextual origins of trauma lost and silenced, but the "treatment" itself silences clients as only the "dysfunctional" symptoms are discussed. This fractured attention to specific symptoms shifts the focus to individualized pathological behaviors, thoughts or memories and the traumatic precipitating event(s) are absent from the conversation. A more recent iteration of the biomedical approach is the trauma-informed approach. This approach seeks to increase public awareness of the prevalence of symptoms of traumatic harm by providing education on the symptoms of trauma and encouraging responses to clients to be less punitive and more sympathetic (Lee, E., Faber, & Bowles, 2022; Lee, E., Kourgiantakis, Lyons, & Prescott-Cornejo, 2021). This approach specifically suggests that inquiry or examination of the source of traumatic injury could be harmful and could result in retraumatization, so there is a specific directive to avoid contextualization.

Tseris (2020) challenges the biomedicalization of trauma, stating that while trauma is experienced internally on an individual level, it is triggered by external events that are usually person-made. Furthermore, she asserts, in creating a typology of the psychological effects of trauma, the DSM-5 describes the symptoms of trauma as decontextualized psychological occurrences, thus presenting a template for individual victim-based interventions, and invisibilizing the triggering event(s). In her study of trauma, women's mental health and social justice, Tseris (2020) identifies that, in the field of gender violence and the aftermath of traumatic injury, these hegemonic psychiatric discourses often disqualify the marginalized voices of the victims (testimonial injustice). This biomedicalization of trauma, where the contextual origins are largely ignored, re-establishes this hermeneutic gap where the cultural and political factors are undertheorized and escape scrutiny. Currently, trauma-informed practices are identified as central issues in constructing mental health services (Lee, E., Kourgiantakis, Lyons, & Prescott-Cornejo, 2021). While heightened recognition of the harm experienced by trauma is a welcome addition to mental health understanding, this application of a decontextualized disorder, which casts trauma as an individual pathology rather than as a phenomenon of social dysfunction and violence, has wider implications. The precipitating dysfunctional cultural patterns, such as patriarchy, misogyny, racism and rape culture, are hidden from scrutiny and the person diagnosed is subject to testimonial, hermeneutic and contributory injustice. The wider social and political inequities that triggered the traumatic experience remain unaddressed and this maintains a status quo of privilege. We suggest that a biomedical model addresses a very narrow understanding of trauma as individual pathology and overlooks that we are mediating a human response to overwhelming events, so we are dealing with something that begins on the outside not the inside and, unlike a disease, is something that cannot be fixed or cured or changed, but rather, like other universal life events such as loss, death and isolation, the person must learn how to live with and manage these occurrences, in order to re-establish a sense of well-being.

At the base of all trauma experiences is the problem of violence, as trauma is the harm that results from violence. Bandy Lee (2019) is a critical psychoanalytic psychiatrist and has written an introductory text, *Violence. An Interdisciplinary Approach to Causes, Consequences and Cures*, in which she applies an interactionist integrative approach to the complex topic of violence. In her book, she synthesizes current knowledge across a broad range of disciplines and advocates for pooling what we know and working collectively to generate approaches and next steps. B. Lee (2019) views violence broadly as a spectrum from the commonly understood phenomenon of individual violence to the wider context of structural violence and environmental violence. She includes the resulting harms as social and economic deprivation, social and political diminution in addition to the more commonly understood psychological injury or trauma. Her final working definition of violence is as follows:

> Intentional or threatened human action, either direct or through structural neglect and diminution of others, that results in or has a high likelihood of resulting in human deprivation, injury, or death, or contributes to the extinction of the human species.
>
> *(Lee, B., 2019, p. 6)*

B. Lee observes that "the mind as a subject of study is vastly complex, and it is clear that our knowledge is miniscule" (2019, p. 47). She observes that theories about the mind have changed many times since psychology became an academic discipline just over a hundred years ago. B. Lee traces the significant shifts between early leading psychologists from Wilhelm Wundt and William James, who were known as fathers of psychology and debated how to understand human minds and human functioning. In 1897, Wilhelm Wundt made psychology an experimental science and broke the mind down into components for study which began the behavioral revolution in psychology; and in 1890, William James (1890) challenged this reductionist approach and said that the mind must be examined holistically. Psychodynamic approaches began in in the 1890s with Sigmund Freud, who began psychoanalysis, which applied theories of the mind into interventions to treat mental distress. While a succession of psychoanalytic thinkers and practitioners added to psychoanalytic knowledge, the field was eclipsed by the rise of behaviorism (following the direction set by Wilhelm Wundt) in 1930 in the United States with John Watson and later in 1976 with B.F. Skinner, where conditioned responses became the focus rather than the mind. The rise of cognitivism renewed an interest in mental processing and cognitive behavior therapy (CBT) emerged as a treatment to teach coping and emotional regulation. B. Lee (2019) observes that "this can be a practical tool for finding relief in the absence of an ability or adequate support to get to 'the source' of the problem, it does not deal with the deeper layers that play an important role in violence" (p. 48).

From the epistemic injustice perspective, cognitivism denies testimonial justice because the lived experience that surrounded the traumatic precipitating event is minimized, if not ignored, and replaced with an exclusive focus on the resulting dysfunctional cognitive patterns. Hermeneutic injustice is implicit in such an approach as there is no opportunity given to the client to make meaning of what has happened and to begin to make sense of it. Atkinson used a trauma genogram to collectively plot the course of trauma generationally, which then assisted the group to begin creating a collective hermeneutic resource. We wonder how we can get to the source of the problem and address the traumatic experiences of individuals and communities without falling into an endless search for technical tools while perpetuating epistemic injustice. By examining the findings and experience of an Indigenous approach to trauma, developed and trialed in Queensland, Australia, we will explore the implications of the diagnosis of trauma and the ensuing approaches to healing. We will contrast this with the implications for treatment arising from a biomedical approach and we will use the theoretical conceptualization of epistemic injustice to tease out the features of each approach.

## Case Study: An Indigenous Approach to Generational Trauma and Healing

In this case study we discuss the findings of Judy Atkinson (2002), an Indigenous scholar of Jiman and Bundjalung descent, who has worked for many years as a trauma therapist with Aboriginal peoples in Australia. Atkinson's work is informed by an understanding of the contextual origins of the generational trauma she is studying. Unlike the biomedical approach, which begins with the presenting symptoms of an individual, Atkinson begins with the known impact and course of colonization in Australia and examines how these violences caused community trauma. She identifies three distinct phases of colonization: (1) invasion and frontier violence; (2) the intercession of paternalistic philanthropic and religious groups; and (3) and the establishment of government responsibility for Indigenous affairs. Atkinson (2002) observes that since the imposition of the ongoing violence of colonial-enforced dependency in Australia, police powers over Indigenous lives have increased, despite inquiries into police brutality that revealed gross police misconduct, and so the violence of family fragmentation, economic deprivation and political diminution has steadily increased, with rising rates of Aboriginal incarceration and child apprehension. Atkinson adopts a sociological perspective on community trauma with the work of Kai Erikson (1976), who documented how a small mountain community in West Virginia was devastated when their tightly knit community was destroyed by an industrial flooding disaster. The subsequent government support response was minimal and short-lived, and Erikson described how the people became disoriented and apathetic and were plagued by distrust, fear and a sense of powerlessness that persisted over time. The biomedical model of trauma provides a timeline for recovery of one month, and if symptoms persist longer the conclusion is that there is a deeper underlying disorder. This diagnostic interpretation of recovery maintains individual responsibility and blames the persons who "failed" to be cured without critiquing the effectiveness of the cure, but also, more importantly, shifts attention away from causative structural factors to individual deficit.

Implicit in Atkinson's work is her understanding of epistemic injustice. She develops healing strategies that honor the voices of her clients (e.g., testimonial justice), by providing a safe space for full disclosure, opportunities for group sharing of lived experience of trauma and facilitates the building of a hermeneutic resource pool, which could be the foundation for challenging contributory epistemic injustice. Indigenous scholar Eve Tuck (2009) notes that Western approaches to Indigenous communities have historically been damage-centered with a focus on "portraying our neighborhoods and tribes as defeated and broken" (p. 412). She observes that ascribing damage-centered identities to Indigenous people (pathological biomedical trauma diagnoses) assists in justifying the occupation of Native lands, genocide and colonization, as it positions the problem of a community in trauma as people who are unable to function effectively. Furthermore, she observes that these individually oriented pathologizing analyses are then used to fund social reform and humanitarian agendas of service delivery, providing employment for White people, while the causative structural issues remain unaddressed. In some instances, these damaged identity symptoms become transmuted into risk assessments and are used as evidence to justify child apprehension, proof of criminality and grounds for the denial of credibility (e.g., testimonial injustice) should a person with a known "damaged identity" attempt to describe their lived experience as shaped by the oppressive violence of colonization, which then led to hermeneutic and contributory injustice.

In her book *Trauma Trails. Recreating Song Lines,* Atkinson (2002) describes the process and results of her doctoral study on the transgenerational effects of trauma in Indigenous Australia. She asked the following research questions: (1) What is the experience of violence? (2) How does violence influence child development, family and community fragmentation, alcohol and drug misuse, race and gender injustice, criminal behavior, and poverty? (3) How do experiences of violence contribute to intergenerational and transgenerational trauma? And finally, (4) How do people heal? Atkinson recruited her participants from Aboriginal people in Queensland, Australia, in an area where there was a history of massacres and displacement and where there were current high rates of violent crime, alcohol and drug abuse, poor health and mental illness. To arrive at a culturally safe way of interviewing, she was guided by Freire's (1972) principles that oppressed people have the most knowledge of their oppression and can often generate the most credible solutions. This is an approach that follows the principles of epistemic justice, as it honors the lived experience of the participants. Atkinson states that "insensitive and unethical research is characterized by the belief that that the researcher can and will know more than the researched about their own experience or their own lives" (p. 14). This position is in direct opposition to the medical model and evidence-based social work, which claims expert (scientifically tested) knowledge is held by them and that it is in the best interests of the client if treatment decisions are rooted in that expert knowledge.

The feminist psychological insights of Judith Herman (2015) were used by Atkinson to inform her understanding of the psychological dimensions of trauma.

Herman identified trauma as an "affliction of powerlessness" (p. 33) and she outlined a healing process that is holistic and relational, beginning with the establishment of a sense of safety through a therapeutic trusting relationship, which provides a safe platform to support the remembrance of traumatic events or circumstances. Remembering is followed by learning how to accept and live with a history of trauma reconnected to daily life. The goal is not the erasure of the trauma and all the associated symptoms but rather a movement toward acceptance of what happened, understanding that the individuals were not able to control the events that occurred. This then allows freedom from a sense of guilt and endless reliving by the individuals to try to discover what they could have done differently; rather, it encourages a forward-looking goal of well-being and a better quality of life. Atkinson echoes Herman when she states that she sets out to enable the "the creation of safe places for sharing where the unspeakable can be given voice, where feelings can be felt, and where sense can be made out of what previously seemed senseless" (Atkinson, 2002, p. 145).

Atkinson used the Western methodological practices of consciousness raising, participatory action and phenomenology to inform her use of *dadirri*, which is an Aboriginal process of listening to one another:

> The principles and functions of *dadirri* are: a knowledge and consideration of community and the diversity and unique nature that each individual brings to community; ways of relating and acting within community; a non-intrusive observation, or quietly aware watching; a deep listening and hearing with more than ears; a reflective and non-judgmental consideration of what is being seen and heard; and, having learned from the listening, a purposeful plan to act, with actions informed by learning, wisdom, and the informed responsibility that comes from knowledge.
>
> *(p. 16)*

The foundational values of *dadirri* are consistent with the principles of epistemic justice as they center testimonial justice by facilitating opportunities for each participant to share their lived experience in a climate of acceptance, i.e., not questioning but believing a story being told, thus communicating respect and credibility. Fricker (2010) states that epistemic injustice is "a wrong done to someone specifically in their capacity as a knower" (p. 1), and that when there is a gap in the hermeneutic resources then that "puts someone at an unfair disadvantage when it comes to making sense of their social experiences" (p. 1). The Indigenous concept of *dadirri*, which is part of Australian Aboriginal lore, supports this important form of justice by institutionalizing listening to the stories of others. In Western society, justice is conceptualized in the law as an adversarial process, which does not accommodate non-judgmental listening, as there is an overriding quest for accountability and punishment of wrongdoing. Rebecca Tsosie, an Indigenous legal scholar, comments that "the principle of Indigenous self-determination depends upon the ability of an Indigenous people to express its own identity as an autonomous group and to negotiate the terms of its political relationship with the given nation-state" (Tsosie, 2012, p. 1154).

This recognition that Indigenous peoples have been involuntarily subjected to colonial rule and harmed through gross epistemic injustice means that a hermeneutic meaning-making process needs to precede the quest for contributory epistemic justice. In discussing Western law and hermeneutical injustice, Tsosie further identifies serious *omissions* in the legal assessment of harm, which raise:

> issues of hermeneutical injustice because the harms asserted include cultural and spiritual claims that do not fall within an available category of experience or thought within the Western legal system. However, the harms are felt by Indigenous people. This is their experience, and it is shared among many different Indigenous groups because they possess a different understanding of the world.
>
> *(Tsosie, 2012, p. 1132)*

This observation is relevant to the assessment of trauma in the mental health system, where hermeneutic injustice issues with respect to the course of traumatic injury and the associated harms remain unknown, as the exploration of the traumatic event or occurrence is minimized or absent and patients have no voice during treatment. The biomedical model of trauma perpetuates epistemic injustice by imposing an expert DSM-based diagnosis on patients and by ignoring or minimizing the lived experience (full personal account of lived experience) of the patient. Alongside many feminist therapists' critiques, the Mad Movement (LeFrancois, Menzies, & Reaume, 2013) and the Hearing Voices Network are good examples of promoting testimonial justice and creating hermeneutic resources to construct contributory justice for people who are diagnosed with a psychotic illness and have uncommon experiences (Johnstone, 2021).

Atkinson (2002) observed that while she facilitated groups of exploration and sharing using *dadirri* it became evident that for the participants that there were numerous "interconnections and interdependencies between people in kinship and other affiliations" (p. 215). But the study also revealed that: "Violence as trauma fragments people's sense of self, identity, family, and community, and fractures the loving and enduring connections of family and community that provide structure to human lives. The key finding was that healing, while hard work, is possible" (p. 216).

Atkinson observed that stories of violence were "crying out to be told" (p. 218) and that often, after sharing experiences of tragedy and indescribable violence, participants would report feeling better and feeling relieved. Herman (2015) has noted that disempowerment and disconnection are core experiences of trauma and that reconnection and empowerment occur when people share their stories and make meaning of their experience (p. 133). An important finding from Atkinson's work was the frequent reporting of the impact of removals on families and in family histories. Atkinson noted that: "the Aboriginal sense of belonging to families and to community and cultural group has been shattered and often feels irretrievable, and this creates deep grief and anger in the individuals and in groups as a whole" (p. 224).

Furthermore, Atkinson observed that the deep rage experienced by abuse survivors was often directed at persons or communities who did not listen or believe, or who were not available to listen, rather than the actual abuser. This observation echoes Fricker's assertion that testimonial injustice is a denial of a person's fundamental humanity and central membership in the world as a knowing person. The harm from not being listened to or being believed reported by these participants is the harm of testimonial injustice. Herman (2015) notes that traumatized people are often involved in risk-taking and recklessness. Atkinson observes that a person expressing anger and hate in violence is detached and unfeeling, and that this acting out then becomes a way of reattaching to the original feelings of anger and hate generated by the original violence of abuse. Atkinson observed that through this process of *dadirri* (testimonial justice) some relief is experienced and some tenuous sense of reconnection to community and kin is achieved.

Herman (2015) noted that traumatized people often have difficulty verbalizing their experiences and that the accounts given are often fragmented and contradictory. Atkinson worked with several generations of the same family and noticed that there was not always correspondence between the differing memories but that these events had not been shared openly and talked about before. This is a description of hermeneutic injustice where the traumatic past has remained unspoken and has not been conceptualized and understood in its full contextual reality. This corresponds to Dotson's (2012, 2014) description of epistemic oppression where there is a deficiency in social knowledge and there is no collective epistemic resource for the community to draw on. It also echoes Kai Erikson's work on community trauma response, which identified how people collectively experienced disorientation, distrust, fear and a sense of powerlessness after the traumatic event if there was no support and no opportunity to share and conceptualize the experience.

Atkinson devised her own participation process to move forward with her work and she blended Herman's analysis of trauma and recovery process with the principles of *dadirri* listening. She organized non-hierarchical circle formations as the structure for sharing experiences, a structure which facilitated egalitarian learning from each other and there were no experts. Storytelling, dance, theatre and reflective discussion were used to "bring to the front the painful stories of trauma and provide experiences of being listened to, of being acknowledged, of reconnecting with others for healing" (p. 241). This process embodied the principles of epistemic justice with a platform for telling each person's story and for shared meaning-making of the experience. As the facilitator, Atkinson brought the colonial contextual factors that surrounded the lived experiences of trauma to the fore, thus enabling hermeneutic epistemic justice as the individual distress of the participants became a shared contextualized experience.

In the words of one of the participants in Atkinson's study, healing is:

> Healing is a very confusing word. When I first thought of it, I thought I would go along and all this pain was going to be healed and at the finish I would just walk away and I would be healed, but now I know that it means learning. Learning about yourself – learning about looking at things in a different way. Understanding how those things came to be. Owning your own things, but not taking on board other people's things. Being responsible for what you are responsible for, but not for other people's responsibilities. Learning how to deal with different situations – how to interact with people – how to lessen conflict – seeing your own things differently.
>
> *(Atkinson, 2002, p. 140)*

## Conclusion

The biomedical approach to trauma uses an individualized approach that focuses exclusively on the impact of a violent event of the psychological functioning of that person. The DSM-5 lists a detailed description on the areas of functioning that are impaired because of the original traumatic event. Treatment responses focus on reducing or eliminating these symptoms and pharmaceutical treatments are supported by coping and controlling cognitive behavior therapies to further advance symptom control. The assumption is that pre-trauma functioning will be restored if the symptoms are gone. This approach places little value on the testimony of the experience from the patient, does not see the precipitating factors of the trauma as having any relevance to treatment, and similarly it does not consider meaning-making or hermeneutic justice as related to recovery. In contrast to this, the approach adopted by Atkinson begins outside the client and considers the collective and individual impact of violence on individual and community well-being. From this perspective, she spends no time on individual assessment and diagnosis but uses a collective platform where there is shared individual testimony and careful, attentive listening. This approach harnesses the strength of epistemic justice and enables the participants to experience membership, commonality and the validation of being believed. Moving beyond testimonial justice, the examples we shared from Atkinson's study then facilitate group exploration and discussion of the material disclosed, and a process of hermeneutic justice is initiated. While discussing the meaning of these past experiences, new understandings and ways of coping can emerge, thus facilitating a healing process and respecting the human dignity of people with trauma experiences.

## References

American Psychiatric Association. (2013). *Diagnostic and statistical manual of mental disorders*. (5th ed.) American Psychiatric Association Publishing.

Atkinson, J. (2002). *Trauma trails. Recreating song lines. The transgenerational effects of trauma in Indigenous Australia*. Spinifex Press.

Dotson, K. (2012). A cautionary tale. On limiting epistemic oppression. *Frontiers*, 33(1), 24–47. https://doi.org/10.5250/fronjwomestud.33.1.0024.

Dotson, K. (2014). Conceptualizing epistemic oppression. *Social Epistemology*, 28(2), 115–138. https://doi.org/10.1080/02691728.2013.782585.

Erikson, K.T. (1976). *Everything in its path. Destruction of community in the Buffalo Creek Flood*. Simon and Schuster Paperbacks.

Freire, P. (1972). *Pedagogy of the Oppressed*. Penguin.

Fricker, M. (2010). *Epistemic injustice. Power and the ethics of knowing*. Oxford University Press.

Herman, J. (2015). *Trauma and recovery. The aftermath of violence – from domestic abuse to political terror*. Basic Books.

James, W. (1890). *The Principles Of Psychology Volume II By William James (1890)*.

Johnstone, M. (2021). Centering social justice in mental health practice: Epistemic justice, narrative social work and the hermeneutic gap. Special edition in *Research in Social Work Practice*, 31(6), 634–643. https://doi.org/10.1177/10497315211010957.

Johnstone, M., & Lee, E. (2018). State violence and the criminalization of race: Epistemic injustice and epistemic resistance as social work practice implications. *Journal of Ethnic & Cultural Diversity in Social Work*, 27(3), 234–252. https://doi.org/10.1080/15313204.2018.1474826.

Lee, B. (2019). *Violence. An interdisciplinary approach to causes, consequences, and cures*. Wiley Blackwell.

Lee, E., Faber, J., & Bowles, K. (2022). A review of trauma specific treatments (TSTs) for post-traumatic stress disorder (PTSD). *Clinical Social Work Journal*, 50, 147-159. Doi.org/10.1007/s10615-021-00816-w.

Lee, E., Herschman, J. & Johnstone, M. (2019). How to convey social workers' understanding to clients in everyday interactions? Towards epistemic justice. *Social Work Education: International Journal*, 38(4), 485–502. https://doi.org/10.1080/02615479.2018.1539070.

Lee, E., Kourgiantakis, T., Lyons, D., & Prescott-Cornejo (2021). A trauma-informed approach to Canadian mental health policies. A systematic mapping review. *Health Policy*, 125, 899–914. https://doi.org/10.1016/j.healthpol.2021.04.008.

Lee, E., Tsang, A.K.T., Bogo, M., Johnstone, M., & Herschman, J. (2019). Clients and case managers as neoliberal subjects? Shaping tasks and everyday interactions with severely mentally ill (SMI) clients. *European Journal of Social Work*, 22(2), 238–251. https://doi.org/10.1080/13691457.2018.1529662.

Lee, E., Tsang, A.K.T., Bogo, M., Johnstone, M., Herschman, J., & Ryan, M. (2019). Honoring the voice of the client in clinical social work practice: Negotiating with epistemic justice. *Social Work*, 64(1), 29–40. https://doi.org/10.1093/sw/swy050.

LeFrancois, B., Menzies, R., Reaume, G. (Ed.) (2013). *Mad matters. A critical reader in Canadian mad studies*. Canadian Scholars Press.

Polhaus, G. (2011). Relational knowing and epistemic injustice: Toward a theory of willful hermeneutical ignorance. *Hypatia: A Journal of Feminist Philosophy*, 27(4), 715–735.

SAMHSA. (2014). Substance abuse and mental health services administration (SAMHSA) concept of trauma. https://store.samhsa.gov/sites/default/files/d7/priv/sma14-4884.pdf.

Tseris, E. (2020). *Women's mental health, and social justice. Pitfalls and possibilities.* Routledge.

Tsosie, R. (2012). Indigenous peoples and epistemic injustice: Science, ethics and human rights. *Washington Law Review*, 87(4), 1133–1202.

Tuck, E. (2009). Suspending damage: A letter to communities. *Harvard Educational Review*, 79(3), 409–427. https://doi.org/10.17763/haer.79.3.n0016675661t3n15.

# 3

# THE MYTH OF TRAUMA-INFORMED MENTAL HEALTH SERVICES

*Emma Tseris*

## Introduction

I felt very tricked ... being grabbed by all my limbs, and then being sedated. I think ... that immobilization, in itself, was quite traumatic. [Woman describing a recent experience of police and paramedic intervention in response to crisis and distress]

I'm the only one who can know if I feel safe ... I'm telling you this is harmful, I'm telling you this isn't ok, I'm telling you I'm ok at home but no matter what I say, it doesn't matter ... [Mental health workers are] terrified of liability ... [They're] willing to traumatize me and really affect the rest of my life ... don't want to deal with any degree of risk, so just chuck [me] in a psych ward. [Young woman describing the harms of involuntary mental health treatment in a contemporary Australian context]

Where am I? How did I get here? Why am I here? How is this going to help me? ... You've just got to live in limbo ... Basically, they wanted me to stop saying I'd kill myself so that they could discharge me. I just didn't really see the benefit. It just made me feel like wanting to try to run away. [Woman describing a recent experience of inpatient treatment in a locked ward during a time of suicidal distress]

Although we are living in an era of de-institutionalization, mental health service responses to emotional distress and differences continue to be shaped by coercion and carceral logics (Wahbi & Beletsky, 2022). As noted by Ben-Moshe (2020,

DOI: 10.4324/9781003379591-4

p. 282), de-institutionalization is not a completed project, but must be understood within the context of "the shifting contours of the carceral state". The opening quotes of this chapter, from a research project exploring women's experiences of involuntary mental health treatment in Australia, offer first-hand accounts that demonstrate the bleak, violent and humiliating impacts of psychiatric coercion in women's lives within a contemporary context. To some readers, such testimonies of institutional violence may seem to be outdated or to represent "outlier" experiences. The silence around psychiatric incarceration is perpetuated by dominant mental health discourses, which are frequently imbued with sanitized accounts of "recovery" following mental distress and positive experiences of mental health services (Daya, Hamilton, & Roper, 2020). As a result, while mental health is being talked about more than ever, only certain perspectives are being invited to contribute to the growing mainstream conversation, which is reinforcing a benevolent view of mental health professional power (Daley, Costa, & Beresford, 2019). Even when psychiatric harm is acknowledged, it is usually within the context of a narrative of progress, which positions psychiatry as a once harmful but now reformed profession. Consequently, within a contemporary paradigm of mental health "awareness-raising", which focuses on the need to talk openly about mental health difficulties, the voices of people who have been harmed by psychiatry and who have had their rights taken away in the name of "care" have been largely subjugated and silenced (Sweeney et al., 2019). Indeed, mental health campaigns implore women to disclose distress and to actively seek formal support services, with almost no reference to the multiple, gendered risks that women experience when they come to be understood within the constraints of a psychiatrized identity (Taylor, 2022).

It is therefore the purpose of this chapter to disrupt sanitized narratives of mental health services and to engage with less comfortable first-person accounts about the system harms that occur within spaces that aim to offer "care" and "protection" in response to distress, crisis and suffering. The gender and psychiatric coercion project (Tseris, Bright Hart & Franks, 2022) has focused on women's experiences (adopting a trans-inclusive definition of women), acknowledging that women often experience heightened and specific harms within psychiatric spaces as a result of highly gendered assumptions and practices. A gender lens enabled us to see the ways in which psychiatric coercion intersects with patriarchal oppression to disrupt and undermine women's rights and well-being, leading us to develop four preliminary themes within our project.

1) Mental health treatment replicates the dynamics and tactics of violence against women
2) Mental health treatment involves significant deprivations and losses, with potential enduring impacts across the life course
3) Mental health treatment disrupts and undermines mothering

4) 'Recovery' (acknowledging that this is a contested concept) is usually found outside coercive mental health systems.

*(Tseris, Bright Hart, & Franks, 2022)*

Expanding on this analysis, the present chapter explores the chasm that often exists between how mental health services describe themselves (with a particular focus on the now-pervasive discourse of trauma-informed care) and the experiences of women on the receiving end of involuntary mental health treatment. This analysis is necessary, as mental health services have become increasingly adept at drawing upon trauma discourses as a way of demonstrating an openness to addressing power imbalances and working toward systemic change. Indeed, trauma-informed care has become a pervasive discourse within mental health services across many countries in the Global North (Becker-Blease, 2017), and rhetorical commitments to trauma sensitivity provide an alluring picture of reform. Trauma-informed care has been defined as existing within an organization or system that:

> realizes the widespread impact of trauma and understands potential paths for recovery; recognizes the signs and symptoms of trauma in clients, families, staff, and others involved with the system; and responds by fully integrating knowledge about trauma into policies, procedures, and practices, and seeks to actively resist re-traumatization.
>
> *(SAMHSA (Substance Abuse and Mental Health Services Administration), 2014, p. 9)*

The turn to trauma in mental health service settings could be labeled as a great achievement and evidence of immense progress. I want to be clear that the work of feminist trauma scholars in the latter part of the twentieth century should be commended as groundbreaking (Birnbaum, 2019). However, a narrative of progress is only one, limited way of understanding the contemporary shift toward trauma awareness among mental health professionals. From a critical perspective, we can ask: What kind of service provider needs to be reminded to treat people with dignity and respect, to take into account what people might want as they seek support, and to actively do things to ensure that the support that is being provided is helpful? Indeed, in a different kind of world, where mental health services truly valued the perspectives of people experiencing distress, it might not be necessary to talk so endlessly about trauma-informed care, as we do now. This is not because trauma-informed care is irrelevant or without value. Rather, such services would already be well along the path to prioritizing the subjugated knowledges and experiences of people experiencing distress and emotional suffering. Within such a world, the dominance of biomedical reductionism, which reduces human suffering to a set of "symptoms" situated within supposedly "disordered" individuals, would be untenable.

Returning to the present world, where mental health systems routinely fail to engage with experiential expertise (or do so only reluctantly or in highly tokenistic ways) and where coercive practices, including dehumanizing practices and the denial of human rights, are common (Daley, Costa, & Beresford, 2019), we can pose the question: If a system is predicated on violence and unequal power relations, what changes are made possible when what is essentially been requested is that individual workers or organizations try to do less harm within the existing status quo? Few genuine changes seem possible. Moreover, even when trauma discourses are in use, our understandings of trauma are deeply embedded in neoliberal influences (Hendrix, Barusch, & Gringeri, 2021). This means that there is a continued focus on "symptoms" and individual "dysfunctions" rather than a connection to the feminist movement and collective efforts to challenge patriarchal structures (Woodlock, Salter, Conroy, Burke, & Dragiewicz, 2022).

This chapter, then, is about the impossibility – or the myth – of trauma-informed mental health services. It arises out of a concern that the espoused principles of trauma theory are inconsistent with coercion, which underpins all involuntary mental health services, but which is also present across most mental health services, even if they are voluntary, due to power imbalances between professionals and the people who access the services, and the elevation of "psy"-thinking as a grand narrative for understanding human experiences, in ways that undermine the legitimacy of all other kinds of knowledge and worldviews. Therefore, an analysis of the disconnect between seemingly benevolent trauma rhetoric and the experiences of people on the receiving end of mental health services is required. This chapter draws upon excerpts from the first-person accounts of psychiatrized women, in combination with the perspectives of people with professional mental health identities who have experienced moral injury within carceral mental health systems. Such accounts demonstrate a range of harmful psychiatric practices occurring, in spite of, or perhaps even because of, the rollout of trauma-informed discourses.

## Mental Health Systems, Gaslighting, and Violence

Through persuasive mental health campaigns, we are all being strongly encouraged to seek professional support for distress (Holland, 2022). Yet, the harms that people experience within acute mental health settings are often immense, to the point where the impacts of system harms may in fact outweigh the original distress. There is now extensive literature identifying the inability or unwillingness of mental health workers to draw connections between distress and injustices, including poverty, violence and social isolation (Neill & Read, 2022). Indeed, some women described the refusal by mental health services to acknowledge gender inequality as a key driver of mental distress as *gaslighting*. The secondary harms caused by engagement with mental health services are deeply troubling, as they represent a mismatch between the promise of support and the reality of further oppression:

I started to think how much of this is trauma [which] then is diagnosed [as] mental illness and the issues [are] located within the individual and not within the context ... that was really apparent to me ... how much trauma there was ... for women. And there was a lot of sexual abuse ... people are having flashbacks, you could just – you could hear it. I found that quite hard. A couple of women that I was in there with had been experiencing domestic violence, and when the police had come, they'd been taken, not looking at what had happened. It's kind of like they were "hysterical" by the time they asked for help, and so the problem was, again, located within them. [Woman with direct experiences of involuntary inpatient mental health treatment]

Mental health services are underpinned by a continuum of coercion (Bentall, 2009). Services are often conceptualized in terms of a binary between voluntary and involuntary interventions, but the lived experience of coercion is often not so clear-cut. For example, "voluntary" support may be comprised of controlling and policing the thoughts and emotions of women (including their responses to gendered violence) within interventions such as cognitive behavior therapy; while there is no use of overt force, the interventions can still involve significant power imbalances. Within involuntary treatment, coercive practices, such as seclusion and restraint, which involve much more blatant deprivations of liberty, may still be obscured by discourses of "care" and "protection".

Mental health services are rarely held to account for injustices, acts of violence and breaches of human rights. Reasons for this include limited community knowledge about coercive practices in an era of de-institutionalization (Blanchette, 2019) and mainstream narratives about mental health that focus on mostly positive accounts of services experienced by people with social privilege (Holland, 2022), meaning that it is rare to connect mental health services to a conversation about human rights or social justice. The social privilege that medical professionals enjoy in comparison to people with psychiatrized identities is another important factor. Indeed, mental health workers receive status and esteem from their professional identities, and mental health services are imbued with assumptions about benevolence and "presumed prudence" (van Daalen-Smith, Adam, Breggin, & LeFrançois, 2014). As a result, it can be very difficult for people to speak out about their experiences of violence within the mental health system, to feel safe to do so and to feel that it will be worthwhile. Consequently, it can be very surprising for people who have not been on the receiving end of mental health services to learn that professional interventions may make things worse, rather than better:

Life has been hard, there's no doubt about that, and it was hard because of childhood trauma and complex childhood trauma, but the mental health system exacerbated that trauma. [Woman recounting the effects of involuntary mental health treatment]

This is not to say that mental health systems are uncritically considered to meet people's needs or even to offer a reasonable level of care; indeed, inadequate systems are routinely scrutinized for their limitation in providing appropriate support to address emotional suffering. However, when people talk about problems within the mental health system, commonly used words such as "complexity", "insufficient resources", and a "broken system" can lead to certain types of questions being asked, while diluting more uncomfortable conversations. Such neutral terms deflect attention from the substantial risks and negative consequences that can eventuate for a person who comes to the attention of mental health services during a time of crisis or despair. It is deeply concerning that negative impacts can accumulate across the life course as a result of mental health system involvement, and that people often discuss that they have recovered not *because* of mental health systems, but *in spite* of them (Tseris, Bright Hart, & Franks, 2022). As described by participants in our project, the current system involves power imbalances that pathologize distress and undermine people's rights and liberty, combined with a short-term perspective that is focused on discharge and reducing "length of stay", all to the detriment of people on the receiving end of services:

> Where do you start? … It's a just a completely flawed system from top to bottom … it is still a completely biomedical model … you might have a little bit of scope to your practicing in your own way, but at the end of the day the bottom line is with the doctor. And is very, very, very focused on symptom resolution, risk reduction, risk minimization and then moving along to not clog up the system. And that's really the premise of the system. It's not … a meaningful recovery or support for a person. [Social worker with experience in an inpatient mental health setting]

This is a dire account of contemporary mental health service provision, speaking of the ways in which trauma-informed care can act as an empty signifier – a tokenistic signal that things are changing, while allowing dehumanizing and neoliberal practices to continue.

## Trauma as Pathology?

In response to the silencing of violence against women by mental health services, efforts have been made to enhance the skills and confidence of mental health workers in asking about experiences of violence and abuse. Nevertheless, the recognition that women who come to the attention of mental health services have often (usually) experienced abuse and trauma is not enough, and can lead to other problems. For example, trauma-informed care can be used as a way of viewing women's distress as stemming from past experiences of violence or abuse alone. This can obscure the serious deprivations and violations occurring within the mental health system itself:

> Everything just gets blamed on the trauma … [Professionals say], "That's just because of [trauma] and your poor coping mechanisms" … It's weaponized! [Survivor of psychiatric coercion]

Trauma-informed care can therefore be problematically used in ways that reflect the inherent othering of mainstream diagnostic practices, whereby those with a traumatized identity are positioned as distinct, and lesser (less resilient, less capable), in comparison to those without. Here, trauma is used as a way of categorizing women as problematic, in a similar way to how diagnostic categories are used to render women as "problematic Others". Assessing for women's "trauma" has become less about providing support in the aftermath of violence and abuse, and more about introducing another avenue for pathologizing women and rendering their voices less valid. In other words, it is as though there is something specific about women who have experienced gendered violence in how they experience and respond to involuntary mental health treatment, that takes the gaze away from psychiatric harm and onto the *perceptions* of individual women. Participants in this research project have strongly contested this position, demonstrating the inherently violent aspects of psychiatric coercion, which would humiliate and terrify any person who is subjected to it:

I think that if most of the Ministers [in the government] or anybody stood inside a high dependency unit and seriously thought about how that might feel for them, they would surely have to understand that putting someone in that environment is just going to make them more distressed. [Mental health worker with experience in inpatient services]

This is not to say that patriarchal violence and psychiatric coercion do not have cumulatively devastating effects. Women who have experienced gendered violence report that involuntary mental health treatment repeats the same dynamics of power, control and violation (Tseris, Bright Hart, & Franks, 2022). Indeed, government officials with swipe cards allowing them to exit a locked ward at any time are very unlikely to experience the setting in the same way as psychiatrized women who have already experienced violence and abuse at other times in their lives. That women who have already experienced violence are placed in a treatment setting that is likely to invoke yet more trauma is truly unjust (Ross, 2018). At the same time, it is concerning to see the ways in which women are experiencing trauma assessments as yet another form of pathologization (in addition to psychiatric labels), whereby an assessment of a trauma history can become a way to undermine women's accounts of the human rights violations occurring within mental health settings as able to be dismissed or minimized due to "a trauma history".

Women have also described the ways in which trauma has been integrated by mental health workers into mainstream assessment processes that seek to identify deficits and pathology within women. Thus, while diagnoses such as borderline personality disorder are in some instances being replaced by the language of trauma, this is not necessarily evidence of progress, as it may be a way of doubling down on the assumptions of diagnostic psychiatry and pathologizing women through using different, more "politically correct" terminology:

> The system devalues and categorises trauma as something that shouldn't exist, and that you're lesser than because you have the effects of trauma. [Woman with direct experiences of involuntary mental health treatment]

Consequently, there are significant limitations of a trauma discourse that reduces the experience of gendered violence to a set of psychological deficiencies, located within individual women. This paradigm re-inscribes trauma into the psychiatric paradigm, making way for status quo actions, such as not believing women, not taking women seriously and undermining women's rights and autonomy. Such an approach presents a stark contrast to a feminist commitment to understanding gendered violence as a structural issue, never ignoring the ways in which trauma is experienced uniquely by individual women but always seeking to located violence against women within social and political structures. As described by Moulding, Franzway, Wendt, Zufferey, & Chung (2021), gendered violence can be more usefully understood outside the bounds of individual pathology, as an "ontological insecurity wrought by a sexual politics that undermines their rights as persons and citizens". This is more than a theoretical move – such conceptualizations allow us to acknowledge the very real impacts of violence on women's lives, while also politicizing it and elevating the analysis beyond the constraints of medical discourses and diagnostic assessment.

## Changes to Rhetoric Rather than to Practice

Our project has found that there is often a substantial disconnect between what mental health services say they do, and the experiences reported by people on the receiving end of mental health services. This means that not only do mental health services enact harm in the name of "care", but also that women experience a further act of betrayal when they are advised that the service they have received is "trauma-informed". The research found that women provided incisive analysis of the overuse and misuse of the trauma concept by mental health workers and services as a way of escaping critique and avoiding meaningful reform. During action research groups, women were scathing about the rhetoric of "trauma" in the context of ongoing biomedical dominance:

> Everyone says they're trauma-informed … even though they use the word so much, services really don't appreciate how pervasive trauma, particularly childhood trauma, is among service users …

It's just absurd ... Trauma-informed can't just be a label or attitude that individuals adopt – if it's truly what's on the box, it needs to be systemic, cultural thing ... Some people are very set in their ways, you can educate them as much as you want, give them the training, but are they actually going to do it? No. ...

Trauma-informed care, it's this label and people think you can take the label and whack it on something, then you've done trauma-informed care ... it's not like you can set up a "trauma-informed care committee", whack trauma-informed care posters around the place, and you're done. You need to constantly be evaluating things and acknowledging trauma and working things out ... it's just a label, it's devoid of the context ...

Trauma itself is a buzzword ... there are different types of trauma, people react to trauma in different ways, everyone's so unique, why are we not using other words besides the word trauma?

It individualizes it as well – it's seen as the person is responding to an individual issue, whereas so much of trauma is structural ... there's not enough structural analysis about what's going on in society ... We are pathologizing normal experiences ... it is completely normal and healthy and natural to be anxious ... you've lost your job ... it's normal to be really stressed and anxious, sad and despairing, they are normal human experiences, not an illness ...

[Collective conversation in an action research group with women who have survived psychiatric incarceration]

Mental health services respond to critique by doubling down on trauma rhetoric, while failing to address the underpinning paradigm of medicalized coercion. In this way, mainstream trauma discourses are complicit in the ongoing perpetuation of intersecting patriarchal violence and psychiatric harms:

We throw around the term, trauma-informed care a lot. I don't actually know if many people really know what that means. [Mental health social worker]

The proliferation of individual-focused notions of trauma is powerfully analysed by Helbich & Jabr (2022, p. 314):

[T]rauma theory has reached an impasse worldwide: it has developed into a medical, symptom-oriented approach that produces methods of therapy that stubbornly disregard sociopolitical discourses and that disguise social and political problems as pathological disorders.

The turn to a depoliticized trauma concept therefore echoes Garrett's (2021, p. 7) recent caution that:

Dissent and social critique are always vulnerable to becoming diluted and incorporated into the mainstream: words and concepts can be slyly abducted and taken to places they are not supposed to be taken!

## Where to From Here?

This chapter has outlined the ways in which the proliferation of trauma-informed care has been a process of myth-making within coercive mental health services, in which a radical idea has been co-opted by conservative policymakers in order to obscure mental health system violence in a contemporary context and to curtail further critique and protest. Consequently, a seemingly relentless tide of trauma-informed discourses (Becker-Blease, 2017) sits uncomfortably alongside the testimonies of people on the receiving end of carceral mental health treatment. The inability of mental health services to meaningfully acknowledge and address the despair and suffering that is inherent to involuntary mental health treatment has placed substantial limits on the possibilities for meaningful reform.

There are several questions that can be posed, following on from this critique: Has trauma theory become so co-opted that it is no longer useful to producing radical and feminist practices in response to abuse and violence? Should efforts be directed toward rebuilding a trauma paradigm that centers survivor voices, or are they best directed elsewhere? Debates and different perspectives exist in response to such questions (Sweeney & Taggart, 2018). What is clear is that in the context of a depoliticized trauma concept, which is disconnected from the priorities of people with lived experience, it is necessary to make space for feminist, social justice, survivor-centered and demedicalized responses to women's distress and suffering – we must reject the notion that mainstream psychiatric responses are the only possible responses to distress, even if we are still in the process of imagining alternatives (Kafai, 2021). As noted by Judith Herman, harm always occurs if it reproduces the dynamics of abuse or injustice and takes power away from a survivor (Sweeney et al., 2019).

It is clearly insufficient for a trauma understanding to sit alongside psychiatric practices, due to the inconsistency between diagnosis, coercion and a biomedical paradigm; to attempt to reconcile these contradictory discourses means to collude with a system that pathologizes and discredits women (Taylor, 2022). A feminist perspective can make space for diverse perspectives on the impacts of diagnosis, while also moving beyond the simplistic narrative that diagnostic processes are helpful for accessing services and support after violence and gendered oppressions. Despite "good intentions", trauma discourses have professionalized mainstream understandings of the impacts of violence against women, encouraging the integration of survivor perspectives into mental health discourses, sometimes denying people with psychiatrized identities the right to speak (May, 2022). Too often, the feminist movement has uncritically drawn upon mental health discourses as a way of making sense of distress. There is a need for feminism to engage in solidarity with critical mental health movements and to reconceptualize distress outside the purview of biomedical explanations. In addition, there can be a renewed focus on addressing the social drivers of distress in women's lives, reconsidering the value of community-based strategies and resources, and developing collective responses to gendered violence rather than a focus on diagnosing and "treating" individuals.

## Conclusion

Reconstructing language has been an important component of challenging biomedical neoliberalism in mental health contexts, for example, questioning the pervasive "illness" model of distress through adopting more expansive ways of describing experiences, including reclaiming the once pejorative term, "madness" (Blanchette, 2019). At the same time, social justice cannot, and should not, be reduced to a mere rhetorical exercise, where we do little other than change the words that we use while continuing unjust and harmful practices (Lee & Johnstone, 2023). I have argued elsewhere that the uncritical uptake of trauma discourses undermines feminist concerns regarding naming and eliminating violence against women and children, through the turn to more sanitized and psychological language (Tseris, 2019).

As women have told us in the gender and psychiatric coercion project, trauma-informed care can offer a dishonest and almost meaningless approach to mental health 'reform':

> The frameworks they're operating in [are] still the old school frameworks, so how can they apply trauma-informed care which is contradictory to those frameworks? It's not going to work, and so they're only misleading themselves and the people that they hope to serve, or purport to serve. So, it's definitely not possible unless they change it. [Woman with direct experiences of involuntary mental health treatment]

Notwithstanding the ways in which knowledge about "trauma" has improved the practices of some individual workers, it is clear that, within the context of institutional psychiatry, trauma-informed care has largely created a mirage of progress while continuing to undermine women's rights and to amplify, rather than alleviate, distress. This is a dire outcome and forces women into making the difficult decision as to whether accessing mental health services is worthwhile or whether the risks outweigh any potential benefits. It is important to note also that the implications of our study's findings extend beyond the bounds of formal involuntary mental health treatment, as coercion remains an accepted practice across mainstream mental health services, undermining the rights, autonomy and choices of psychiatrized people, sometimes overtly but sometimes in more subtle ways that may not be recognized due to how coercive practices have been normalized within biomedical psychiatry (Bentall, 2009). Critical scholars, human service workers and policymakers must therefore guard against the uncritical uptake of trauma-informed care across the full range of mental health spaces that are premised upon power imbalances supported by legislative structures, biomedical imperialism and patriarchal oppression. The first-person accounts by psychiatrized women (alongside mental health workers who have experienced moral injury) demonstrate that the co-option of feminist trauma theory has expanded to such an extent that the trauma concept can invite complacency about patriarchal social structures, emphasize a woman's problematic "symptoms" after violence, and undermine women's credibility when reporting on either psychiatric harm or gendered violence – the very practices that trauma theory seeks to critique (Herman, 2015). Unfortunately, this means that the promise of reform offered by trauma-informed discourses in mental health settings might be evaluated as largely illusory. Even more concerningly, the language of trauma-informed care can be elicited as a "defence mechanism" (Birnbaum, 2019) to shut down any attempt to engage in a discussion about mental health system harms. Rhetorical commitments to trauma-informed practices, in the absence of concerted efforts to enact emancipatory outcomes for women through non-coercive and non-pathologizing forms of support, must therefore be viewed as an impediment rather than a resource in the feminist movement to eliminate violence against women.

## Acknowledgments

This chapter draws upon findings from a research project funded by the Australian Research Council. I acknowledge and thank my project colleagues, Scarlett Franks and Eva Bright Hart, for their invaluable contributions to knowledge-building around women's experiences of psychiatric incarceration in the contemporary context.

## References

Becker-Blease, K.A. (2017). As the world becomes trauma-informed, work to do. *Journal of Trauma & Dissociation*, 18(2), 131–138.

Ben-Moshe, L. (2020). *Decarcerating disability: Deinstitutionalization and prison abolition*. University of Minnesota Press.

Bentall, R.P. (2009). *Doctoring the mind: Is our current treatment of mental illness really any good?*. NYU Press.

Birnbaum, S. (2019). Confronting the social determinants of health: Has the language of trauma informed care become a defense mechanism? *Issues in Mental Health Nursing*, 40(6), 476–481.

Blanchette, S. (2019). A feminist bioethical and mad studies approach to resisting an increase in psychiatric paternalism to competent mental health users/refusers. *Journal of Ethics in Mental Health*, 10, 1–19.

Daley, A., Costa, L., & Beresford, P. (Eds.). (2019). *Madness, violence, and power: A critical collection.* University of Toronto Press.

Daya, I., Hamilton, B., & Roper, C. (2020). Authentic engagement: A conceptual model for welcoming diverse and challenging consumer and survivor views in mental health research, policy, and practice. *International Journal of Mental Health Nursing,* 29(2), 299–311.

Garrett, P.M. (2021). *Dissenting social work: Critical theory, resistance and pandemic.* Routledge.

Helbich, M., & Jabr, S. (2022). A call for social justice and for a human rights approach with regard to mental health in the occupied Palestinian territories. *Health and Human Rights,* 24(2), 305–318.

Hendrix, E., Barusch, A., & Gringeri, C. (2021). Eats me alive! Social workers reflect on practice in neoliberal contexts. *Social Work Education,* 40(2), 161–173.

Herman, J.L. (2015). *Trauma and recovery: The aftermath of violence – From domestic abuse to political terror.* Hachette.

Holland, K. (2022). Marketing mental health: Critical reflections on literacy, branding and anti-stigma campaigns. In *Communication and health: Media, marketing and risk* (pp. 165–187). Springer.

Kafai, S. (2021). *Crip kinship: The disability justice and art activism of Sins Invalid.* Arsenal Pulp Press.

Lee, E., & Johnstone, M. (2023). Critical pedagogy to promote critical social work: Translating social justice into direct social work practice. *Social Work Education,* 1–14.

May, M. (2022). Can people diagnosed as chronically mentally ill speak? *Social Work & Society,* 20(2).

Moulding, N., Franzway, S., Wendt, S., Zufferey, C., & Chung, D. (2021). Rethinking women's mental health after intimate partner violence. *Violence Against Women,* 27(8), 1064–1090.

Neill, C., & Read, J. (2022). Adequacy of inquiry about, documentation of, and treatment of trauma and adversities: A study of mental health professionals in England. *Community Mental Health Journal,* 58(6), 1076–1087.

Ross, D. (2018). A social work perspective on seclusion and restraint in Australia's public mental health system. *Journal of Progressive Human Services,* 29(2), 130–148.

SAMHSA. (2014). SAMHSA's concept of trauma and guidance for a trauma-informed approach. Retrieved from: https://ncsacw.acf.hhs.gov/userfiles/files/SAMHSA_Trauma .pdf.

Sweeney, A., & Taggart, D. (2018). (Mis)understanding trauma-informed approaches in mental health. *Journal of Mental Health,* 27(5), 383–387.

Sweeney, A., Perôt, C., Callard, F., Adenden, V., Mantovani, N., & Goldsmith, L. (2019). Out of the silence: towards grassroots and trauma-informed support for people who have experienced sexual violence and abuse. *Epidemiology and Psychiatric Sciences,* 28(6), 598–602.

Taylor, J. (2022). *Sexy but psycho: How the patriarchy uses women's trauma against them.* Hachette.

Tseris, E. (2019). *Trauma, women's mental health, and social justice: Pitfalls and possibilities.* Routledge.

Tseris, E., Bright Hart, E., & Franks, S. (2022). "My voice was discounted the whole way through": A gendered analysis of women's experiences of involuntary mental health treatment. *Affilia,* 37(4), 645–663.

van Daalen-Smith, C., Adam, S., Breggin, P., & LeFrançois, B.A. (2014). The utmost discretion: How presumed prudence leaves children susceptible to electroshock. *Children & Society*, 28(3), 205–217.

Wahbi, R., & Beletsky, L. (2022). Involuntary commitment as "carceral-health service": From healthcare-to-prison pipeline to a public health abolition praxis. *Journal of Law, Medicine & Ethics*, 50(1), 23–30.

Woodlock, D., Salter, M., Conroy, E., Burke, J., & Dragiewicz, M. (2022). "If I'm not real, I'm not having an impact": Relationality and vicarious resistance in complex trauma care. *British Journal of Social Work*, 52(7), 4401–4417.

# 4

# ETHICS AND THE CONCEALMENT OF EPISTEMIC AND INSTITUTIONAL VIOLENCE IN MENTAL HEALTH AND ADDICTIONS SERVICES

*Norma Jean Profitt*

## Introduction

In this chapter I critically analyze my tenure in women's services at a Canadian provincial rural mental health and addictions center. Established in addictions services in 2002 with the aim of enhancing responsiveness to women's specific needs, women's services positions across the province were groundbreaking and fostered a political and regional analysis of the sexism and misogyny shaping women's substance use and emotional distress. These trauma- and violence-informed posts had two complementary and synergistic components – the provision of therapeutic support for women (individual and group) and community development (such as education, health promotion and coalition advocacy). I worked alongside generalist addictions therapists until the amalgamation of mental health and addictions services.

Under the restructuring of mental health and addictions services through the establishment of the Choice and Partnership Approach (CAPA), introduced to reduce waiting lists and provide "evidence-based treatment", addictions services quickly became assimilated into mental health, underpinned by the dominant biomedical model of psychiatric diagnosis, the *Diagnostic and Statistical Manual of Mental Disorders* (5th edition) (DSM-5) (American Psychiatric Association, 2013). Under CAPA, shaped by biomedical psychiatry and a neoliberal efficiency model, the historical, more justice-based, biopsychosocial and spiritual lenses of addictions were erased. Any vestigial understanding of substance use as rooted in the socio-structural context of women's lives was expunged. The amalgamation had significant repercussions for service users and for women's services, leading to the elimination of the positions across the province. I argue that the current conceptualization of substance use and emotional distress obscures and

DOI: 10.4324/9781003379591-5

individualizes gender violence, trauma and structural oppression and is itself a form of epistemic and institutional violence against women.

In my role as women's advocate, I resisted the treatment of women as a collection of symptoms with alleviation as the goal. In resistance, I was deluged with emotions, somatic experiences and insights that eventually demanded articulation through the language of feminism. My analysis here is rooted in my observations as well as the experience of service users whom I attended. The majority of women were survivors of patriarchal violence such as childhood sexual abuse, woman abuse, sexual assault, including rape and gang rape, sexual harassment and non-state torture. Many, by their own assessment, lived with trauma although they were not formally diagnosed with post-traumatic stress disorder (PTSD). Service users were primarily White, with a mix of working-class, low-income, and professional earners; Acadian, Indigenous, and Black women were underrepresented despite the composition of the region.

First, I briefly review the connections between women's substance use and emotional distress and their experiences of gender-based violence, trauma and intersecting structural oppressions. Second, I discuss my experience at the center by highlighting what the current paradigm obscures and omits about women's realities and the political context of oppression in order to make the case that it constitutes epistemic and institutional violence against women. I then problematize the ethics of such a narrow and impoverished conceptualization and suggest directions for change.

## Making Connections: Structural Violence, Emotional Distress and Substance Use

A robust and long-standing body of evidence across many countries establishes that social inequalities of power and access to material resources play a powerful role in shaping the quality of people's integral physical, mental, emotional and spiritual health (Marmot, 2010; Raphael, 2012; World Health Organization, 2000). The social determinants of health or structural violence are crucial in illuminating how social, economic, political and material conditions engender and maintain psychological, emotional and behavioral distress. Social determinants now encompass systemic social oppression, such as sexism, racism, colonialism and legislated poverty (McGibbon & McPherson, 2013); and some argue that violence against women and trauma (Native Women's Association of Canada, 2007) and capitalism (Ferguson, 2017) are major determinants of health and mental health.

As relevant today as when she wrote *Toward a Radical Understanding of Trauma and Trauma Work*, Bonnie Burstow (2003) identifies the centrality of structures of oppression in the traumatizing of human beings, communities and the Earth itself. Two examples suffice: violence against women and girls is the most pervasive, yet least recognized human rights violation in the world (World Health Organization, 2021). As a public health issue, it saps women's spirit, constricts their freedom, compromises their health, and impedes their flourishing in all spheres of life. Across the globe, Indigenous peoples have been collectively traumatized by colonization, genocidal practices and enforced disconnection from the land (Brave Heart, 2003; Duran & Duran, 1995), therefore, emotional and spiritual distress is a result of "human beings living under conditions of severe and prolonged oppression" (Chrisjohn, n.d., 2nd para.). In Canada today, Indigenous women experience staggering rates of violence, which reflect the history of colonization, genocide and ongoing racism toward Indigenous peoples (National Inquiry into Missing and Murdered Indigenous Women and Girls, 2019).

The ways in which structural violence and traumatizing conditions shape people's lives are complex and profound. Systemic and structural domination disproportionately traumatize oppressed groups (Burstow, 2003; McGibbon, 2012) and subject people to the insidious traumatization of everyday racism and sexism (Root, 1992), which are manifestations of institutionalized oppression. The interface between structural inequalities and people's inner worlds, pain and suffering (Frost & Hoggett, 2008) is often compounded by income inequity and policy-created poverty.

Researchers have substantiated ineluctable connections between substance use and emotional distress and gender violence and trauma. Women often experience long-term violence and abuse rather than a single traumatic "event" and the specificity of the trauma resulting from gender violence depends on contextual factors. Compelling research shows that women's experiences of violence and trauma often precede their substance use and/or mental distress (Canadian Women's Foundation & BC Society of Transition Houses, 2011). Research also documents that substance use and mental health distress frequently co-occur in women survivors of violence (British Columbia Centre of Excellence for Women's Health, 2016). As many as two-thirds of women living with substance-use problems report concurrent mental health problems such as anxiety, depression and PTSD (Canadian Women's Foundation & BC Society of Transition Houses, 2011).[1] Violence against women results in injuries, depression, anxiety, PTSD, suicide attempts and overall poor health (World Health Organization, 2021).

Gender violence and trauma always occur in the traumatizing context of structural oppression, which shape women's responses to violence including both how and if they seek help and their forms of expressing resistance (Women's Aid, 2021) . Not only do social inequalities create emotional distress but they also maintain and exacerbate it (Mental Health Commission of Canada, 2009). Structural social conditions and institutional elements such as racism contribute to mental ill-health and affect women's access to mental health services (Thiara & Harrison, 2021). Further to this, professional responses to gender violence, such as victim-blaming language, pose a significant barrier to disclosing victimization and seeking help (Humphreys & Thiara, 2003). Not surprisingly, the intersections of the social determinants of health, which include intersecting forms of oppression such as gender, race, class, sexual orientation and where we live geographically, and which together create barriers in accessing services, considerably affect mental health outcomes (McGibbon, 2012).

There are many critiques of the limitations of the biomedical model and dominant trauma theory (Burstow, 2005; Brown, C., 2020; Caplan, 1995; Davis, 1999; LeFrançois, Beresford, & Russo, 2016; Tseris, 2013, 2019; Ussher, 1991). Recent research in Canada on the implementation of CAPA in mental health care reveals how neoliberalism, biomedicalism and managerialism work in tandem to commodify mental health service delivery and promote medicalized, efficiency-based, short-term approaches that individualize, pathologize and decontextualize emotional distress and obliterate social inequity and diversity (Brown, C., 2021; Brown, C., Johnstone & Ross, 2021; Brown, C., Johnstone, Ross, & Doll, 2022; Johnstone, Brown, C., & Ross, 2022).

## Individualizing and Pathologizing Women's Pain

As the implementation of the Choice and Partnership Approach progressed, mental health slowly absorbed addictions services. In my position in women's services, I felt a seismic shift in culture as I encountered the language of biomedical psychiatry. In a state of shock, I began to perceive how the medicalization of oppression was accomplished. Medical language wholly removed from view the social relations of power and material circumstances that shape the development and maintenance of women's pain. The funneling of the power dynamics inherent in adversities such as childhood sexual abuse, racism and income inequity into "mental disorders" adroitly relocates oppression from the public collective arena to a private individual mental space (Summerfield, 2012).

Andrea Daley and colleagues (Daley, Costa and Ross (2012) call this excision of social context, including women's meaning-making about their distress, "de-contextualization" (p. 8). It is a strategy and process that transforms "subjective suffering as a socially, culturally, and historically situated phenomenon to an object of medicine" (Coker, 2003, p. 908). The richness and diversity of subjective experience are descriptively reduced to categories of illness. Thus, the psychiatrization and biomedicalization of injustice and trauma conceal larger, enduring social inequities like heterosexism, colonialism and ableism and situates them in women's minds and bodies that are lifted "out of socio-political relations" (Thompson, 2021, p. 12). In my experience, any recognition of social, political, economic and cultural arrangements was "a neglected afterthought" (Daley, Costa, & Ross, 2012, p. 9). This omission has serious ramifications for women, communities and progressive social change.

In my position in women's services, I observed that the psychiatric gaze would almost always land on women's "coping skills", yet another reductionist means to individualize and pathologize pain. Under CAPA, the push to teach women skills grew exponentially. Women's coping skills appeared to be viewed as either inadequate or calcified into discrete, static entities divorced from any contextual understanding of how they came to be or what purpose they served. Nurses referring to women's services would sometimes state the reason as "lacks coping skills". Such language conveyed the lament: "If only women were better able to cope." Unfortunately, for example, coping skills do little to change the social landscape of misogyny in the "post" of PTSD.

Bonnie Burstow (1992) reframes women's mental health "symptoms" as coping skills that allow us to survive unbearable situations. Coping skills and survival mechanisms such as substance use are understood as "intelligible or understandable in their particular personal, social and cultural context" (Johnstone et al., 2018, p. 24). With the exception of feminist colleagues, I rarely heard that the diagnostic process acknowledged women's coping skills as remarkable feats: how they sought natural spaces outside or in the woods as a place of relative safety away from abusers at home or how depression served to dampen their resistance in the face of ongoing violence while still longing for a better life. The ingenuity with which women "coped" with adversity throughout their lives, either with conscious intent or unconsciously, astounded me; yet the deficit paradigm of psychiatric diagnosis rarely spoke about issues of context, subjectivity and meaning-making (Tseris, 2013).

In peer supervision and clinical discussions with staff, I also noted that the biomedical model rarely attended to sex- and gender-specific factors in women's lives, such as instances of heteropatriarchy, among others. "De-contextualisation works to accomplish the erasure of women as particularly gendered, sexualised and racialized in relation to their experiences of madness while underscoring their visibility as biological entities of mental illness" (Daley, Costa, & Ross, 2012, p. 11). Although the DSM-5 includes a chapter on trauma- and stressor-related disorders that require a triggering external event, very little import is assigned to present circumstances that would evoke or maintain suffering. Such circumstances include disproportionate caregiving responsibilities, social isolation, gendered income inequity and lack of employment, intellectual and restorative opportunities. Helpers' ignorance about the role of gender in mental health "symptoms", a form of institutionalized oppression, can exacerbate substance use and emotional distress by adding to women's disempowerment, frustration and the sense that they are alone.

As I experienced the crushing weight of the language of biomedical psychiatry that burgeoned under CAPA, I had a piercing insight: there is nothing wrong with the women I serve. I had never thought there was, but the insight was a response to feeling pressure to view them as wanting. CAPA and the biomedical model worked in tandem to narrow the field for building trust. The CAPA instruments of neoliberal efficiency – the push to move service users in and out as quickly as possible, the first line "treatment" of cognitive behavioral therapy, the one-size-fits-all approach, the mainstream (read White dominant culture) depoliticized trauma protocols, the pressure to "let go" of service users to promote their "self-reliance" – all converged to violate my feminist relational ethics and the therapeutic space as a place of relative freedom for service users.

In the McDonaldization of social work under CAPA (Johnstone, Brown, C., & Ross, 2022), I felt coerced into becoming an automaton carrying out a technical activity rather than fully engaging as an embodied interbeing (Powell, 2003). In response to time-limited sessions, women commented that those making decisions at the top understood nothing about their experiences of violence and the time required to mitigate the pain. Yet human connection is the crucible for learning and the enlargement of possibility, and not incidentally, the ground for exploring coping strategies in therapy. Exploration of patterns of habitual responses to threat or perceived threat demands trust. The emphasis on skills as if they sprout in a vacuum is counterproductive to the therapeutic purpose and is often direly disconfirming of women's capacity.

## Cleaving Women from Their Social World

Given that gender violence, trauma and oppression are fundamentally sociopolitical and relational issues, what is the place of meaning-making in forging more effective coping skills? In my practice, women's meaning-making about their experience has been indivisible from their ability to better meet life's hardships. I observed that women drew upon wider social and cultural discourses imbued with relations of power to make meaning of their suffering. They sought to understand their responses to adversity in the context of the confluence of elements in their lives; for example, how they turned to alcohol to numb their pain or dissociated to survive violence. Service users anticipated what was possible for them despite demoralizing social norms and messages; for example, a woman raped by her brother-in-law wanted her community to know about his wrong action and her resistance. They worked to reach an interior place of peace where their assessment of their responses in the face of violence and adversity was kind. I believe that they wanted to be known as moral equals and moral agents.

Among many things, women desired both alternative ways of interpreting their experience and "something beyond recognition" of their socially devalued identity and the fact of their pain. Kelly Oliver (2004) challenges the position that the social struggles manifest in feminist theory and social movements are "claims for recognition" (Fraser, 2003). She suggests that victims of violence and oppression seek "witnesses to horrors beyond recognition" (Oliver, 2004, p. 79) alongside "another level of meaning and truth, the truth of suffering" (p. 85). Proposing witnessing as an alternative to recognition, reconceiving subjectivity and, thereby, ethical relations, she insists that:

> subjectivity is the ability to address oneself to others combined with the ability to respond to others ... At its core, subjectivity is relational and formed and sustained by addressability (the ability to address others and be addressed by them) and response-ability (the ability to respond to others and oneself).
>
> *(Oliver, 2004, p. 84)*

For many service users, the "something beyond recognition" that they sought was a witness to their witnessing of the violence and injustice against them and of their capacity for engagement with suffering.

Making meaning of their lives, punctuated but not defined by adversity, women unspooled their narratives with the authority of lived experience. Attuned to verbal and non-verbal experiential connection, they carefully gauged whether a witnessing of their agency and resistance might occur. According to Vikki Reynolds (2010), the act of witnessing speaks to a hoped-for connection ... of *being held up* collectively, experiencing ourselves as alongside others (p. 161). Witnessing as an ethical stance and performance of solidarity identifies the actions of the narrator to maintain connections to humanity (Reynolds, 2010). Acknowledgment of injustice and resistance to oppression are crucial aspects of this practice (Wade, 1997). As an act of presence of spirit, witnessing addresses power in the sociopolitical world while decentering the therapist's activism (Reynolds, 2010).

The biomedical paradigm reflects deeply rooted Western philosophical assumptions such as "the separation of mind from body, thought from feeling, the individual from the social group, and human beings from the natural world" (Johnstoneet al., 2018, p. 5). Such assumptions severely impair the ability to witness connections between oppressive environments and distress.

> One of the most damaging effects of medicalized and individualized narratives is the marginalizing of meanings that potentially link distress with adverse life experiences ... Overall, then, medical narratives of distress have profound implications for agency, subjectivity, construction of the self, and the links between all these and issues of social justice.
>
> *(Johnstone et al., 2018, p. 89)*

The practice of "treating" service users one at a time functions to obscure the roots of women's pain from themselves and their communities. In this imposed partialization of experience, women are isolated from each other and often plunged further into shame. They are robbed of opportunities for meaning-making about experiences of adversity alongside sources of support, spirit and community.

Long-standing evidence from women's movements, collective organizing and community survival affirms the importance of socially shared vocabularies for everyday experience; benefits include mutual learning, self-recognition of agency and resistance, ethical accountability for actions, development of self-compassion, and politicization. Yet despite global evidence about the power of community, CAPA management planned to terminate the feminist women's therapy group since it was deemed to be not "evidence-based." Feminist alternatives centered in relational components often fall outside the realm of what is held to be "evidence-based" (Tseris, 2013). To the detriment of service users, alternative understandings or interpretations are not imagined or considered within medicalization processes (Daley, Costa, & Ross, 2012).

The psychopathological framework of psychiatry is therefore unable to recognize women as social agents who engage in advocacy and social action. Situating troubles in the fabric of their existence, I found that service users do articulate the social roots of their suffering. Woven into women's narratives were calls for deep changes in society – ideological, symbolic, structural and material. For example, they imagined a living wage so they could pursue their interests and fill the oil tank without worry; male partners who listened to their feelings without dismissing them; just divorce settlements instead of injustice where partners hid thousands in assets from lawyers; judges who took domestic violence into account in custody arrangements; and non-hierarchical organizational structures that engaged them as workers. With a keen sense of social organization, they knew what would enrich the quality of their lives, materially, emotionally and spiritually.

## Naming Epistemic and Institutional Violence Against Women

Through the practices of medicalizing, individualizing and pathologizing, psychiatry constructs others as "mentally ill" and abnormal. Brenda LeFrançois describes psychiatrization, legitimated through unequal power relations, as "a violent state of being objectified through diagnosis" (LeFrançois, as cited in Mills, 2014, p. 79). The "historical production of a knowledge of others as different" is a form of epistemic violence that naturalizes difference (MacDonald, 2002, p. 20). Similarly, Maria Liegghio (2013) uses the concept of epistemic violence to describe how the DSM-5 reinterprets and reduces people's experiences and perspectives to labels that represent them. Epistemic violence attempts to eliminate the knowledge possessed by oppressed groups (Dotson, 2011) or disqualify them as legitimate knowers through institutional practices (Liegghio, 2013). The refusal to recognize women's knowledge of the social world, whether intentional or unintentional, also constitutes a form of violence against women as social beings and agents of their own interiors.

These "relations of ruling" (Smith, 1996) reproduce and perpetuate misogyny, gender violence and oppression by privatizing trauma and social and relational violence against women (Thompson, 2021). Violence against women was never explicitly named as patriarchal violence at the center, except by feminist colleagues. On the occasions when violence was noted (for example, child sexual abuse), the violence of both individual aggressors and structural violence remained something nebulous, thereby concealing the violence, obfuscating perpetrators' responsibility, concealing victims' resistance and blaming and pathologizing victims (Coates & Wade, 2007). What then does the biomedical model of psychiatric diagnosis, with its "inherently political position of neutrality" (Reynolds, 2010, p. 165), communicate to women about their human rights?

When CAPA was well underway, I went on a hiking trip vacation. Entering the front door of the center after immersion in natural beauty, I grasped in a flash that mental health and addictions services masked the damage done to people from unjust and inequitable structures such as heteropatriarchy, colonization, ableism and so forth. Social issues such as the devastating effects of capitalism are individualized and pathologized, "removed from public debate and their social, political, and ethical elements hidden" from view (Johnstone et al., 2018, p. 31). Lucy Johnstone and colleagues (2018) give the example of economic austerity measures in the United Kingdom that have resulted in higher reported rates of distress, suicide and prescriptions of psychiatric medication, all of which stem from factors such as increasing inequality and privatization of health care and social services but fall under the purview of mental health and addictions. The ubiquity of the Western disease model primes the public to accept notions of women's "bad nerves" rather than entertain the notion that the political economy and patriarchal violence are sources of depression and anxiety.

As I have argued, biomedical psychiatry violates women's social being by depoliticizing distress. Sociopolitical relations of domination and subordination, such as White supremacy and heterogender are systematically (re)produced in economic, political and cultural institutions through the everyday practices of people who are generally well-intentioned (Young, 1990). Like all institutions, the institution of mental health and addictions is "a complex assembly of socially negotiated power relations" (Thompson, 2021, p. 14) in which the power dynamics of oppression are embedded in ideology, discourse and social practices. Institutions therefore can be understood as "*methods* of power" for the reproduction of trauma (Thompson, 2021, p. 16) and oppression. Since the biomedical paradigm of expert knowledge is integral to mental health and addictions services, it both represents and perpetuates systemic violence by framing social suffering as individual psychiatric illness.

In Western liberal democratic societies, social institutions are generally considered to be trustworthy and benevolent, or benign at best, even though there is ample evidence to the contrary: for example, institutionalized racism and sexism and the retraumatization that marginalized and racialized people experience in health care systems. The biomedical model of psychiatric diagnosis, far from being benevolent or benign, constitutes a form of institutional violence against women. "In this world, violence is an organizing practice through which power relations are sustained and identities are organized" (Thompson, 2021, pp. 16–17). Institutional adherence to this model sanctions the erasure of patriarchal and structural violence. Service users are epistemologically resourceful, deciding what to accept and what to dismiss or refuse in terms of support, but that does not annul the violence of the institution that forms part of the taken-for-granted violence so endemic in our social world.

## Ethics, Power and Politics: In Whose Interests?

As CAPA became fully implemented, I experienced significant moral distress (Profitt, 2021, 2022). Finally, I left because the institutional limits to practice violated my personal and professional values. The violence done to service users could have been done to me; it was not done to me – and yet, it was also done to me. That such violence can be concealed in the guise of helping is partly due to the way that ethics is conceptualized in the professions. A critical social justice ethics, an ethic of solidarity as a political ethic (Fraser, 1986), can offer an understanding of ethics as structural rather than individual.

The traditional view of ethics in mainstream social work situates ethics primarily within the parameters of the social worker-client relationship, where the structural dimensions of power are all too readily perceived as peripheral rather than central to ethical practice (Weinberg, 2010). The Western liberal modernist tradition that underpins the profession is rooted in a conception of power that emphasizes individualism and personal responsibility (Ferguson & Lavalette, 2007). This "often unacknowledged dominant cultural bias" (Jani & Reisch, 2011, p. 14) works to mask from view the ideologies, social structures and power relations in society that oppress along the lines of gender, racialized identities, sexuality, ability and so forth. This tradition reduces social relations of power to an interpersonal level (Ferguson & Lavalette, 2007); however, relationships are not just personal "but deeply embedded in the way our institutions, cultures, and structures are arranged" (Powell, 2003, p. 124). Thus, moral and ethical relations with others cannot be separated from cultural, social, political and economic ones (Jani, Ortiz, Pierce, & Sowbel, 2011; Young, 1990). This view of ethics and power has implications for thinking about relations with service users in the context of relations of ruling.

The traditional view of ethics as an individual responsibility is consistent with the Western hegemonic professional distance model (Greenspan, 1995). Mental health professionals are socialized to ignore the big picture through "the application of a diagnosis which imposes a powerful expert narrative of individual deficit and medical illness" (Johnstone et al., 2018, p. 201). Where caring has become an institutional responsibility, this narrative functions "to relieve the individual from the obligation to critically appraise the structural causes of whatever problems are addressed via institutional support" (MacDonald, 2002, p. 3). The alleviation of this obligation can work together with epistemic differences related to social, economic, racial and gender positioning (Dotson, 2011) and the structural social production of types of epistemic ignorance, such as willful ignorance (Alcoff, 2007), to maintain the status quo view of the origins of distress.

Willful ignorance by dominant social groups is the active denying or ignoring of social oppression and one's place in it. This raises an ethical question of what is the responsibility of helping professionals to examine dominant views that do not acknowledge their power, especially in the face of "countervailing evidence on a daily basis that is at least potentially visible to everyone in the society" (Alcoff, 2007, p. 48). Movement from willful ignorance to a position of solidarity necessarily entails understanding one's political location in social relations of power, continuously examining one's ethical positioning (Reynolds, 2010), and moving beyond hearing survivors' pain to a collective response-ability to act for justice and against injustice (Wade, as cited in Reynolds, 2010, p. 162).

An alternative view to "ethics as individual" is "ethics as structural". Ethics are constructed within relations of power, reflecting a divergence of values, interests and power among groups (Rossiter, Walsh-Bowers, & Prilleltensky, 2002). Ethics, always shaped by power, sit "at the center of conflictive social relations" with competing views of what is right and desirable (Chambliss, 1996, as cited in Prilleltensky, Valdés, Rossiter, & Walsh-Bowers, 2002, p. 246). With the view that dominant notions of ethics often reflect structural power, the claim that the DSM is objective, neutral and outside social influence obscures its political location, Eurocentricity and discursive power, not to mention its lack of validity and reliability (Johnstone et al., 2018; McGibbon & McPherson, 2013). Although contested by many, DSM proponents cement its legitimacy through a web of social relations, bolstered by corporate interests such as the pharmaceutical industry, which unduly influences diagnostic and treatment guidelines.

Accordingly, the narrow and impoverished conceptualization of women's substance use and emotional distress, paramount in mental health and addictions, is able to conceal the violence it harbors under the guise of helping. Such a conceptualization harms women as well as hinders the development of policies that would improve people's lives. Johnstone and colleagues (2018) affirm that "A cumulative and synergistic model of the impact of adversities does not support the individualisation of distress, either medically or psychologically. Instead, it implies the need for action, primarily through social policy" (p. 197). Apart from my appraisal of biomedical psychiatry as epistemically and institutionally violent, it is also ethically indefensible on these grounds.

Ethics can be defined as "the principles and values guiding thinking and action" (Rossiter, Walsh-Bowers, & Prilleltensky, 2002, p. 231). Ethical principles for a critically just society could include equity, participation, human rights, access to social and material resources (including health care and education), diversity, freedom and ecological integrity. Personal and professional ethics rooted in these aspirations would: take into account the sociopolitical, economic and cultural context in which ethics are lived; consider democratic values and social justice as preconditions for individual well-being; understand professional practice as an expression of social and political values that contribute to creating a better society rather than solely a practice of alleviating individual distress; and practice respect and compassion as part of relations of solidarity in service of the public good (Rossiter, Walsh-Bowers, & Prilleltensky, 2002).

Ethics mobilized to concretize social justice principles is politics; ethics and politics are interrelated and interdependent (Fraser, 1986). Politics is the use of power to create and maintain a particular vision of life (Spretnak, 1982). The need to infuse mental health and addictions as a public institution with a culture of critical social justice is all the more urgent in the face of neoliberalism as a political strategy aimed at: wealth accumulation for corporations and the rich; rising far-right extremism and hatred; the growing impoverishment of people across the globe; and the colonial psychiatrization of global mental health (Cosgrove, Mills, Karter, Mehta, & Kalathil, 2019).

## Directions for Change

Shifting thinking about the philosophical, ontological and epistemological assumptions of biomedical psychiatry is a monumental task since they form part of the fabric of Western culture (Ashcroft & Van Katwyk, 2016). However, alternatives to functional psychiatric diagnosis do exist (Johnstone et al., 2018; Ussher, 2005). Politically informed social and structural determinants of a health/structural violence framework suggests that policy changes to radically reduce economic and social inequity would be a crucial step in improving people's well-being. In my experience at the local level, one of the most potentially transformative steps that management of mental health and addictions could take, if they had the political will, would be to learn from service users. The "personal is structural" (Ahmed, 2017, p. 30) and political.

An ethical approach to learning from women's lived experience could entail critical appreciative inquiry (Cockell & McArthur-Blair, 2012) into the needs of women and their communities and historical and cultural forms of support that have long nurtured belonging and well-being. The diversity and complexity of women's experiences of violence, trauma and intersecting oppressions must be taken into account in the framing of policy alternatives and recommendations for change. Such an approach could also be utilized with staff, instead of perpetuating top-down anti-intellectual hierarchical structures that silence workers and intensify moral distress. Clear structures and processes for service users' and workers' participation in institutional functioning must apportion power rather than be regarded as instances of "consultation".

Social work as a profession has been "almost wholly complicit" as a participant in the *psy-complex*, "an expansive and overarching system that informs and intersects with other neoliberal systems of oppression" (LeFrançois, Beresford, & Russo, 2016, p. 1). Composed of allied professions such as psychiatry, psychology and social work that deal with matters of the psyche, it is implicated in the control and regulation of the conduct of citizens through shaping social issues and human experience in psychological terms. Social workers can educate themselves about their participation in this complex and interrogate how institutional thinking and practice narrows their understanding of ethics. They can integrate social justice and intersectional analyses into practice with service users and broaden their framework of mental health to include anti-oppressive practice (Joseph, 2017) and critical clinical social work (Brown, C., 2021).

Feminist research suggests that women who have experienced gender violence and struggle with substance use and emotional distress benefit from a range of supports (Canadian Women's Foundation & BC Society of Transition Houses,

2011; Women's Aid, 2021), such as women's groups, accompaniment and advocacy, peer support, empowerment resources, outreach and follow-up programs after shelter stays. This is important because women are scrutinized by authorities such as child protection and consequently they risk losing custody of their children, particularly Indigenous women, poor women and women of colour (Canadian Women's Foundation & BC Society of Transition Houses, 2011). Spaces where women can collectively engage in making meaning about their experiences, build reciprocal relationships, and rebuild self are pivotal to relational, intellectual and spiritual well-being. Such spaces position women as knowers and social actors, and some provide opportunities for activism (MacDonnell, Dastjerdi, Khanlou, Bokore, & Tharao, 2016). Furthermore, informal networks of support can nurture a sense of personhood in community, opening up opportunities for normalizing experience and finding joy in the companionship of others.

## Conclusion

Based on my experience in women's services in a provincial rural mental health and addictions center, I have shown how biomedical psychiatry and the neoliberal efficiency model of CAPA work to erase and individualize women's oppression, gender violence and trauma, thus constituting a form of epistemic and institutional violence against women. A critical social justice view of ethics as structural reveals the violence of biomedical psychiatry concealed under the guise of helping and suggests alternative ways of attending to social suffering.

Clearly, a liberating approach to women's emotional distress and substance use is desperately needed in mental health and addictions. A social justice framework emphasizes women's human rights, such as a viable livelihood/livable income, decent working conditions, adequate food, water and shelter, sexual and reproductive rights, sovereignty and connection to the land, the right to live without violence, the right to culture, and participation in community. These must be at the forefront of change rather than repudiated in the philosophical, ontological and epistemological commitments of biomedicine that are ingrained in Western power dynamics and dominant ways of responding to emotional, physical, and spiritual distress.

## Note

1  To avoid determinism, it is important to note that not all women who experience violence will develop mental health or substance-use problems, and not all distressed women will have experienced violence since not all mental distress is rooted in oppression.

**84** Norma Jean Profitt

## References


Ahmed, S. (2017). *Living a feminist life*. Duke University Press.

Alcoff, L. (2007). Epistemologies of ignorance: Three types. In S. Sullivan & N. Tuana (Eds.), *Race and epistemologies of ignorance* (pp. 39–57). State University of New York Press.

American Psychiatric Association. (2013). *Diagnostic and statistical manual of mental disorders* (5th ed.). American Psychiatric Association Publishing.

Ashcroft, R., & Van Katwyk, T. (2016). An examination of the biomedical paradigm: A view of social work. *Social Work in Public Health*, 31(3), 140–152. https:///doi.org/10.1080/19371918.2015.1087918.

Brave Heart, M.Y.H. (2003). The historical trauma response among natives and its relationship to substance abuse: A Lakota illustration. *Journal of Psychoactive Drugs*, 35(1), 7–13. https://doi.org/10.1080/02791072.2003.10399988.

British Columbia Centre of Excellence for Women's Health. (2016). Coalescing on women and substance use: Trauma-informed online tool. https://yourexperiencesmatter.com/wp-content/uploads/2016/01/R_181.pdf.

Brown, C. (2020). Feminist narrative therapy and complex trauma: Critical clinical work with women diagnosed as "borderline", In C. Brown & J. MacDonald (Eds.), *Critical clinical social work: Counterstorying for social justice* (pp.82–109). Canadian Scholars Press.

Brown, C. (2021). Critical clinical social work and the neoliberal constraints on social justice in mental health. *Research on Social Work Practice*, 31(6), 644–652. https://doi.org/10.1177/1049731520984531.

Brown, C., Johnstone, M. & Ross, N. (2021). Repositioning social work practice in mental health in Nova Scotia. Nova Scotia College of Social Workers Report. NSCSW-Repositioning-Social-Work-Practice-in-Mental-Health-in-Nova-Scotia-Report-2021.pdf.

Brown, C., Johnstone, M., Ross, N., & Doll, K. (2022). Challenging the constraints of neoliberalism and biomedicalism: Repositioning social work in mental health. *Qualitative Health Research*, 32(5), 771–787. https://doi.org. 10.1177/10497323211069681.

Burstow, B. (1992). *Radical feminist therapy: Working in the context of violence*. Sage.

Burstow, B. (2003). *Toward a radical understanding of trauma and trauma work. Violence against Women*, 9(11), 1293–1317. https://doi.org/10.1177/1077801203255555.

Burstow, B. (2005). A critique of post-traumatic stress disorder and the DSM. *Journal of Humanistic Psychology*, 45(4), 429–445. https://doi.org/10.1177/0022167805280265.

Canadian Women's Foundation & BC Society of Transition Houses. (2011). *Report on violence against women, mental health and substance use*. PDF-VP-Resources-BCSTH-CWF-Report_Final_2011_-Mental-Health_Substance-use.pdf (canadianwomen.org).

Caplan, P. (1995). *They say you're crazy. How the world's most powerful psychiatrists decide who's normal*. Addison-Wesley.

Chrisjohn, R. (n.d.). Excerpts of a speech delivered in Edmonton, Alberta. Transcribed by J. Craven and posted on September 1, 1998. http://sisis.nativeweb.org/resschool/chrisjohn.html.

Coates, L., & Wade, A. (2007). Language and violence: Analysis of four discursive operations. *Journal of Family Violence,* 22(7), 511–522. https://doi.org/10.1007/s10896-007-9082-2.

Cockell, J., & McArthur-Blair, J. (2012). *Appreciative inquiry in higher education: A transformative force*. Jossey-Bass.

Coker, E.M. (2003). Narrative strategies in medical discourse: Constructing the psychiatric "case" in a non-Western setting. *Social Science & Medicine*, 5(5), 905–916. https://doi .org/10.1016/S0277-9536(02)00459-8.

Cosgrove, L., Mills, C., Karter, J.M., Mehta, A., & Kalathil, J. (2019). A critical review of the Lancet Commission on global mental health and sustainable development: Time for a paradigm change, *Critical Public Health*, 30(5), 1–8. https://doi.org/10.1080/09581596 .2019.1667488.

Daley, A., Costa, L., & Ross, L. (2012). (W)righting women: Constructions of gender, sexuality and race in the psychiatric chart. *Culture, Health & Sexuality: An International Journal for Research, Intervention and Care*, 14(8), 955–969. https://doi.org/10.1080 /13691058.2012.712718.

Davis, H. (1999). The psychiatrization of post-traumatic distress: Issues for social workers. *British Journal of Social Work*, 29(5), 755–777. https://doi.org/10.1093/bjsw /29.5.755.

Dotson, K. (2011). Tracking epistemic violence, tracking practices of silencing. *Hypatia*, 26(2), 236–257. https://doi.org/10.1111/j.1527-2001.2011.01177.x.

Duran, E. & Duran, B. (1995). *Native American postcolonial psychology*. State University of New York Press.

Ferguson, I. (2017). *Politics of the mind: Marxism and mental distress*. Bookmarks.

Ferguson, I., & Lavalette, M. (2007). "Dreaming a great dream". Prospects for a new, radical social work. *Canadian Social Work Review*, 24(1), 55–68.

Fraser N. (1986). Toward a discourse ethic of solidarity. *Praxis International*, 5(4), 425–429.

Fraser, N. (2003). Rethinking recognition: Overcoming displacement and reification in cultural politics. In B. Hobson (Ed.), *Recognition struggles and social movements: Contested identities, agency and power* (pp. 21–32). Cambridge University Press.

Frost, L., & Hoggett, P. (2008). Human agency and social suffering. *Critical Social Policy*, 28, 438–460. https://doi.org/10.1177/0261018308095279.

Greenspan, M. (1995). Out of bounds. *Common Boundary*, 13(4), 51–58.

Humphreys, C., & Thiara, R. (2003). Mental health and domestic violence: "I call it symptoms of abuse". *British Journal of Social Work*, 33(2), 209–226. https://doi.org/10 .1093/bjsw/33.2.209.

Jani, J.S., Ortiz, L., Pierce, D., & Sowbel, L. (2011). Access to intersectionality, content to competence: Deconstructing social work education diversity standards. *Journal of Social Work Education*, 47(2), 283–301. https://doi.org/10.5175/JSWE.2011.200900118.

Jani, J.S., & Reisch, M. (2011). Common human needs, uncommon solutions: Applying a critical framework to perspectives on human behavior. *Families in Society: The Journal of Contemporary Social Services*, 92(1), 13–20. https://doi.org/10.1606/1044 -3894.4065.

Johnstone, L., Boyle, M., Cromby, J., Dillon, J., Harper, D., Kinderman, P., Longden, E., Pilgrim, D., & Read, J. (2018). *The power threat meaning framework: Towards the identification of patterns in emotional distress, unusual experiences and troubled or troubling behaviour, as an alternative to functional psychiatric diagnosis*. British Psychological Society. https://www.bps.org.uk/member-networks/division-clinical -psychology/power-threat-meaning-framework.

Johnstone, M., Brown, C., & Ross, N. (2022). The McDonaldization of social work: A critical analysis of mental health care services using the Choice and Partnership Approach (CAPA) in Canada. *Journal of Progressive Human Services*, 33(2), 1–21. https://doi.org/10.1080/10428232.2022.2050117.

Joseph, A. (2017). Pathologizing distress: The colonial master's tools and mental health services for "newcomers/immigrants". In D. Baines (Ed.), *Doing anti-oppressive practice: Social justice social work* (3rd ed.) (pp. 233–251). Fernwood.

LeFrançois, B., Beresford, P., & Russo, J. (2016). Editorial: Destination mad studies. *Intersectionalities*, 5, 1–10.

Liegghio, M. (2013). A denial of being: Psychiatrization as epistemic violence. In B. LeFrançois, R. Menzies, & G. Reaume (Eds.), *Mad matters: A critical reader in Canadian mad studies* (pp. 122–129). Canadian Scholars Press.

MacDonald, K.I. (2002). Epistemic violence: The body, globalization and the dilemma of rights. *Transnational Law and Contemporary Problems*, 12(1), 65–87. https://tspace .library.utoronto.ca/bitstream/1807/9932/1/Epistemic%20Violence.pdf.

MacDonnell, J.A., Dastjerdi, M., Khanlou, N., Bokore, N., & Tharao, W. (2016). Activism as a feature of mental health and wellbeing for racialized immigrant women in a Canadian context. *Health Care for Women International*, 38(2), 187–204. https://doi .org/10.1080/07399332.2016.1254632.

McGibbon, E.A. (2012). Oppression and mental health: Pathologizing the outcomes of injustice. In E.A. McGibbon (Ed.), *Oppression: A social determinant of health* (pp. 123–137). Fernwood.

McGibbon, E., & McPherson, C. (2013). Stress, oppression and women's health: A discussion of the health consequences of injustice. *Women's Health & Urban Life*, 12(2), 63–81.

Marmot, M. (2010). *Fair society, healthy lives: Strategic review of health inequalities in England post 2010*. Institute of Health Equity.

Mental Health Commission of Canada. (2009). *Toward recovery & well-being: A framework for a mental health strategy for Canada*. Mental Health Commission of Canada.

Mills, C. (2014). *Decolonizing global mental health: The psychiatrization of the majority world*. Routledge.

National Inquiry into Missing and Murdered Indigenous Women and Girls. (2019). *Reclaiming power and place: The final report of the National Inquiry into Missing and Murdered Indigenous Women and Girls* (Volumes 1a & 1b). Canada. https://www .mmiwg-ffada.ca/final-report/.

Native Women's Association of Canada. (2007). Social determinants of health and Canada's Aboriginal women. Ottawa: NWAC. http://www.nwac.ca/wp-content/uploads/2015/05 /2007-Social-Determinants-of-Health-and-Canada%E2%80%99s-Aboriginal-Women -NWAC-Submission-to-WHO-Commission.pdf.

Oliver, K. (2004). Witnessing and testimony. *Parallax*, 10(1), 78–87. https://doi.org/10 .1080/1353464032000171118.

Powell, J.A. (2003). Lessons from suffering: How social justice informs spirituality. *University of St. Thomas Law Journal*, 1(1), 102–127.

Prilleltensky, I., Valdés, L.S., Rossiter, A., & Walsh-Bowers, R. (2002). Applied ethics in mental health in Cuba: Part II – Power differentials, dilemmas, resources, and limitations. *Ethics & Behavior*, 12(3), 243–260. https://doi.org/10.1207/S15327019EB1203_3.

Profitt, N.J. (2021). The political language of moral distress. *Connection Magazine*, 4(2), 17–18.

Profitt, N.J. (2022). Moral distress and collective advocacy. *Connection Magazine*, 5(2), 16–17.

Raphael, D. (2012). Critical perspectives on the social determinants of health. In E.A. McGibbon (Ed.), *Oppression: A social determinant of health* (pp. 45–59). Fernwood.

Reynolds, V. (2010). Doing justice: A witnessing stance in therapeutic work alongside survivors of torture and political violence. In J. Raskin, S. Bridges, & R. Neimeyer (Eds.), *Studies in meaning 4: Constructivist perspectives on theory, practice, and social justice* (pp. 157–184). Pace University Press.

Root, M. (1992). Restructuring the impact of trauma on personality. In L. Brown & M. Balfour (Eds.), *Personality and psychopathology* (pp. 108–118). Guilford.

Rossiter, A., Walsh-Bowers, R., & Prilleltensky, I. (2002). Ethics as a located story: A comparison of North American and Cuban clinical ethics. *Theory & Psychology*, 12(4), 533–556. https://doi.org/10.1177/0959354302012004298.

Smith, D.E. (1996). The relations of ruling: A feminist inquiry. *Studies in Cultures, Organizations and Societies*, 2(2), 171–190.

Spretnak, C. (Ed.). (1982). *The politics of women's spirituality: Essays on the rise of spiritual power within the feminist movement*. Anchor Press/Doubleday.

Summerfield, D. (2012). Afterword: Against "global mental health". *Transcultural Psychiatry*, 49(3–4), 519–530. https://doi.org/10.1177/1363461512454701.

Thiara, R.K., & Harrison, C. (2021). *Reframing the links: Black and minoritised women, domestic violence and abuse, and mental health – A review of the literature*. Women's Aid.

Thompson, L. (2021). Toward a feminist psychological theory of "institutional trauma". *Feminism & Psychology*, 31(1), 99–118. https://doi.org/10.1177/0959353520968374.

Tseris, E.J. (2013). Trauma theory without feminism? Evaluating contemporary understandings of traumatized women. *Affilia: Journal of Women and Social Work*, 28(2), 153–164. https://doi.org/10.1177/0886109913485707.

Tseris, E.J. (2019). *Trauma, women's mental health, and social justice: Pitfalls and possibilities*. Routledge.

Ussher, J.M. (1991). *Women's madness: Misogyny or mental illness?* Harvester Wheatsheaf.

Ussher J.M. (2005). Unravelling women's madness: Beyond positivism and constructivism and towards a material-discursive-intrapsychic approach. In R. Menzies, D.E. Chunn & W. Chan (Eds.), *Women, madness and the law: A feminist reader* (pp. 19–41). Glasshouse Press.

Wade, A. (1997). Small acts of living: Everyday resistance to violence and other forms of oppression. *Contemporary Family Therapy*, 19(1), 23–39. https://doi.org/10.1023/A:1026154215299.

Weinberg, M. (2010). The social construction of a social work ethics: Politicizing and broadening the lens. *Journal of Progressive Human Services*, 21(1), 32–44. https://doi.org/10.1080/10428231003781774.

Women's Aid. (2021). Mental health and domestic abuse: A review of the literature. Women's Aid, Bristol. https://www.womensaid.org.uk/wp-content/uploads/2021/12/FINAL-WA-literature-review.pdf.

World Health Organization. (2000). *Women's mental health: An evidence-based review*. Department of Mental Health and Substance Dependence, World Health Organization.

World Health Organization. (2021). *Violence against women*. https://www.who.int/news-room/fact-sheets/detail/violence-against-women.

Young, I.M. (1990). *Justice and the politics of difference*. Princeton University Press.

# 5

# FEMINIST THERAPY, COMMUNITY MENTAL HEALTH AND TRAUMA

*Heather Gaskill*

## Introduction

What defines the most severe and damaging traumatic experiences is the doubt they often instill about our basic human worth, due to the feelings of powerlessness and humiliation that so often accompany trauma in its worst forms. This often involves a complete disregard for the person, their emotional needs and their well-being, and it communicates to the person that they do not matter at all. The complete lack of meaningful cultural and social response with which trauma is so often met exacerbates the traumatic impact, indeed it is *re*traumatizing. When we have an experience that teaches us that we are nothing, disposable, less than human, and that experience is then met with skepticism, disbelief, or outright blame, there is little chance that our basic view of ourselves and of the world will not be profoundly negatively affected. In my psychotherapy practice with trauma clients, I always begin by asking if they trust themselves, and if they ever feel safe. These two questions often reveal the extent to which their core beliefs may have been shaped by the damage they have experienced. The answer to both of these questions is invariably "no".

Mainstream approaches to trauma treatment, in pursuit of a reliably effective formula to follow, have long reflected poorly conceptualized post-traumatic stress as only a misfiring nervous system; for example, polyvagal theory (Porges & Dana, 2018); faulty cognition (cognitive processing therapy) (Resick, Monson, & Chard, 2016); disordered personality (dialectical behavior therapy (Dimeff & Linehan, 2001); or as a problem with memory storage and processing (Eye Movement Desensitization and Reprocessing (EMDR)) (Oren & Solomon, 2012). Techniques designed only to correct these symptoms fail to address the root of what is damaged by trauma: core beliefs about oneself and about the world. Trauma clients

DOI: 10.4324/9781003379591-6

present with the narrative that they are worthless, weak and failing as human beings, and believe wholeheartedly that the world is a fundamentally dangerous place and holds no shelter for them, no justice for the wrongs they have experienced, and that they can always expect the worst of circumstances to befall them. These beliefs shape every decision they make, amplify every emotional response they experience and infect every relationship they attempt to forge.

In this chapter, I will use my experience of working as a psychotherapist in the public health care system (mainly in community mental health and addictions) to describe the failure of mainstream mental health to adequately assess for and treat trauma. I will argue that the typical conceptualization of trauma-as-an-illness that has been individualized, depoliticized, and seen as separate and unrelated to other "mental health issues" – prevents clinicians from providing effective treatment, and in fact often results in resources being wasted on standardized and formulaic interventions that do not address the root causes of people's distress. I will further assert that trauma cannot be adequately treated outside of the sociopolitical context that so often creates and maintains it, and that a feminist, narrative lens is essential to doing this work.

## The Powerful Impact of Trauma

Technique-based approaches encourage clinicians to place trauma in a silo to be treated by specialists, thus isolating it from a person's general mental health, much in the same way that our culture treats substance use issues as distinct and separate. This separation further encourages mainstream clinicians to view trauma as divisible from any general psychotherapeutic process, lessening the likelihood that initial attempts at counseling might identify the main issues. Given the research on how adverse childhood experiences create vulnerability for difficulties with mental health and addictions in adulthood, and in fact predispose people to develop post-traumatic stress disorder (PTSD) due to events later in life, this is a dangerous omission (Crandall et al., 2019).

Trauma at its most devastating teaches powerful lessons about our value, and for those who are most frequently targeted, these lessons reflect what we already know about the social and cultural construction of our worth. This construction is based in oppression, and assigns the right to basic safety, autonomy, protection and justice to some groups, and not to others. To find oneself outside of these basic rights is devastating. Post-traumatic stress is as much about the cultural response we receive following trauma as the traumatic event itself. Treatment that ignores or omits the damage done at this core level of meaning is a missed opportunity of heartbreaking proportion.

## Lessons as a Trauma Therapist

My education in trauma began in rape crisis work, and through feminist activism. It continued through work as a psychotherapist in addictions, community mental health and finally work with the military. The theoretical foundation I gained at the beginning – as a feminist therapist – still defines the work I do with any population.

Ten years of working in sexual assault centers familiarized me not only with the issue of sexual violence from a political perspective, but also with the average presentation, which surprised me. My first counseling position was intake: for a year I did every initial assessment that came through the door, which required a full assessment for trauma, mental health and addictions. I discovered almost immediately that a tiny fraction of the women presenting for services had experienced only one sexual assault as an adult, Western culture's classic portrayal of a "rape victim". Virtually all of the clients had been assaulted by someone they knew. Most women would offer a single experience of sexual violence at the outset of the interview, either in adulthood or more frequently in childhood, but I learned to ask follow-up questions that generally revealed additional experiences of having been victimized. The most frequent presentation in that context was a woman who had been sexually abused as a child, been raped by either acquaintances or boyfriends as an adolescent, and then had experienced abuse in relationships as an adult. This presentation was often accompanied by the lack of a secure attachment with a caring, attentive parent or caregiver in childhood. My observation was that the less love, care and attention a child receives, the more vulnerable she is to abuse. This observation is supported by research (Briere, Runtz, Eadie, Bigras, Godbout, 2017).

These women typically displayed some or all of what I learned to view as the hallmark symptoms of trauma: anxiety with panic, severe depression with suicidality and a history of attempts, a compromised or negligible ability to regulate emotion, difficulty with setting boundaries and being assertive, and, perhaps the most damaging, pervasive and severe, self-loathing and self-criticism. They often had a history of or were currently struggling with one or more coping mechanisms, such as cutting, problems with eating and body image (e.g., anorexia, bulimia or binge-eating) or substance-use problems, which often both provide relief and cause additional difficulties. I later learned that in mainstream mental health settings each of these symptoms was often viewed and treated independently of the others. I saw more than one woman at Addictions Services in Halifax, Nova Scotia, who in addition to seeing me had a therapist at the sexual assault center, the eating disorders clinic and community mental health, giving a total of four mental health clinicians. This baffled me, both in terms of the gross waste of public resources due to redundancy, but also the perspective that each of these issues was somehow distinct and separate from the others and required its own specialist. This separation also failed to provide clients with the precious opportunity to understand the connections between their histories of trauma and their attempts at coping. Instead, this made them feel further pathologized by "needing four different therapists" due to a host of apparently unrelated issues.

By the time I started working in the mainstream mental health system, I had already spent several years learning to work with each of these symptoms as predictable outcomes of a larger whole. I observed that the more severe and sustained the damage had been, the worse the symptoms would be. Like many before me (Flores, 2004), my resulting conceptualization of mental health symptoms, including substance use, was essentially based on attachment. We learn much of our emotional and relational skill through modeling our caregivers (Karreman, van Tuijl, van Aken, & Deković, 2006). If this learning process is shaped by trauma, abuse or neglect, our "skills" will look more like trauma adaptations and, worse, boundary violations will become normalized, thus leaving us vulnerable to being additionally victimized (Alexander, 2009). Without intervention, this situation then perpetuates itself, and we are left to manage severe and complicated symptoms with essentially no tools.

What I discovered following my work at sexual assault centers and when I was working in the women's program at addictions services in Halifax was even more striking. Given what I knew about the statistics around women, addictions and sexual violence (Liebschutz et al., 2002), I was perplexed by women denying any experiences of assault or abuse in their initial screenings with me. They also tended to minimize any childhood abuse or neglect, and were careful to inform me that they were not blaming their mistakes on anyone but themselves. I learned quickly to change my language: instead of using the term "sexual assault", I began to ask women if they had ever had anything sexual happen while using or drinking that they were not comfortable with. I then received a deluge of stories. Very frequently, the women's stories were characterized by self-blame, minimization and uncertainty (Brown, C., 2013).

These women were not being intentionally deceptive or secretive. Mainstream approaches to addictions, particularly those asserted by Alcoholics Anonymous (AA) and Narcotics Anonymous (NA) (which were designed by White men), hold a primary focus on accountability and personal responsibility (Houston, 2014). These women were holding themselves accountable for the rape and sexual assault they had experienced because they had been drinking or using at the time, and so did not feel entitled to use the term "assault", or to think about their experiences as victimization. This view did not change the reality of what they had experienced. The same principle applied to their experiences of childhood or adolescent traumas: they glossed over the details and focused instead on the ways that they had placed themselves in dangerous situations, acted irresponsibly or perceived themselves to be failing in recovery. It was a paradigm shift for many of them, when I explained to them that alcohol is the most frequently used "rape drug".

Speaking with me was often the first time these women had ever had assistance in reframing their experiences in a way that did not make them the authors of their own demise. Some of them fought me on it. One woman left my office at the sexual assault center in outrage because I had gently tried to suggest that the people responsible for her gang rape were the four men involved, not her and her drinking. All I had done in this regard was to ask her what her perpetrators might have been thinking during the assault, and whether it could be possible that they had planned her attack. This was enough to essentially end that counseling session. She told me in no uncertain terms that I clearly "didn't understand addiction", and how important it was for her to take responsibility for the damage she had caused herself and others through her use of alcohol.

This is a crucial question for trauma therapists: What shaped the meaning she was making of her trauma experience? Why would a woman who was gang-raped while barely conscious due to the effects of alcohol, feel so responsible for having been attacked? How can we use trauma therapy to dismantle the self-blame that is so strongly defended? I would argue that we cannot responsibly offer trauma therapy that does not directly address the story of self-blame that a woman holds onto. Self-blame has a powerful impact on how survivors of trauma think and talk about their experiences, greatly reducing the chances that they might receive adequate or relevant treatment, particularly by those without awareness and concern around the complexities of trauma and how women cope with it. The woman above had been seen by multiple clinicians at community mental health and addictions centers, had participated in inpatient programming, and had for several years been attending AA, which discourages self-reflection and instead encourages people to view themselves as "powerless" and to cede control to a "higher power". Given the centrality of issues of power in trauma this is particularly dangerous. The primary and generally singular goal of AA is to abstain from alcohol, while little effort is made to explore why one is drinking to cope and the history and meaning of a person's alcohol use. Participants are encouraged to view themselves as having no power or control over their drinking, which is framed not as a choice they are able to make (or not to make) but instead as a disease with which they are permanently afflicted. There is no attention paid to how alcohol use could be adaptive to someone with extreme levels of distress and no other coping skills, a line of inquiry useful in dismantling the considerable shame that so often accompanies addictions. Often clinging to the thin strand of hope around the promise of "recovery", people can understandably become quite threatened by the idea of exploring *why* they are drinking. Until we worked together, this woman's narrative around self-blame and its accompanying shame, despair and self-loathing remained intact.

This phenomenon is by no means limited to women. When I was working at an inpatient addictions treatment center for men, I had a client initially explain to me that his main issue was that he was "a pathological liar". Upon careful exploration he revealed that he was only lying to his wife, and this was because when he told her the truth, she would escalate into violence that had involved at least once advancing on him with a knife in front of their children. Prior to meeting with me he had been seen by several psychiatrists and at least two psychologists, but his wife's violence and controlling behavior had "never come up". Our culture maintains a strong narrative that men cannot be victims, they cannot be vulnerable and feel powerless, which likely discouraged these clinicians from fully exploring that aspect of his story.

Mainstream mental health and addictions, at least for the ten or so years when I was working there (ending in 2018), was plagued with this problem. In my experience, the majority of clients I worked with in that context for any significant period of time had a trauma history. This was not limited to sexual trauma, although that was frequent on my caseload given my background in sexual assault work and the relative dearth of clinicians who identified as having that skill set, given that it was viewed as separate from "regular" mental health issues. At the very least, the clients I saw had attachment traumas and/or adverse childhood experiences (Felitti et al., 1998). There were virtually no exceptions to this. I was, therefore, continually confused by the steady stream of clients I met with for initial assessments who had often been assessed several times at community mental health in the decade prior to meeting with me. No one had asked them about experiences of trauma. Twenty minutes into their appointments these clients were relating repeated and severe trauma histories, no detail of which could be found documented anywhere on their files. I asked one woman, in particular, who was too anxious to leave her house most of the time, why she had not chosen to share her considerable history of abuse at any of those appointments. She shrugged: "They never asked. Is that important?" A review of her chart revealed that she had been diagnosed with generalized anxiety disorder, treated with cognitive behavioral therapy for ten sessions, and then discharged. This treatment loop had happened at least three times in a period of about seven years, without any significant clinical improvement.

While I think it was quite possible that at least one of the clinicians with whom this woman met over a period of years asked her about an abuse history, a crucial point demonstrated by her case is one that has repeatedly arisen during my work as a psychotherapist, both in the public system and private practice. She, herself, did not see her history of abuse as a particularly relevant factor to her panic and inability to leave her house. The idea that growing up in an inherently unsafe environment might make her feel that the world is too dangerous to engage with had not occurred to her, in the same way that it had not to many of the clinicians she had met with. In fact, like many clients with whom I have worked, she was quick to declare her reluctance to "blame" her childhood for what she perceived as her own mistakes and weakness of character. This left her feeling helpless and stuck.

This is a critical moment in any assessment process. We know that the stories humans tell about themselves are at best biased and incomplete and at worst damaging, and that the process of psychotherapy should seek to reinterpret clients' experiences into a more strengths-based and sustainable narrative (White, 1998). However, this process is entirely dependent on our theoretical framework as clinicians. Every time we meet with someone new, deliberately or not, we decide what the problem is and how to address it, regardless of how collaboratively we approach our work. We hold beliefs on what trauma looks like, who experiences it, and its relationship to mental health and substance-use issues. These beliefs affect our basic ability to recognize trauma, and we cannot work with something that we cannot see.

Self-reflection is an ethical obligation for mental health professionals. The ability to identify which forces and ideas have shaped our perspectives is essential, as our perspectives shape how we offer treatment. Our thinking as clinicians is subject to at least some of the same cultural influences as the clients we see, which may increase the danger that we will accept without question their narratives around self-blame and shame. In psychotherapy we regularly have to decide whether to endorse a client's self-assessment, no matter how skewed and self-punishing. Reflecting a narrative therapy framework, we need to explore how their story emerged the way that it did. All stories are shaped within a social context and hence socially constructed, and that is very clear when we acknowledge the power and politics of violence and trauma in women's lives. From this feminist narrative view, there is no one single author of a story, and certainly no objective stance. People often tell stories about themselves that are negative, injurious and self-blaming: our stories can cause us serious ongoing harm. It is crucial to collaborate with clients to uncover a more helpful counterstory that will support their healing and recovery. Our individual conceptual framework will guide every question we ask as we practice, and drive every intervention we offer.

## Inadequate, Injurious, and Oppressive Social Responses

Both clients and clinicians face an uphill battle against the influence of mainstream culture's basic response to trauma, which is denial. This denial shapes both our collective thinking and how the public health care and judicial systems respond. The current "trauma-informed" language follows on previous decades of feminist work, which sought to advocate for social and legal changes around violence and trauma as well as developing distinct psycho-educational and psychotherapeutic strategies for clinical work. Today, the presence of the #MeToo movement and the mobilization of a "trauma-informed" discourse within the health care system obscures the depth and scope of the problem. There seems to be little acknowledgment of the lack of services and training for trauma work, alongside lengthy waiting lists, an insistence on short-term biomedicalized work and an overall lack of funding and programming. Multiple high-profile cases have arisen in recent years, including those of Gian Ghomeshi and Steven Galloway in Canada, Bill Cosby and Harvey Weinstein in the US, and more recently the Donald Trump civil lawsuit in which the jury awarded E. Jean Caroll approximately US $5 million in damages for sexual abuse and defamation, but not rape, as she had alleged. Despite the furor on social and conventional media, it took literally dozens of women coming forward to produce convictions for Weinstein and, in Cosby's case, only one conviction, which was later overturned on a technicality. In the cases of Galloway and Ghomeshi, there were no convictions, and Galloway is now pursuing civil suits against the women who made complaints against him. Trump continues to publicly malign E. Jean Caroll in an overtly misogynist way.

Even when women repeatedly came forward to speak openly about consistent patterns of repeated, predatory behavior and risked public humiliation and defamation, all these men except Weinstein refused to acknowledge sexual assault and rape. These examples reflect a much larger cultural phenomenon: literally millions of women have spoken about their experiences of having been raped. They do not tell police, but they tell their doctors and sisters and friends and counselors and spiritual leaders. They tell other women. Despite their numbers, and the fact that many of them are struggling to function with severe symptoms of post-traumatic stress, our society has concluded that instead of having a serious problem with sexual violence, we have a problem with women who lie.

Legally speaking, there is still virtually no consequence for committing rape or sexual abuse for most offenders. I have worked with literally hundreds of women (and men, and non-binary folk) who have been raped or sexually abused and almost none of them reported their experiences to the police. They simply did not see it as a process likely to improve their circumstances, and in fact, often asserted their belief that it would only make things worse. Conviction rates for sexual assault and abuse cases that are brought forward remain abysmally low (Statistics Canada, 2017), and my experiences accompanying women to court have revealed a slow, grueling, humiliating and retraumatizing process that I can definitely say I would not want to engage in if I was raped tomorrow. I would do what most people do – try to forget about it and move on.

To further muddy our collective thinking, unfortunately we live in a culture where it is still a political act to make the statement that the person solely responsible for a rape is the person who committed it. Despite decades of statistics it is also severely controversial to name the gendered reality of sexual violence. It is a crime predominantly perpetrated by men and experienced by women and girls (McCloskey & Raphael, 2005), and yet to make this statement publicly is to face accusations of being discriminatory. These accusations now arise both from the conservative right and the liberal left, and have backed feminism into a corner of silence that invisibilizes women's experiences once again. There is now significant pressure not to talk about how our culture's construction of gender contributes to trauma, despite the fact that the gendered nature of sexual violence has not changed.

Perhaps the most devastating aspect of our cultural construction of rape that influences dominant cultural narratives is that it continues to be conflated with sex. Prevention messages now bring a laser-like focus to consent, as though the only difference between rape and sex is the word "no". Feminists have been pointing to this fallacy for decades without success. This conflation perpetuates the idea that it could be possible to "accidentally" rape someone, and that the whole thing is just too confusing and murky for men to figure out. Adoption of this idea means that professionals responding to disclosures of sexual assault may automatically feel that it is somehow biased and unfair to respond with unequivocal belief and support.

It is not a coincidence that trauma frequently targets the most vulnerable: those with the smallest measure of social, political and economic power. In a painful irony, vulnerability heavily influences who we view as credible: the more vulnerable a person is, the less credibility they tend to be assigned. Groups that are oppressed and marginalized experience much higher rates of assault and abuse, and yet these are the folk who tend to evoke the most suspicion when they attempt to get help. This creates a situation where it is essentially open season for abuse with certain groups, as has long been the case for Indigenous women in Canada. The same goes for women with (dis)Abilities, who are four times more likely to be sexually assaulted in their lifetimes (Martin et al., 2006). Children fall into this category, because they essentially have no voice and are often completely dependent on the people who harm them.

In the absence of any critical analysis, these ideas shape how our culture (including the mainstream mental health system) responds to trauma, and this applies not only to women and sexual assault. The last five years of my social work career prior to entering private practice were spent working almost exclusively with men, and the last three years were spent at a military base, where I was further exposed to military culture around war trauma. I was in no way surprised to hear stories from women service members who had been sexually assaulted while serving who were struggling with the same lack of systemic response that I had so long witnessed in the civilian system. I was, however, surprised to hear military members who were clearly struggling with service or combat-related post-traumatic stress and were refusing to be assessed or sufficiently treated for fear of being perceived as "that guy".

"That guy", in military and first responder circles, refers to an individual who falsely claims to have PTSD for secondary gain (usually financial), and is generally viewed with the height of disdain and revulsion. It quickly became clear to me that, in this military context, people who were coming forward with symptoms of post-traumatic stress were subject to similar skepticism as are women who have been sexually assaulted. The same questions were being asked: *Did it really happen the way that you say that it did? Was it really that bad? Are you sure these symptoms aren't just you being dramatic?*

When I make the observation to clients that I have never actually met "that guy" and gently question his existence, everyone is able to give me at least one example of a person who was almost certainly faking PTSD and besmirching the names of "legitimate" survivors. There was a pervasive narrative associating symptoms with weakness and a resulting social isolation and shame that was consuming and often led to explosive anger, addictions and the breakdown of intimate relationships. Our culture's ongoing mainstream gender socialization was impossible to miss in this context. This was the other side of the coin, and these men were also struggling with deep questions about their own worth. Our requirement that men be invincible, emotionally unaffected, and without relational needs was and is wreaking havoc on men trying to recover from legitimate responses to violence. In this sense, patriarchal society is not serving anyone.

## The Need for Feminism and Gender Politics in a Postfeminist Era

Feminism questions traditional power structures, refuses to blindly accept oppression and injustice and insists that how we are socialized by gender is relevant to how we experience ourselves and the world. It provides an effective antidote to much of the blindness around trauma with which mainstream mental health and addictions has suffered, and yet feminism continues to be wildly unpopular. My experience is that it is largely viewed by the mainstream as irrelevant and clinically weak, despite its considerable contribution to the field. It appears that much of the history of this contribution has been lost, despite continuing to be directly relevant to how we think about and treat trauma today.

Prior to my decision to pursue social work, I was involved in feminist activism, and was exposed to a perspective on trauma very much in opposition to the mainstream view. I was the Atlantic regional representative for the Canadian Association of Sexual Assault Centers (CASAC) in 2001/2002, and the unofficial leadership of that collective organization was then fighting to prevent the professionalization of sexual assault services in Canada, an argument that arose both from the anti-psychiatry movement of the 1970s and 1980s and also from the belief that when women are raped or battered they need consciousness-raising and empowerment, not counseling (Burstow, 1992). Professional counseling was viewed in those circles as being in direct opposition to empowerment, and in the context of trauma a process that turned a social and political issue into a medical one.

These feminist women activists believed that the answer to sexual violence was to get organized and to fight back (Lakeman, 2000). It is difficult to quote these women in an academic context as many of them never published in this setting. They were adamantly opposed to the idea that academic credentials were required to lend credibility to their descriptions of their own oppression, but their ideas both reflect and stem from aspects of the works of bell hooks, Gloria Steinem, Audre Lorde and others. Many of them never attended university, perhaps first due to economic circumstances but then as a stance on class. They asserted that oppressed people should be empowered to speak for themselves, and to drive their own emancipation. These ideas were not unique to these women, but they were unpopular. Then, as now, there was great pressure to cede authority to credentialed professionals.

The view asserted by these women was that stopping rape, sexual abuse and domestic violence was a far more efficient and effective (not to mention just and fair) strategy than continually trying to stem the bleed of post-traumatic stress. There was a basic recognition that these crimes were not a random phenomenon and that we live in a culture that creates and maintains rape and abuse, perpetrated by those in power against those without. These were the women who started the first transition houses in Canada, were publicly calling out the justice system for its lack of action on sexual violence, were confronting perpetrators of abuse and were organizing "Take Back The Night" marches. They are the reason we now have sexual assault services and a #MeToo movement.

Perhaps the argument by these feminist advocates most salient to this chapter is the idea that physical, spiritual, cognitive and emotional responses to trauma are not a "mental illness" (Burstow, 1992). Being affected by having been brutalized and humiliated is normal. It is not a disease, and it does not arise out of an inherent weakness or pathology of the individual. Post-traumatic stress, to use this umbrella term, is a series of predictable symptoms typically arising in proportion to the severity of the meaning associated with the trauma experienced. Feminists wanted to prevent survivors of trauma being cast into the role of "patient", as a sick or disordered person needing medical treatment.

To some extent, feminism was co-opted into the "trauma-informed" language of the day that tends to embrace the medicalization of trauma and a focus on the individual. Post-traumatic stress is now firmly entrenched as a mental disorder in the *Diagnostic and Statistical Manual of Mental Disorders* (5th edition) (DSM-5), and the past several decades have revealed an ongoing series of trendy techniques in trauma treatment, each one promising to have finally uncovered a cure for post-traumatic stress. Techniques at their worst, in untrained or insufficiently skilled hands, can cause major damage. I have worked with clients who returned to me feeling much worse after poorly administered exposure and EMDR protocols. The new vanguard of trauma treatment, psychedelic therapy, is now ironically mired in allegations of sexual assault, perpetrated by clinicians against participants in clinical trials (McNamee, Devenot, & Buisson, 2023). Psychedelic therapy also raises some ethical questions regarding how in control of sessions clients can be when they are drugged, to what extent no coercion is ensured, and what the implications are for people who are already struggling with substance-use issues. While some of these techniques have garnered some evidence and have made their way into mainstream usage (Resick, Monson, & Chard, 2016; Shapiro, 2014), most lack any political analysis or focus on meaning that might help survivors locate their experiences in the broader context of a culture that allows abuse and blames and disbelieves survivors. Without this analysis survivors are left to make sense of their experiences in the context of the mainstream medical model.

Further to this model, many survivors of trauma receive diagnoses of borderline personality disorder (BPD), which shares many of the same diagnostic criteria as PTSD but erases the experience of trauma completely (American Psychiatric Association, 2013). Politics aside, telling survivors of trauma that their symptoms are a defining component of their personality seems extremely unlikely to inspire confidence in their ability to change and heal. Women are diagnosed with BPD at three times the rate of men (Skodol & Bender, 2003). Very strong critiques have been advanced by feminists around who gets diagnosed with BPD and why (Brown, C., 2020; Herman, Perry, & van der Kolk, 1989; Shaw & Proctor, 2005).

Feminist critiques of mainstream approaches to trauma are valid, but the rejection of the professionalization of trauma services failed to acknowledge the depth and complexity of damage inflicted on survivors and what might be required to adequately address it. The idea that survivors need only empowerment and crisis intervention was simply not accurate. In the early 2000s, sexual assault centers, many of which were primarily staffed by volunteers, were being overwhelmed by clients whose needs outstripped the services available. At one of the national meetings for CASAC, of which I was part, I listened to center after center talk about how women who clearly needed complex and ongoing care were repeatedly calling rape crisis lines and speaking to volunteers who were woefully under-equipped for the task. I was one such volunteer in the late 1990s, and often felt frustrated and helpless when faced with clients whose clinical symptoms reached far beyond my depth of understanding or skill set. Research has clearly and repeat-edly demonstrated that trauma changes our bodies and our brains, both of which need to be addressed in recovery (Solomon & Heide, 2005).

Despite strong resistance from the national organization (CASAC), the most well-funded and well-organized sexual assault center in my region conducted a needs assessment with women who had been accessing their services. The over-whelming outcome was a demand for professional counseling. It is important to note that these clients wanted counseling from a sexual assault center: an agency organized and run by women governed by feminist principles. It was very clear that women had been trying to be seen and heard by the mainstream medical system, which was overwhelmingly ineffective at meeting their needs. Something was happening at rape crisis centers that was not happening anywhere else.

## The Value of Feminist Therapy

When we begin conversations about feminist therapy, there appears to be an assumption that this will somehow involve a lecture on feminism, or a revisitation of what was once referred to as "consciousness-raising". Most of my clients have no idea that I am a feminist. I am not interested in teaching them about feminism. I want them to learn to love themselves. "Empowerment", is a term much beloved by social work students and academics, but the feedback I repeatedly received as a teaching assistant in social work and later as a clinical supervisor often con-sisted of confusion and frustration about how to actually implement it in a clinical context. I have also found myself in professional situations where management complained that this or that crop of new graduates is too political and lacking in actual clinical skill, as though the two were divisible. If my experiences in mental health and addictions are any indication, they are not.

Given what we know about efficacy in psychotherapy generally speaking, a lecture on anything (including evidence-based concepts) is likely to be a rapport-destroying waste of time. The quality of the relationship between therapist and client is the strongest determinant of therapeutic satisfaction (Ardito & Rabellino, 2011). Information is obviously an important component in therapy: we go to counseling because we want to feel, think and relate differently. However, in psychotherapy, the medium is the message. Feminist relational work is explicit about this. We use the therapeutic relationship as a platform *to teach relationship*, which is a key area of injury for folk with relational trauma. The reason infants need a secure attachment is because it teaches essential lessons about self-regulation, what to expect from the world, and also about their worth. Together these form a foundation for coping in the world. Folk who have never experienced a secure attachment will have to learn one, and the therapeutic relationship can and should be a vehicle for this (Mallinckrodt, 2010).

If our culture teaches us to doubt and minimize our experiences of trauma, suggests that we are culpable, and encourages us to feel shame for "failing" to recover, feminism asserts that we can trust ourselves, that we are not responsible for the behavior of people who hurt us, and that we need and deserve care and attention and justice in order to heal. Where the mainstream medical model pathologizes symptoms of post-traumatic stress and encourages us to see ourselves as flawed and sick, feminism asserts that there is nothing wrong with us: the problem is with what has been done. In a world that refuses to acknowledge that systemic oppression has created an epidemic of trauma that targets the most vulnerable, feminism refuses to ignore this, and perhaps more importantly, refuses to accept it.

To be seen as outwardly feminist or to describe our therapeutic approach as such in the mainstream has unfortunately become a serious professional liability. When I was working in mainstream mental health and addictions, I and the colleagues with whom I shared perspective and values generally maintained a quiet and benign diplomacy. We also received most of the trauma referrals and were typically overloaded with complex cases while many of our colleagues were not even full. Feminist approaches to psychotherapy are effective, and they are particularly effective for treating trauma. Other than sexual assault centers in the non-profit sector, none of the public agencies for whom I have worked have ever acknowledged this, despite the fact that much of their complex work was being done by feminists.

## Conclusion

While I have provided an in-depth exploration of feminist principles in psychotherapy for trauma – in this chapter I have offered my experiences as a feminist practitioner working within the mainstream system of care and highlighted a number of central issues of concern. Our approach as clinicians to trauma, mental health and substance-use problems, should challenge the assumption that we can be neutral or objective when working with violence and trauma. We should be clear about our own positionality and seek to be intentional in counterviewing and counterstorying injurious dominant narratives with which survivors of trauma suffer. These narratives often include self-blame along with stories of low self-worth and the belief that they, the traumatized, are unlovable and that other people cannot be counted on to care for them. These stories are also present within experiences of hopelessness, sadness, depression and anxiety and the subsequent effort people make to cope with those experiences. Individually and biologically centered, technique-based approaches have limited effectiveness overall. Principles of practice established by feminist activists in the 1970s and 1980s provide a clear path to connection, recovery and healing with the emphasis on the social context shaping experiences of violence and trauma within a collaborative relationship that emphasizes emotional safety and is sensitive to issues of power and control. These principles are much needed in the context of a mainstream mental health system that is still struggling both to understand and to effectively treat post-traumatic stress.

## References

Alexander, P.C. (2009). Childhood trauma, attachment, and abuse by multiple partners. *Psychological Trauma: Theory, Research, Practice, and Policy*, 1(1), 78–88. https://doi.org/10.1037/a0015254.

American Psychiatric Association. (2013). *Diagnostic and statistical manual of mental disorders* (5th ed.). https://doi.org/10.1176/appi.books.9780890425596.

Ardito R., & Rabellino, D. (2011). Therapeutic alliance and outcome of psychotherapy: Historical excursus, measurements, and prospects for research. *Frontiers in Psychology*, 2. https://www.frontiersin.org/articles/10.3389/fpsyg.2011.00270.

Briere, J., Runtz, M., Eadie, E., Bigras, N., & Godbout, N. (2017). Disengaged parenting: Structural equation modeling with child abuse, insecure attachment, and adult symptomatology. *Child Abuse & Neglect*, 67, 260–270. https://doi.org/10.1016/j.chiabu.2017.02.036.

Brown, C. (2013). Women's narratives of trauma: (re)Storying uncertainty, minimization, and self-blame. *Narrative Works*, 3(1), 1–30.

Brown, C. (2020). Feminist narrative therapy and complex trauma: Critical clinical work with women diagnosed as "borderline". In C. Brown & J. MacDonald (Eds.), *Critical clinical social work: Counterstorying for social justice* (pp. 82–109). Canadian Scholars Press.

Burstow, B. (1992). *Radical feminist therapy: Working in the context of violence*. Sage.

Crandall, A.A., Miller, J.R., Cheung, A., Novilla, L.K., Glade, M., Novilla, B., Magnusson, B., Leavitt, B.L., Barnes, M.D., & Hanson, C.L. (2019). ACEs and counter-ACEs: How positive and negative childhood experiences influence adult health. *Child Abuse & Neglect*, 96. https://doi.org/10.1016/j.chiabu.2019.104089.

Dimeff, L., & Linehan, M.M. (2001). Dialectical behavior therapy in a nutshell. *The California Psychologist*, 34(3), 10–13.

Felitti, V.J., Anda, R., Nordenberg, D., Williamson, D., Spitz, A., Edwards, V., Koss, M., & Marks, J. (1998). Relationship of childhood abuse and household dysfunction to many of the leading causes of death in adults: The adverse childhood experiences study. *American Journal of Preventative Medicine*, 14(4), 245–258.

Flores, P.J. (2004). *Addiction as an attachment disorder*. Jason Aronson.

Herman, J.L., Perry, J.C., & van der Kolk, B.A. (1989). Childhood trauma in borderline personality disorder. *The American Journal of Psychiatry*, 146(4), 490-495, https://doi.org/10.1176/ajp.146.4.490.

Houston, John. (2014). Friendship, accountability, and mutual growth in virtue. In J.A. Miller (Ed.), *Sobering wisdom: Philosophical explorations of twelve step spirituality.* University of Virginia Press.

Karreman, A., van Tuijl, C., van Aken, M.A.G., & Deković, M. (2006), Parenting and self-regulation in preschoolers: A meta-analysis. *Infant and Child Development,* 15, 561–579. https://doi.org/10.1002/icd.478.

Lakeman, L. (2000). Why law and order cannot end violence against women and why the development of women's (social, economic, political, and civil) rights might. In *Canadian Woman Studies/Les cahiers de la femme,* 20(3), 24–33.

Liebschutz, J., Savetsky, J.B., Saitz, R., Horton, J.H., Lloyd-Travaglini, C., & Samet, J.H. (2002). The relationship between sexual and physical abuse and substance abuse consequences. *Journal of Substance Abuse Treatment,* 22(3),121–128. https://doi.org/10.1016/S0740-5472(02)00220-9.

Mallinckrodt, B. (2010). The psychotherapy relationship as attachment: Evidence and implications. *Journal of Social and Personal Relationships,* 27(2), 262–270. https://doi.org/10.1177/0265407509360905.

Martin, S.L., Ray, N., Sotres-Alvarez, D., Kupper, L.L., Moracco, K.E., Dickens, P.A., Scandlin, D., & Gizlice, Z. (2006). Physical and sexual assault of women with disabilities. *Violence Against Women,* 12(9), 823–837. https://doi.org/10.1177/1077801206292672.

McCloskey, K.A., Raphael, D.N. (2005). Adult perpetrator gender asymmetries in child sexual assault victim selection: Results from the 2000 National Incident-Based Reporting System. *Journal of Child Sexual Abuse,* 14(4), 1–24.

McNamee, S., Devenot, N., & Buisson, M. (2023). Studying harms is key to improving psychedelic-assisted therapy: Participants call for changes to research landscape. *JAMA Psychiatry,* 80(5), 411–412.

Oren, E., & Solomon, R. (2012). EMDR therapy: An overview of its development and mechanisms of action. *European Review of Applied Psychology,* 62(4), 197–203.

Porges, S.W., & Dana, D. (2018). *Clinical applications of the polyvagal theory: The emergence of polyvagal-informed therapies* (Norton series on interpersonal neurobiology). W.W. Norton & Company.

Resick, P.A., Monson, C.M., & Chard, K.M. (2016). *Cognitive processing therapy for PTSD: A comprehensive manual.* Guilford Publications.

Shapiro, F. (2014). The role of eye movement desensitization and reprocessing (EMDR) therapy in medicine: Addressing the psychological and physical symptoms stemming from adverse life experiences. *The Permanente Journal,* 18(1), 71–77. https://doi.org/10.7812/TPP/13-098.

Shaw, C., & Proctor, G. (2005). I. Women at the margins: A critique of the diagnosis of borderline personality disorder. *Feminism & Psychology,* 15(4), 483–490. https://doi.org/10.1177/0959-353505057620.

Skodol, A.E., & Bender, D.S. (2003). Why are women diagnosed borderline more than men? *Psychiatric Quarterly,* 74(4), 349–360.

Solomon, E.P., & Heide, K.M. (2005). The biology of trauma: Implications for treatment. *Journal of Interpersonal Violence,* 20(1), 51–60. https://doi.org/10.1177/0886260504268119.

Statistics Canada. (2017). From arrest to conviction: Court outcomes of police-reported sexual assaults in Canada. *The Daily.* https://www150.statcan.gc.ca/n1/daily-quotidien/171026/dq171026b-eng.htm.

White, M. (1998, August). Narrative therapy. In *Workshop presented at Narrative therapy intensive training.* doi: 10.3389/fpsyg.2011.00270. ISSN: 1664-1078.

# 6

# TALKING TRAUMA TALK AND THE DANGERS OF SPEECH

## Feminist Narrative Therapeutic Conversations for Complex Trauma

*Catrina Brown*

## Introduction

In this chapter I emphasize an ethical stance on critical discursive feminist practice, which involves equalizing power in the therapeutic context by stressing safety, client power and control over their own choices, and transparency throughout the work. This chapter will outline an approach to addressing issues of power in therapeutic conversations through exploring how power and resistance play out in everyday life, as people cope with issues of trauma and violence and in the problem stories people tell about themselves. Clients' stories are contextualized and this collaborative approach emphasizes clients' strengths and agency alongside their vulnerability, marginalization and pain.

Through adopting a feminist narrative lens, I illustrate critically based direct practice with a focus on gender and mental health counseling, drawing on a case example from the substantive practice areas of co-occurring trauma and subsequent mental health issues. As stories emerge in social, cultural, political and historical contexts, they can challenge or reify harmful and unhelpful ideas. Women with histories of trauma often end up with unhelpful pathologizing diagnoses alongside internalized critical stories of self. Trauma stories are often difficult to tell, in part because they can be painful, because others have threatened the person, and because existing frameworks often fail to capture people's experiences, making it dangerous to speak. Taken together, this is enforced silence. As such, speaking of trauma often requires fearless speech (Foucault, 2001), as speaking often involves risk to oneself. A feminist narrative lens will challenge pathologizing diagnoses and refocus the therapeutic conversations on unpacking the meaning and construction of women's stories of trauma, the influence of the stories on their lives, and the creation of more helpful, less fearful counterstories.

DOI: 10.4324/9781003379591-7

Feminists have critiqued, for example, the diagnosis of women with complex trauma as "borderline" and rejected the pathologization of their lives (Brown, C., 1993a, 1993b, 2007a, 2007b, 2011, 2019, 2020b; Brown,C. Johnstone, & Ross, 2021; Brown, L., 1992, 2004; Burstow, 2003; Herman 1992; Herman, Perry, van der Kolk, 1989; Lafrance & McKenzie-Mohr, 2013; Moulding, 2015; Ross, Brown, C., & Johnstone, 2023; Tseris, 2013, 2019; Ussher, 2010). I explore the constraints and dangers of telling a trauma story, the influence of dominant trauma discourses and the importance of double listening. The therapeutic conversation will center on the importance of the therapeutic alliance and unpacking the experience of being in relationships within trauma work. I will do this by delving into Rosa's story of complex trauma and the coping strategies she has used to deal with this. I chose to discuss Rosa's story in this chapter because, while it is critical that a therapist working with Rosa is able to be compassionately involved, their own reactions to Rosa's ways of coping may obstruct attentive listening and being helpful. It is easy to see how her expressions of complex trauma are likely to be pathologized and misunderstood. Rosa's most important influential relationships have been very injurious. Throughout, I am emphasizing the importance of the therapeutic relationship and its importance when there has been relational injury. According to Herman (2015),

> the alliance of therapy cannot be taken for granted; it must be painstakingly built by the effort of both patient and therapist. Therapy requires a collaborative working relationship in which both partners act on the basis of their implicit confidence in the value and efficacy of persuasion rather than coercion, ideas rather force, mutuality rather than authoritarian control.
>
> *(p. 136)*

The development of a healing relationship is critical to trauma work. Herman states:

> I must practice with these beliefs as my foundation, especially in association with trauma work as the traumatic experience has oftentimes fractured these very beliefs in survivors.
>
> *(Herman, 2015, p. 136)*

What is completely clear is that stories are not straightforward. They can be unspeakable, almost too painful to tell. Stories are often uncertain, contradictory, partial, hinted at and even silent. Unpacking narrative metaphors can reveal the indirect ways people often tell their stories. Metaphors like coping strategies are invitations to explore meaning. Like many people with histories of violence and trauma, Rosa's self-harm through cutting tells a story. For Rosa, blood itself is a powerful metaphor and central to her story.

## Making Connections Through Counterviewing Coping

When double listening, we can see that coping strategies are often entry points to trauma stories (White, 2004, 2007). According to White (2000, 2007), double listening involves listening for the absent but implicit. Listening for what is not immediately apparent reflects the understanding that things are not always as they seem, and that most stories, however ambivalent or not one is in telling them, can only ever be partial. People often speak their distress and struggles through "symptoms" and their ways of coping, therefore we need to explore what they mean. Rather than pathologize them, I argue we need to listen to how they make sense (Brown, C., 2017, 2018, 2020b; Brown, C. & MacDonald, 2022).

Critical feminist approaches have reframed "symptoms" as "coping skills" (Brown, C., 2019, 2020a, 2020b; Brown, L., 1992, 2004; Burstow, 2003). Because trauma and violence are so commonly connected with mental health and substance-use struggles, we should routinely explore the possibility of current and/or historical trauma and violence when working with these issues. I am interested in how and why co-occurring coping strategies exist and whether they are related to dominant story lines in people's life experiences, in particular those of abuse and trauma. Counterviewing allows for the unpacking of dominant discourses, noting the effects of trauma and violence itself, and encouraging the subsequent creation of more helpful stories. Trauma-based practice unpacks trauma experiences. In doing so, trauma work counterviews stories of trauma to allow the creation of counterstories that are less minimizing, self-blaming and pathologizing. Women's trauma stories often reflect and reinforce negative unhelpful identity conclusions. According to narrative therapist Michael White, "distress as an outcome of trauma can be understood as a tribute to the maintenance of an ongoing relationship with what a person holds precious, and as refusal to surrender to this" (2004, p. 61).

In the Canadian National Film Board film *To a Safer Place*, Shirley Turcotte describes the intrusive fear and dread of impending abuse and her efforts at coping with the abuse through dissociation or constriction:

> Night after night I lay there afraid to sleep. Wondering when his hand would reach for me next. I always went to bed with my clothes on, hoping to protect myself. But I couldn't. It's there that I learned how to leave my body on the bed and to take myself to a safer place where he couldn't get me. I would hide in the wall. A place too hard and too cold for him to touch. But when he took me upstairs and put me in a chair, I had no place to go, and he took me until there was almost no me left.
>
> *(Shaffer, 1987)*

After deliberately returning to the basement where the abuse occurred as a child she states: "I always felt a part of me was missing, but in that basement, I recovered the child who had been hiding in the wall. She was the survivor in me. She had always been there. She has made me feel strong" (Shaffer, 1987).

While I critically engage with therapeutic conversations that explore women's trauma experiences, subsequent mental health struggles and co-existing coping strategies, I concur with Tseris (2013, 2019) that we must be cautious to avoid abandoning the feminist contributions that situated women's experiences of violence and trauma in the patriarchal and intersectional context of their lives and that emphasized the "personal is political". We need to remain committed to the pioneering feminists who brought gender-based violence and trauma into the public sphere: drawing attention to and integrating the need for addressing the political and social context alongside personal are political feminist approaches to working with women who have struggled with the effects of trauma. As such, we cannot simply adopt a psychocentric approach that decontextualizes and depoliticizes mental health and trauma by locating the problem within the individual or as a biomedical disorder. While there has been a growing social attention to "trauma-informed" care, it frequently fails to move the conversation outside of the individual and often maintains conventional "medical model" approaches to practice. Too often there is little said about the actual trauma work.

### The Challenges of Telling Trauma Stories: Injurious Speech

Women reveal in their efforts to story their experiences of rape and depression a *"linguistic incongruence"* (McKenzie-Mohr & Lafrance, 2011, 2014). The dominant discourse available to talk about experiences of violence and trauma are deeply limiting and often incongruent with women's experiences (DeVault, 1990; McKenzie-Mohr & Lafrance, 2011, 2014). Butler (1997) argues that forcing experience into such dominant discourses produces injurious speech. According to Butler (1997), dominant social discourse – for instance, in this case, "you caused the violence" or "it wasn't as bad as you say it was", or "it did not really happen" is injurious speech. The injurious linguistic incongruence may be reflected in partial disclosure, partial talk or hints of the yet-to-be-spoken ways of telling without telling (Brown, C., 2014). Indeed, when women begin to disclose trauma stories, their stories are often fraught with uncertainty, contradiction and minimization (Brown, C., 2013). bell hooks (1990) states that:

> moving from silence into speech is for the oppressed, the colonized, the exploited, and those who stand and struggle side by side a gesture of defiance that heals, that makes new life and new growth possible. It is that act of speech, of "talking back", that is no mere gesture of empty words, that is the expression of our movement from object to subject – the liberated voice.
>
> *(p. 211)*

For hooks, fighting oppression requires liberating voices – moving from silence to speech – engaging in what Foucault (2001) calls fearless speech. And, while bell hooks argues that oppressed people must *move from silence to speech*, holocaust survivor Eli Weisel reminds us not to underestimate the dangers of speech. In his book *Night* he describes the *difficulty of speaking the unspeakable*:

> And yet, having lived through this experience, one could not keep silent no matter how difficult, if not impossible, it was to speak. And so, I persevered. And trusted the silence that envelops and transcends words. Knowing all the while that any one of the fields of ashes in Birkenau carries more weight than all the testimonies about Birkenau. For, despite all my attempts to articulate the unspeakable, "it" is still not right.
>
> *(Weisel, 2006, p. x)*

In therapeutic conversations, the process of moving from silence to speech is important. Our work is to assist that process. We are challenged to listen carefully, to listen to silence itself, as it often reflects subordination, oppression and abuse. The telling of one's stories in encouraged, however at the same time we need to pay close attention to silence. We are double listening in the process of people moving from silence to speech (Morgan, 2000). The double listening continues when people begin to talk about the trauma – we still need to listen beyond the words. This is especially true as the frameworks available to talk about trauma are already constraining, making it even more difficult to put one's experiences into language. There are many obstacles in both the telling and the hearing of stories.[1] And, of course, if one risks sharing painful traumatic stories and they are not acknowledged, believed or heard, this is often retraumatizing or revictimizing. Putting all this together helps us to understand that trauma work is often "messy". Yet, when trauma experiences are profoundly unspeakable, silence becomes an ordinary part of everyday life as one finds ways to cope (Warin & Dennis, 2008). We need to be comfortable and respectfully patient in the speech spaces that are partial, indirect and uncertain. According to Foucault:

> Silence itself – the things one declines to say, or it is forbidden to name, the discretion that is required between speakers – is less the absolute limit of discourse, the other side from which it is separated by a strict boundary, than an element that functions alongside the things said, with them and in relation to them within overall strategies. There is no binary division to be had between what one says and what one does not say; we must try to determine the different ways of not saying such things, how those who can and those who cannot speak of them are distributed, which types of discourse are authorized, or which forms of discretion is required in either case. There is not one but many silences and they are an integral part of the strategies that underlie and permeate discourse.
>
> *(Foucault, 1980, p. 27)*

Narrative therapeutic conversations unpack what is said and not said. We are interested in what has not made it into the story, what has become disqualified knowledge (Brown, C. & Augusta-Scott, 2007, p. xxv). Exploring the parts of one's experience that have been pushed underground may be important in challenging dominant, unhelpful pathologizing stories about oneself.

According to Foucault:

> Discourse transmits and produces power; it reinforces it, but also undermines and exposes it, renders it fragile and makes it possible to thwart it. In like manner, silence and secrecy are a shelter for power, anchoring its prohibitions, but they also loosen its hold and provide for relatively obscure areas of tolerance.
>
> *(1980, p. 101)*

The coercive effect of dominant discourse produces constraints about what can be said, by whom and to whom (Butler, 1997). Women try to find a way to make sense of their experiences within dominant social narratives that provide inadequate accounts of their experiences and tend to reify oppressive dominant discourse, including the blaming of women for rape and abuse. As such, women's uncertainty about speaking may reflect how difficult it can be to story a trauma experience, to find the words, or to fit one's experience within existing discourses. Taken-for-granted, socially constructed master narratives often do not reflect the interests of women and the associated dominant knowledge claims represent a gap or rupture from women's own sense of violence and trauma.

Telling trauma stories may be experienced as dangerous (sometimes for both client and therapist) as they may raise uncomfortable/painful emotions such as anxiety and fear about acknowledging trauma, disclosure, the perpetrator, being blamed or not believed, potential conflict, being judged or thought less of, possible, shame, guilt and lack of trust. This danger may shape the story telling to both oneself and the listener. Caution and self-surveillance may render invisible or disqualify other aspects of the story. In this way we can directly see the politics of emotion and the social grip on regulating them (Ahmed, 2004; Brown, C., 2019). In the silencing of stories is the silencing of pain and suffering. The silencing and dangers of speech are political. As women often rely on the dominant discourses available to them, the stories they tell about themselves and their lives may be unhelpful (Brown, C., 2007c, 2022; McKenzie-Mohr & Lafrance, 2011). These epistemic gaps are referred to as epistemic injustice (Fricker, 2010), as women's experiences are too often left invisibilized, silenced and unheard. Dominant social relations of power are enacted through discourses that fail women.

## Listening Beyond the Words

In listening beyond the words, we can challenge the dominant discourse and work toward the development of alternative and more helpful narratives (DeVault, 1990,

White, 2001). Storytelling is often selective and partial, involving ways of telling without telling – especially when dangerous – which means we need to listen beyond the words (Brown, C., 2018). The practitioner working with trauma stories needs to be comfortable with the uncertainty and partial telling. People do not come to therapy with their trauma stories and coping all worked out. Trauma work requires an appreciation of the dangers of speaking in a culture in which violence against women and children often continues to be normalized and minimized, and for which the women and children are too often blamed. As people rely on the dominant discourses available to them, which often normalize and minimize trauma and violence, they may join with unhelpful pathologizing, deficit-based stories about their lives and experiences (McKenzie-Mohr & Lafrance, 2011).

## Telling and Hearing: Counterviewing Injurious Speech

The task of practitioners working with those who are dealing with the aftermath of trauma is to disrupt injurious speech through counterviewing trauma stories and to collaboratively create more helpful counterstories. The idea that people's reactions to trauma and violence is a reflection of their weakness or lack of resilience is injurious. Internalized dominant unhelpful social discourses and messages need to be counterviewed. Trauma stories are not neutral. The meaning attached is constructed within available social discourses, which means negative identity stories often reflect and reinforce oppressive social ideas and relations. As the meaning attached is constructed within available social discourses, negative identity stories are frequently developed that often reflect and reinforce oppressive social ideas and relations. Trauma practice asks counterviewing questions to disrupt unhelpful internalized ideas (Madigan, 2003).

Dominant social discourses often shape people's stories of experience and can contribute to unhelpful and oppressive identity conclusions. Feminist narrative approaches see people's stories as socially constructed within existing social relations and available social discourses.

There is little doubt that women's trauma stories are constrained by the limited discourses available to them that fit well with their experiences. Women try to find a way to make sense of their experiences within dominant social narratives that provide inadequate accounts of their experiences and tend to reify oppressive dominant discourse, including the blaming of women for rape and abuse.

## The Discursive Politics of Emotion and Trauma

Emotional life is in the grip of cultural practice and never simply subjective (Brown, C., 2014). Within neoliberal emotional regimes, emotions are expected to be tightly controlled and regulated. The dominant culture of self-management shapes the expectations and performance of emotion management. The emotional life that people experience is often driving the narrative thread in their problem stories or struggles. As such it is critical that we unpack and expose the dominant political discourses surrounding both their emotional experiences and stories of trauma. Trauma experiences are filtered through social discourses.

Despite the expectation of tightly controlled emotions within neoliberal emotional regimes, the aftermath of trauma and violence often creates significant difficulty regulating or feeling in control of one's emotions. People create coping strategies to deal with these distressful emotions. They may be trying to numb pain, get relief, give themselves comfort, or, alternatively, to make themselves feel something other than emptiness or pain. The dominant social context that requires a strict or "totalitarian" disciplining and regulating of subjectivity is impossible for most to adhere to (Brown, C., 2007b). This expectation shapes how people respond to their own emotional suffering and pain related to trauma. Indeed, this socio-emotional context is often damaging, dangerous and oppressive. It forces life experiences into tightly constraining and limiting boxes through tactics such as responsibilizing, minimizing, pathologizing, retraumatizing, invisibilizing, silencing and gas-lighting. The politics of emotion and the social grip on regulating them (Ahmed, 2004), includes processes of self-surveillance, which may render invisible or disqualify parts of one's story and silence talking about trauma. As such, critical approaches to understanding the social creation of trauma and the associated suffering it creates must involve resistance to neoliberal, psychocentric framing that is likely to exacerbate rather than helpfully respond to and reduce these negative effects.

The meaning that individuals make of their trauma experiences is central to therapeutic work. This must involve counterviewing dominant discursive influences that contribute to a social context in which violence and trauma exist, to the unhelpful self-blaming and minimizing meaning that people often attach to their experiences, and to how people can meaningfully create counter-notices of their experience.

Through exploring the case example of Rosa,[2] I will illustrate how difficult it is to tell and hear trauma stories. In this trauma work the telling and hearing of stories involves a critical overlapping process. Through a narrative conversation, stories are unpacked and counterviewed. The intention is to create more helpful meaningful counterstories. There is what Rosa says and what she *does not say* – what I, the therapist, hear and what I *do not hear* – what we discover together that is not yet known to us. My thoughts and interpretations are reflected in intentional unpacking about Rosa's experiences and the meaning she attaches to her struggles. This all leads to counterviewing scaffolding questions that intentionally explore Rosa's story. These questions are not neutral, as they reflect my worldview and subsequent interpretation of what I am hearing. While they are part of shaping the conversation, they in turn are shaped by Rosa's responses.

Part of all therapist's work, especially, in the area of trauma and violence, involves reckoning with our own emotional responses. We may feel outraged, horrified and even wounded by the images of what the person has endured. In this work, we must challenge dominant binary constructions that obstruct the complexity of people's stories. This often involves adopting a "both/and" stance which avoids either/or ways of thinking and encourages complexity. For instance, we need to attend to the coalescing of pain, vulnerability, suffering, helplessness, hopelessness, powerlessness and capacity, creativity, coping, resisting, hopefulness, power and surviving. We cannot only emphasize pain and suffering or only emphasize capacity and resources. When people experience violence and trauma it is rarely helpful to see them as passive victims or simply as resilient survivors. Surviving is a process involving many strategies. How one survives very often reveals the trauma and pain in different ways. It is not as if people are simply resilient and left unwounded from trauma. We must equally attend to the wounds and the efforts at coping, which are likely both helpful and not helpful.

## Rosa

A young woman Rosa, aged 24, was referred to me in private practice. She lives in an apartment on her own and is unemployed. She was referred to me after her psychiatrist refused to see her any further due to an incident where she poured blood over his parking spot. In this referral, I learned she had been given a "borderline personality" diagnosis and that she had a history of self-harm. She cuts herself at times very severely, almost cutting her ear off on one occasion. While self-harm is a coping strategy, I will also highlight that the blood itself is a metaphor of her struggle. It is well known that the effects of chronic abuse are commonly misdiagnosed as indicating "personality disorders" such as borderline (Herman, 2015, p. 116). Given the diagnosis Rosa had been given and the ongoing self-harm, I suspected she had a history of complex trauma and abuse.

In many mental health and substance-use stories of coping we see trauma and the intense human efforts that are made to survive. Herman (1992) reminds us that the child often lives in a climate of domination, terror and shame, over which she has very little control. Children experiencing violence and abuse are often told they must keep the abuse a secret. In these abusive contexts, little attention is given to the needs or feelings of the child. As such, all abuse involves a critical lack of respect and neglect of the emotional well-being of a child. It is not surprising that violence and abuse often has a profound impact on the developing child. While coping strategies are often creative – some produce adaptive/functional coping and others produce unhelpful, negative, problematic effects (Herman, 1992). Usually there is a bit of both. In order for a child to make sense of their situation – in order to survive, to preserve hope and meaning in the face of despair – they may take on a kind of "double think" which allows them to maintain their attachment to their parents or caregivers by blaming themselves (Herman,1992).

Often the child, in particular, will take the blame and responsibility, believing that the abuse is occurring because they are bad.

She must find a way to preserve a sense of trust in people who are untrustworthy, safety in a situation that is unsafe, control in a situation that is terrifyingly unpredictable, power in a situation of helplessness. Unable to care for or protect herself, she must compensate for the failures of adult care and protection with the only means at her disposal, an immature system of psychological defenses.

*(Herman, 1992, p. 96)*

The stories children tell about themselves and others is often continued throughout their lives: they are unworthy and unlovable, their needs do not matter, and people are not to be trusted or depended upon. Moreover, many become adults without ever having told their story. They have remained silent. This is only worsened when, despite many indicators that something is wrong as a child, youth and then adult, no one asks them.

As a result, I asked Rosa from the beginning of our work together whether she had experienced any violence or trauma and she responded with an unequivocal "no". As I was not convinced, I gently returned to the question from time to time where she switched from "no" to "I don't remember – maybe". She began to acknowledge she was emotionally neglected by her mother and eventually that she had been sexually abused by her father. In tracing Rosa's history of self-harm, it seemed clear that cutting provided a release and a way to cope as it does for many people. In my work with Rosa, it was my view that both cutting and blood were also metaphors, which meaningfully represented and communicated her struggle. However, I felt they only partially spoke of what she was unable to yet say directly – they represented the "yet to be spoken" (Brown, C., 2007a, 2014, 2017). So much was still silent, much that was difficult to acknowledge and speak about. As meanings attached to cutting and blood are socially situated, they also produce strong individual and cultural reactions. They are, therefore, able to hint very loudly – they are a way of speaking. As metaphors, they both pull us in and push us away. Blood is commonly associated with harm, hurting, pain, accidents, violence and death. Yet, of course, it is necessary for life and birth.

In addition to self-harm, Rosa also struggled with depression, body image issues, and a tendency to be dissociative. Her eyes revealed at moments deep disconnection and detachment, seemingly flat and blank. Rosa was dealing with co-occurring issues – each significant on its own. Overall, Rosa regulated her emotions through an oscillation of intrusion (blood, cutting) and constriction (depression). People may find themselves experiencing deep numbness, feeling nothing, feeling empty or feeling very depressed. This *constriction* serves to keep the emotional pain at bay – it is protective. Constriction is an important coping strategy. Difficult, powerful and overwhelming emotions are present in *intrusion* and often almost impossibly hard to tolerate. As such, constriction often takes over. Cutting may itself be a way to feel something when in a deep state of constriction. Feeling nothing and feeling too much can both be very difficult to live with. Yet, one state compensates for and reacts to the other. Cutting can be a way to regulate feeling too much and too little.[3] Herman (1992, 2015) described this as the "dialectic of trauma" – the repetitive oscillation between constriction and intrusion, alongside an often steady, overwhelming state of hyperarousal where one is always on the alert for potential danger.

When I began to explore Rosa's social history, I asked her about her first memory in life. She described lying in her crib and hearing her mother vacuuming. She reported a disconnect with her family and that it took significant effort to get the attention she needed. One example she offered was breaking the large living-room window from outside the house to get a reaction – to be noticed. She described feeling her older brother was the "proper golden" child who was more valued, getting most of the desired and needed attention and care.

In the very first session, I learned that Rosa's cutting went beyond the typical descriptions of release and/or the matching of internal emotional pain with physical pain. For Rosa, the blood itself had become very meaningful. In addition to cutting, Rosa wanted to consume the blood from cutting. Further to that, she collected and refrigerated menstrual blood for that purpose, which creatively offered a predictable and painless blood supply. When telling me this, I sensed Rosa was testing how I would react and whether she could trust me to work with her and this hidden aspect of her life. I took note of how she seemed to relish telling me this. I assume she thought I would be shocked. I calmly asked her how she thought I might react to this information. She shrugged – this question seemed to satisfy her. I needed to be conscious of the kind of role I was playing in this relationship. I needed to be very present and engaged with a focus on relationality. I needed to not be pushed away, and to not push her away. I needed to be both collaborative and capable.

I asked her when she first remembered consuming blood. She told me that at the age of 5 she had been playing in her basement with another child who fell off the top of the washing machine, resulting in a bloody nose. Her mother and another adult came and took the injured child upstairs, and Rosa described feeling compelled to lap the blood off the floor. She did not really understand why, but thought she was cleaning it up. Although, she has experienced her mother as emotionally disconnected or absent with her, she observed her mother becoming engaged and caring to her friend with this accident that involved blood. It is possible that Rosa has found that accessing and releasing her blood through cutting is reassuring and that it may be a way to stimulate her mother's caring. She may have been taking in some of the caring by cleaning up the blood. Without question, this experience led her to attach meaning to blood and connection. Blood gets a big reaction.

In the first instance, Rosa's lapping up her injured friend's blood is meaningful. Putting blood on the psychiatrist parking space was also meaningful. Without question the blood was meant to communicate, to express her feelings to him and about him. A layered message of hating him, needing him, listen to me, look at how much pain I am in, and perhaps even meaning to scare him, threaten him. Putting her blood on his parking sign, was a deliberate and powerful expression of both power and powerlessness – it was an act where she had some impact, some power, and importantly power to create a response, a reaction, when most often she felt she did not.

Throughout our work together, she described being interested in both her blood and other people's blood. She was not actively suicidal, but thought about dying. She often felt depressed and disengaged. She described cutting herself regularly for the release experienced and to collect and consume the blood itself. At the same time, she described wanting other people's blood – not necessarily because she wanted to hurt them, but, literally, because she wanted their blood. She was aware she needed to be in control of this urge, this need, but did hint she might not be and thus could potentially be at risk of harming another. It was at the time unclear to me whether she would harm someone or not. She had no history of doing so.

I did, however, move our sessions, for my own safety and hers, out of my private practice in my home to a public office. Similar to her stance while telling me about consuming her menstrual blood, the idea I may fear her desire for my blood seemed to give her satisfaction. I admit, I deliberately sat closest to the door in the room. At the beginning of sessions, she would slowly draw out going into her purse and then pull out a piece of gum for instance. I would wonder if she might bring out a weapon of some sort and she seemed to sense and be amused by this.

When I directly asked Rosa, she confirmed my suspicion that she wanted my blood. My concern about this had been making me anxious. Rosa seemed to be not only aware of this, but her response conveyed satisfaction at causing a reaction. From a critical feminist narrative clinical approach, I am deeply concerned when therapists let their anxiety and fear (or their needs in general) control or determine the therapeutic work. At the same time, I recognize we need to pay attention to our emotional responses and what they may be telling us. Noticing our "countertransference", or, simply put, noticing our own emotional reactions to our clients and their emotional experiences is part of hearing what they are saying and not saying. The therapeutic alliance or relationship and our capacity for empathy is central to doing this work, especially where there has been clear relational injury and a lack of empathy in their lives (Brown, C., 2020b; Herman, 1992, 2015).

Rosa can reasonably anticipate that people might be afraid if they think someone might draw blood from them. She can anticipate that they may become emotionally engaged, not neutral or distant. Perhaps, seeing that a person is afraid or anxious about this reassures her of her power to make someone *feel something in relation to her*. Given her painful sense of her mother's emotional disconnection and abandonment of her, the capacity to create an emotional reaction may bring significant pleasure and satisfaction. It may speak to the significant extent to which she is in need of meaningful, non-abusive recognition, acknowledgement and connection.

I was beginning to develop a stronger sense that her desire for other people's blood was, in part, a form of connection, of closeness and of emotional need. I thought that it potentially involved a conflation of anger/rage and need – and recognized that, depending on the balance of the conflation, this could be dangerous. Rage at her mother's disconnection, yet significant need for her mother's love and affection and connection, seemed to be part of her relationship with blood.

Relatedly, the example of the blood poured on her ex-psychiatrist's parking place may have been an expression of her frustration and anger with the therapeutic disconnection and lack of alliance. Pouring blood on his sign was meaningful, perhaps revealing a deep rage/need conflation. Through our conversations, it seemed this was her way of expressing to him a frustrating conflation of anger and need. I also noticed that she did not have any strong positive relationships in her life and her discussion of the relationships she did have seemed to regularly communicate the anger/need conflation. It seemed we needed to explore how her ordinary human desire for connection with another or needing them in any way simultaneously incited anger and maybe even rage. This seemed to speak to her experience of not getting her needs met, not knowing how to do so, and ultimately not expecting her needs to be met. Need and anger co-existed. One ignited the other. We spent quite a bit of time talking about this.

Rosa was interested in having a session with her parents to communicate what was going on with her and her relationship with her family. It was a very stiff and awkward session, which became very intense when Rosa began to tell the story of how her father would come into her room at night if she had bad dreams or if she thought there were monsters under the bed. In the telling of this story, her demeanor toward her father mirrored her pleasure and amusement when she noticed my anxiety or reactions to her. She watched him very closely for reactions. In this moment, she hinted – telling without telling – provoking reactions as she led the story right to the edge of what seemed was surely going to reveal he had been molesting her. During her telling, he splayed his hands over his mouth and face. He was clearly very anxious and distressed. Rosa's mother, in contrast, barely seemed interested, barely in the room. I could see the manifestation of her mother's profound disconnection and lack of concern, which had clearly had an impact on Rosa, while simultaneously seeing a different manifestation of profound disconnection and lack of concern from her father. Neither parent showed her any concern or care in the session. It was as if her mother was not in the room, and her father seemed concerned about protecting himself.

In our next session alone, I asked Rosa about the bad dreams and monsters under her bed. I asked her how she felt about her father coming into her room. I asked her if she noticed how her father was reacting as she talked about him coming into her room. I said he looked afraid to me, asking directly: What do you think he was afraid of? How do you feel your mother was reacting to this conversation? This led to the disclosure that he had molested her. She suspected her mother knew and did nothing. My brief observation was that of the two parents, despite the incest, her father showed some emotional response to her, where her mother was very shut off. Yet Rosa's needs did not appear to matter to either parent. Taken together, her relationship with both parents seemed to convey the message that she herself did not matter.

The life memories and stories she shared with me spoke of a lack of emotional connection and meaningful positive affirming attention in her family as she was growing up. Again, this part of her story to me involved never quite fully telling. It seemed the attention she did receive was often inappropriate or abusive. She described feeling she was not valued or loved as much as she needed to be by her family. She described needing to express herself very strongly to get a response. When her friend was injured and bleeding, she was taken care of. On the other hand, Rosa, at just five years old, was left behind and left alone with the blood. There was no concern showed to Rosa who was likely disturbed by both her friend being hurt and by the blood. Lapping up the blood was her connection to the friend and cleaning up the mess was somehow symbolic. Perhaps blood had become associated with this early accident, with its conflated mix of aloneness, connection, anger, pain, distress, care and attention.

It had never really occurred to Rosa to make sense of what all of this meant to her. She became quite intrigued in doing so. Unpacking how her relationship to blood had complex meaning and significance, and that it served as a way of coping, seemed to create a sense of relief for Rosa. The unpacking of this experience allowed her to be focused more directly on her needs, on self-compassion, on her emotional pain, on her anger and on her need to cope. Her vulnerability, fragility and need for love and care were more clearly evident to me – and to her. Herman states: "When survivors recognize the origins of their psychological difficulties in an abusive childhood environment, they no longer need to attribute them to an inherent defect in the self" (2015, p. 127). In her book *Trauma and Recovery*, Herman quotes a woman acknowledging this:

> Finally, dreams began unlocking. Spurred on by the fresh, crisp increase of the Still, Small Voice. I began to see what some of those silent unspoken words never said. I saw a mask. It looked like me. I took it off and beheld a group of huddled, terrified people who shrank together to hide terrible secrets.
>
> *(2015, p. 128)*

Too often the legacy of the abuse experienced in childhood is reflected in a person's dominant story and identity, with the conclusions that they unworthy and unlovable. As adults they often continue to see themselves as the problem. For these reasons developing alternative or counterstories that resist these conclusions is important. For Rosa, the act of cutting herself and the need for the blood itself, were her "Still, Small Voice" – a dramatic and powerful symbolic voice that was working hard to be heard despite being small, scared and vulnerable. Through unpacking her experiences, Rosa was able to be more self-compassionate, less self-blaming and more reflective – and relieved from the weight of not understanding what was happening to her. She had little experience of having her needs acknowledged with empathy and understanding from others. She had separated herself from the depth of her pain, betrayal and sense of not mattering to the people she loved.

To reiterate, telling stories is not at all straightforward. They can be unspeakable, almost too painful to tell. As I have stated earlier in this chapter, stories are often uncertain, contradictory, metaphoric, partial, hinted at – telling without telling – and even silent, perhaps leading us to the *yet-to-be-spoken*. Rosa's ways of telling her story through blood is not a common one. That she is telling it metaphorically is much more common. It is understandable that one may focus on the action of self-harm, and perhaps, subsequently and harmfully, ignore exploring Rosa's relationship to the blood itself. This is similar to the bingeing and purging of food where clients and therapists so often focus on the bingeing and fail to consider the significance of purging, which is often at best an afterthought. In Rosa's case, which involves an intense and meaningful relationship to blood, the therapist's discomfort may obscure its importance and the importance of exploring what blood means to Rosa. Indeed, her psychiatrist avoided what it meant. It is understandable that therapists may problematically avoid it altogether if it makes them uncomfortable. And it is also easy to see how therapists may be so distracted by Rosa's relationship to blood that they do not see beyond it. Moving past the surface of the story was important for both Rosa and I to better understand what it meant. This takes us back to Rosa breaking her parents' living-room window. How big an effort does she need to make to have someone listen to her, notice her?

I have argued that the telling and hearing of stories both matter. It is hard for Rosa to tell her story and it is inseparable from her relationship with blood and the meaning that it has for her. However, if the therapist evades this relationship with blood, as it incites fear and anxiety in them, the therapy work will not go very far. It can be very hard for therapists to hear some of the stories we hear. The stories have an impact on us, they imprint on us. This has been written about extensively as vicarious trauma (Hernandez-Wolfe, 2018). Ceccolini said this about her work in pediatric oncology:

> My memories are a blend of witnessing the stories of people's difficult, pain filled traumatic events: blood soaked clothing, shivering bodies, hours of waiting, not knowing, piercing cries of anguish in knowing, floods of tears and angry tirades somehow exist alongside stories of resiliency, of victory … goodbye at the hospital door without a child. It seems to me that to have a conversation about how we are vicariously traumatized by pain and suffering is incomplete without the story of how we experience even the small "V" victories in difficult times.
>
> *( Ceccolini, 2014)*

Ceccolini (2014) emphasizes the importance of exploring both how suffering is managed through coping and through moments of relief. She suggests that the story is incomplete if we only attend to the direct suffering without acknowledging and unpacking the agency and creativity involved in coping and finding relief. Doing so encourages a sense of hopefulness for the future.

Central to this, and critical to trauma work, requires the abandonment of fictitious notions of objectivity and neutrality. When we are working with people who have experienced violence and trauma, we are positioned on the side of the client, as a therapist, an ally and advocate. We are not passive neutral observers, we are active and collaborative in the conversation with a focus on building on the client's preferences and hopes for the present and the future. Empathic engagement calls on us to have a genuine response to another's experience, not buffered or distanced by notions of neutrality. "In our work it is normal to be affected by the events that happen to our clients, their reactions, responses to those events, and the meaning those events hold in their lives" (Cecollini, 2014).

Together, we are trying to make sense of the events that the clients experience in their lives that are often painful and difficult. In these conversations, our reflective questions are intentional in creating opportunities for clients to explore stories of possibilities and preferences. This empathic engagement is a double-edged sword, however, for while it contributes to a strong therapeutic alliance it also creates the possibility for therapists to be harmfully impacted by clients' painful and difficult experiences (Ceccolini, 2014). All told, this means that, when there is a strong empathic engagement in the therapeutic alliance, it is likely vicarious trauma is potentially offset by vicarious resilience in the therapeutic alliance (Hernandez-Wolfe, 2018). In other words, we can, and perhaps should, be deeply affected by our clients.

Research consistently finds that the therapeutic relationship is the strongest determinant of successful helping conversations (Horvath, 2018; Horvath, Del Re, Flückiger, & Symonds, 2011; Lambert & Barley 2001). In a strong therapeutic alliance, clients experience a sense of understanding, acceptance and hope. Someone cares about how they feel. Further to this, feminist therapy has historically and importantly emphasized the importance of a collaborative relationship that emphasizes the client's power, safety and control in the therapeutic process (Brown, C., 1993a, 1993b, 2007c; Brown, C. & Jasper, 1993; Herman, 2015). When women have experienced significant relational injury from people who should love and care for them, not abuse them, the therapeutic alliance is critically important (Brown, C., 2020b).

Trauma-based care should emphasize principles of safety, trust, collaboration, choice and empowerment (Ross, Brown, C., & Johnstone, 2023). Herman (1992) stresses that "no intervention that takes power away can foster her recovery no matter how much it appears to be in her immediate best interest" (p. 135). As disconnection and disempowerment are often central to traumatic experience, the therapeutic alliance involves both empowerment and a sense of reconnection (Herman, 1992). In complex trauma, for healing to occur, there must be both safety and connection.

Australian researchers have found that experiences of complex trauma among women are often overlooked (Salter et al., 2020). They report that in Australia, "one quarter of women subject to gendered violence report at least three different forms of interpersonal victimisation in their lifetime, such as child sexual abuse, domestic violence, sexual assault and stalking." They note that women who have experienced complex trauma are often medicalized without adequate attention to the experiences of trauma and gender-based violence. This invisibilizes the trauma and violence. It arguably serves to silence women's suffering and experiences of pain. Their voices and stories remain subjugated and unheard. Indeed, very often women are never asked about whether they have experienced of trauma or violence. Repeated experiences of violence and trauma are much more common than often realized with a significant impact on the survivors' mental and physical health. In both Canada (Ross, Brown, C., & Johnstone, 2023) and Australia (Salter et al., 2020) there is a lack of appropriate services. It is very difficult for those living with the effects of complex trauma to find services and, specifically, to find ones that address the complexity of their needs. Salter's report documents a series of useful recommendations to begin to rectify this problem, including the development of appropriate services that are designed to offer compassionate care that is not short-term and disjointed. This is necessary for a therapeutic relationship that enables both connection and empowerment to occur.

## Unpacking Rosa's Experience: Thematic Scaffolding Questions

White (2007) describes a process of therapeutic mapping through scaffolding questions that help to unpack of how people's stories have emerged, in what context and what they mean to the person. Through this process the story is externalized, which means it is contextualized and non-pathologized. In exploring the meaning of the story and seeking to understand it, the problem is seen as the problem – not the person themselves. The unhelpful stories being told are counterviewed with the intention of developing preferred counterstories that are more helpful and create a sense of possibility for the future. Generally, these counterstories resist negative identity conclusions, including internalized deficit-based, pathologizing dominant discourse. Stories need to be situated, explored and understood in the context of people's lives, not simply as subjective.

Scaffolding questions will intentionally explore Rosa's story by unpacking her experiences and the meaning she attaches to her struggles. These questions are intentional, with the task of uncovering and unpacking the meaning Rosa attaches to the trauma she has experienced and her subsequent meaningful efforts at coping with the trauma. My questions are not neutral, they reflect my worldview and interpretation of Rosa's story. The telling and the hearing flow back and forth in a collaborative conversation. Scaffolding questions may also move back and forth between dominant themes in a story and help produce a conversational map. For instance, with Rosa, some scaffolding themes include: her childhood family experience, neglectful relationship with her mother, sexual abusive relationship with her father, her history and relationship with blood, coping and trauma, and her therapy history. These questions do not represent all questions, or the order they should be asked in. There is skill in how to ask them, when to ask them, in what tone and order. The tone needs to be emphatic, gentle and non-judgmental. As the client initiates the conversational direction as well, other questions will emerge. Rosa's responses to questions and what she chooses to talk about or initiate will also direct the conversations. These sample scaffolding questions are meant to explore Rosa's traumatic experiences and the meaning of her subsequent efforts at coping through cutting and consuming blood.

### Family

- What is your first memory as a child?
- What do you remember about being a child?
- What was your relationship with your family like?
- When your mother paid very little attention to you how did you feel?
- What message did that give you?
- Did anyone else pay attention to you?
- Do you feel other people are able to meet your needs?
- How did you feel when your father came into your room at night?
- When your father came into your room at night did he care about how you felt?
- Tell me about the monsters under your bed? What were they? Why were they under your bed?
- What was your relationship like with the monsters under your bed?
- Did you feel your needs mattered in your family?
- How did that make you feel about yourself?
- What difference would it have made if you had felt your needs mattered?
- Did you feel alone?
- Can you tell me about relationships you have had where you felt there was a positive sense of connection?
- How did this feel?

### The Blood and Coping

- When do you first remember taking an interest in blood?
- What interested you about it?
- What were you feeling?
- Can you tell me about when your friend fell off the washing machine and got hurt?
- How did you feel about her being hurt?
- How did you feel about adults coming and taking her away to take care of her?

- How did you feel about being left alone?
- What were your feelings about the blood on the floor?
- What did the blood mean to you?
- What do you remember about lapping it off the floor?
- What did you feel when you lapped it off the floor?
- What did you feel after you did that?
- Did it make you feel better about the situation?
- How do you feel when you see blood now?
- How do you feel when you make yourself bleed?
- When you consume blood what do you feel? Is it soothing? Comforting?
- What other feelings do you connect with consuming blood?
- Do you ever feel that blood is connected to feeling anger?
- Does is reduce feelings of need or anger?
- Does it sooth, reduce stress, or create a sense of release ?
- How is wanting blood helpful to you?
- Does it help take care of your needs?
- How might it be helping you cope?
- Are there ways it is not helpful or that you don't like?
- It seems like menstrual blood is a pretty predictable, less painful way of collecting blood. Does that make sense to you?

### Cutting and Coping

- How do you feel before you cut yourself?
- What are you thinking about or feeling before cutting yourself?
- How do you decide to cut yourself?
- How do you decide where to cut yourself?
- What do you feel while you are cutting yourself?
- What is going through your mind?
- How do you collect blood?
- How do you feel after you cut yourself?
- When you cut yourself how does it help?
- Are there ways it does not help?
- What difference does it make?
- Is there anything else that would make you feel this way?
- Are there times you only cut and do not collect and store the blood?
- What's the difference between when you decide to collect blood and when you don't?
- Are you able to control how much you harm yourself?
- How do you do this?
- Is this important to you?
- Can we come up with some ways to make this less harmful to you?

### Coping and Needs

- Do you have a sense of what you feel when you feel like you want blood?
- When are you most likely to want blood?
- What do you feel before you want to have blood?
- What does it feel like when you want to consume blood?
- What does it feel like when you do consume blood?
- What do you feel after you consume blood?
- Does it help you feel better? How?
- Do you ever feel numb? Empty?
- When you feel empty does blood help you to feel less empty?
- What does blood mean to you?
- How do you think consuming blood helps you cope?
- Does it help you when feel depressed or sad?
- Does it help you when feel numb?
- Does it help you when feel alone or disconnected?
- Does it help you when feel angry?

### Other People's Blood

- When are you most likely to want other people's blood?
- What makes you want to have someone else's blood instead of your own?
- Is it a form of connection?
- How does it relate to what you want from people, if at all?
- Who are some of the people whose blood you have wanted?
- How does that come about?
- Other than your friend's blood when you were a child, have you ever consumed someone else's blood?
- If so, how did you get the blood?
- How do you feel this connects to lapping up your friend's blood when you were five?
- What needs or feelings are you aware of having when you feel you want someone's blood?
- How do you feel about having those needs?
- What does wanting and consuming blood say about what you need?
- It seems like there are at least three big parts: (1) cutting, (2) consuming the blood, and (3) consuming someone else's blood.
- What is the difference for you between the cutting process and the consuming blood part?
- What is the difference for you between consuming your blood and the desire for someone else's blood?
- What overall connection do you make between blood and how you feel?

## *Future – Hope and Possibilities*

- What do you want for yourself in the future?
- What do you need to make that happen?
- Would you like to have a greater sense of connection to other people in the future?
- What supports and resource would help make that happen?
- What do you worry might get in the way?
- How might you work with that?

## Conclusion

In trauma work the telling and hearing of stories influence each other. This is a critical overlapping process in unpacking stories and creating more helpful counterstories. There is what Rosa says and there is what she does not say – and also what I, the therapist hear, and do not hear – what we discover together that is unknown or seemingly unknown. My thoughts, impressions and interpretations are reflected in the conversation. When working with people's efforts at coping with violence and trauma, we necessarily reckon with our own emotional responses. As practitioners, we may feel outraged, horrified and even wounded by images of what the person has endured. In this work, we need to attend to the coalescing of pain, vulnerability, suffering, helplessness, hopelessness, powerlessness and capacity, creativity, coping, resisting, hopefulness, power and surviving. We cannot only emphasize pain and suffering, or only emphasize capacity and resources. When people experience violence and trauma it is rarely helpful to see them simply as passive victims or as resilient survivors. We must attend equally to the wounds and the efforts at coping. Coping efforts seek to remedy past and present struggles and are often an effort at survival. We need to appreciate coping as survival, even when it also produces harm, and as critical entry into understanding a person's story. The coping efforts often begin to tell us what the person has yet to fully speak. When we double listen, we may hear that which is difficult and often dangerous to speak. The development of counterstories can be helpful in moving from silence to speech. We must double listen to and counterview the partial or indirect speech seen in both coping approaches and silence to enable the emergence of the often unspeakable. An alternative or counterstory may offer a more compassionate, preferred account that resists negative identity conclusions and allows for a more hopeful future. And, critically, we must seek to from a collaborative meaningful connection that can begin to counter traumatic relational injury.

## Notes

1 Paul Simon (1964) wrote the popular song *The Sound of Silence*. In many ways this chapter is about the reverberating sounds of silence in unspoken trauma stories and the

struggle to tell the story and be heard. Referring to the difficulties people have communicating, Simon writes: *"People talking without speaking, People hearing without listening."* It is risky to challenge silence: *"No one dared. Disturb the sounds of silence."* Yet, Simon recognizes the harm of silence: *"Silence like a cancer grows."*

2 In my discussion of Rosa's case some details have been left out for confidentiality reasons, and some to create a clearer focus in the chapter.

3 In the song "Leave the Light On", award-winning blues singer Beth Hart, who has struggled with mental health issues, substance use and multiple abusive relationships, describes cutting herself. She describes running from herself, her life and everyone around her. She is afraid of being alone. She describes being in a perpetual state of alert and need for self-protection as a child. "I ain't that scarred when I'm covered up / I leave the light on / Little girl hiding underneath the bed was it something I did". She describes cutting as a way to cope. "… I'm all messed up inside / I cut myself just to feel alive…", "I don't know what to do, can the damage be undone". Her experiences fit within Herman's (1992) dialectic of trauma which includes intrusion, constriction and hyperarousal. This song tells the story of living with the fear of being hurt and protecting herself and trying to manage the oscillation of feeling too much and too little (Hart & Lieber, 2004).

# References

Ahmed, S. (2004). *The cultural politics of emotion.* Edinburgh University Press.

Brown, C. (1993a). Feminist contracting: Power and empowerment in therapy. In C. Brown & K. Jasper (Eds.), *Consuming passions. Feminist approaches to weight preoccupation and eating disorders* (pp. 176–194). Second Story Feminist Press.

Brown, C. (1993b). Feminist therapy: Power, ethics, and control. In C. Brown & K. Jasper (Eds.), *Consuming passions. Feminist approaches to weight preoccupation and eating disorders* (pp. 120–136). Second Story Feminist Press.

Brown, C. (2007a). Dethroning the suppressed voice: Unpacking experience as story. In C. Brown & T. Augusta-Scott (Eds.), *Narrative therapy. Making meaning, making lives* (pp. 177–196). Sage.

Brown, C. (2007b). Discipline and desire: Regulating the body/self. In C. Brown & T. Augusta-Scott (Eds.), *Narrative therapy. Making meaning, making lives* (pp. 105–131). Sage.

Brown, C. (2007c). Situating knowledge and power in the therapeutic alliance. In C. Brown & T. Augusta-Scott (Eds.), *Narrative therapy. Making meaning, making lives* (pp. 3–22). Sage.

Brown, C. (2011). Reconceptualizing feminist therapy: Violence, problem drinking and re-storying women's lives. In D. Baines (Ed.), *Doing anti-oppressive practice: Building transformative, politicized social work* (2nd ed.) (pp. 95–115). Fernwood Press.

Brown, C. (2013). Women's narratives of trauma: (Re)storying uncertainty, minimization and self-blame. *Narrative Works: Issues, Investigations & Interventions, 3*(1), 1–30.

Brown, C. (2014). Untangling emotional threads, self-management discourse and women's body talk. In M. LaFrance & S. McKenzie-Mohr (Eds.), *Women voicing resistance. Discursive and narrative explorations* (pp. 174–190). Routledge.

Brown, C. (2017). Creating counterstories: Critical clinical practice and feminist narrative therapy. In D. Baines (Ed.), *Doing anti-oppressive practice: Building transformative, politicized social work* (3rd ed.) (pp. 212–232). Fernwood Press.

Brown, C. (2018). The dangers of trauma talk: Counterstorying co-occurring strategies for coping with trauma. *Journal of Systemic Therapies, 37*(3), 38–55.

Brown, C. (2019). Speaking of women's depression and the politics of emotion. *Affilia: Journal of Women and Social Work*, 34(2), 151–169.

Brown, C. (2020a). Critical clinical social work: Theoretical and practical considerations. In C. Brown & J. MacDonald (Eds.), *Critical clinical social work: Counterstorying for social justice* (pp. 16–58). Canadian Scholars Press.

Brown, C. (2020b). Feminist narrative therapy and complex trauma: Critical clinical work with women diagnosed as "borderline". In C. Brown & J. MacDonald (Eds.), *Critical clinical social work: Counterstorying for social justice* (pp. 82–109). Canadian Scholars Press.

Brown, C. (2022). Postmodern theory: The case of narrative theory in social work. In Hugman, R., Holscher, D., & McAuliffe, D. (Eds.), *Social work theory and ethics* (pp. 79–100). Springer.

Brown, C., & Augusta-Scott, T. (Eds.) (2007). *Narrative therapy. Making meaning, making lives*. Sage.

Brown, C., & Jasper, K. (Eds.) (1993). *Consuming passions. Feminist approaches to weight preoccupation and eating disorders*. Second Story Feminist Press.

Brown, C., Johnstone, M., & Ross, N. (2021). Repositioning social work practice in mental health in Nova Scotia. Report. Nova Scotia College of Social Workers. https://nscsw.org /wp-content/uploads/2021/01/NSCSW-Repositioning-Social-Work-Practice-in-Mental -Health-in-Nova-Scotia-Report-2021.pdf.

Brown, C., & Macdonald, J. (2022). Critical clinical social work. Working in the context of trauma and (dis)Ability. In D. Baines (Ed.), *Doing anti-oppressive practice: Building transformative, politicized social work* (4th ed.) (pp. 118–140). Fernwood Press.

Brown, L. (1992). A feminist critique of personality disorders. In L.S. Brown & M. Ballou (Eds.), *Personality and psychopathology: Feminist reappraisals* (pp. 206–228). Guilford Press.

Brown. L. (2004). Feminist paradigms of trauma treatment. *Psychotherapy: Theory, Research, Practice, Training*, 41(4), 464–471.

Burstow, B. (2003). Toward a radical understanding of trauma and trauma work. *Violence Against Women*, 9(11), 1293–1317.

Butler, J. (1997). *Excitable speech: A politics of the performative*. Routledge.

Ceccolini, J. (2014). Vicarious trauma: An incomplete story. Social Workers Retreat. Powerpoint slides. June 22, 2014, Berwick, Nova Scotia.

DeVault, M. (1990). Talking and listening from women's standpoint: Feminist strategies for interviewing and analysis. *Social Problems*, 37(1), 96–116.

Foucault, M. (1980). *The history of sexuality. Vol 1. An introduction*. Vintage.

Foucault, M. (2001). *Fearless speech*. Semiotext(e).

Fricker, M. (2010). *Epistemic justice. Power and the ethics of knowing*. Oxford University Press.

Hart, B., & Lieber, O.J. (2004). Lyrics. *Leave the Light On.* © Kobalt Music Publishing, Universal Music Publishing Group.

Herman, J. (1992). *Trauma and recovery: The aftermath of violence – From domestic abuse to political terror* (1st ed.). Basic Books.

Herman, J. (2015). *Trauma and recovery: The aftermath of violence – From domestic abuse to political terror* (2nd ed.). Basic Books..

Herman, J., Perry, C., & van der Kolk, B. (1989). Childhood trauma in borderline personality disorder. *American Journal of Psychiatry*, 146, 490–495.

Hernandez-Wolfe, P. (2018). Vicarious resilience: A comprehensive review. *Revista De Estudios Sociales*, (66), 9–17. https://doi.org/10.7440/res66.2018.02.

hooks, b. (1990). *Talking back: Thinking feminist, thinking black.* Routledge.

Horvath, A.O. (2018). Research on the alliance: Knowledge in search of a theory. *Psychotherapy Research*, 28(4), 499–516. doi: 10.1080/10503307.2017.1373204.

Horvath, A.O., Del Re, A.C., Flückiger, C., & Symonds, D. (2011). Alliance in individual psychotherapy. *Psychotherapy, 48*(1), 9–16. https://doi.org/10.1037/a0022186.

Lafrance, M., & McKenzie-Mohr, S. (2013). The DSM and its lure of legitimacy. *Feminism and Psychology*, 23(1), 119–140.

Lambert, M.J., & Barley, D.E. (2001). Research summary on the therapeutic relationship and psychotherapy outcome. *Psychotherapy: Theory, Research, Practice, Training*, 38(4), 357–361. https://doi.org/10.1037/0033-3204.38.4.357.

McKenzie-Mohr, S., & Lafrance, M. (2011). Telling stories without the words: Tightrope talk in women's accounts of coming to live well after rape or depression. *Feminism and Psychology*, 21(1), 49–73.

McKenzie-Mohr, S., & Lafrance, M. (2014). Women's discursive resistance: Attuning to counter-stories and collectivizing for change. In S. McKenzie-Mohr & M. Lafrance (Eds.), *Creating counterstories: Women resisting dominant discourses in speaking their lives* (pp. 191–205). Routledge.

Madigan, S. (2003). Counterviewing injurious speech acts: Destabilizing eight conversational habits of highly effective problems. *International Journal of Narrative Therapy and Community Work*, 1, 43–59.

Morgan, A. (2000). *What is narrative therapy? An easy-to-read introduction.* Dulwich Center Publications.

Moulding, N. (2015). *Gendered violence, abuse and mental health in everyday lives: Beyond trauma.* Routledge.

Ross, N., Brown, C., & Johnstone, M. (2023). Beyond medicalised approaches to violence and trauma: Empowering social work practice. *Journal of Social Work*, 1–19.

Salter, M., Conroy, E., Dragiewicz, M., Burke, J., Ussher, J., Middleton, W., Vilenica, S., Martin Monzon, B., & Noack-Lundberg, K. (2020). *"A deep wound under my heart": Constructions of complex trauma and implications for women's wellbeing and safety from violence* (Research Report, 12/2020). Australia's National Research Organisation for Women's Safety (ANROWS).

Shaffer, B. (1987). Film. *To a safer place.* National Film Board, Canada.

Simon, P. (1964). Lyrics. *The Sound of Silence.*

Tseris, E. (2013). Trauma theory without feminism? Evaluating contemporary understandings of traumatized women. *Affilia: Journal of Women and Social Work*, 28(2), 153–164.

Tseris, E. (2019). *Trauma, women and mental health and social justice. Possibilities and pitfalls.* Routledge.

Ussher, J. (2010). Are we bio-medicalizing women's misery? A critical review of women's higher rates of reported depression. *Feminism & Psychology*, 20(1), 9–35.

Warin, M., & Dennis, S. (2008). Telling silences: Unspeakable trauma and the unremarkable practices of everyday life. *The Sociological Review, 56*(2, suppl.), 100–116. https://doi.org/10.1111/j.1467-954X.2009.00818.x.

Weisel, E. (2006). *Night* (2nd ed.). Farrat, Straus and Giroux. (1958, original Editions de Minuit.)

White, M. (2000). Re-engaging with history: The absent but implicit. In M. White, *Reflections on narrative practice: Essays and interviews* (pp. 35–58). Dulwich Centre Publications.

White, M. (2001). Narrative practice and the unpacking of identity conclusions. *Gecko: A Journal of Deconstruction and Narrative Ideas in Therapeutic Practice*, 1, 28–55.

White, M. (2004). Working with people who are suffering the consequences of multiple trauma: A narrative perspective. *International Journal of Narrative Therapy and Community Work*, 1, 45–76.

White, M. (2007). *Maps of narrative practice*. Norton.

# 7

# TRAUMA, (DIS)ABILITY AND CHRONIC PAIN

## Taking Up Sufferer-Informed Practices

*Judy E. MacDonald, Rose C.B. Singh,
Sarah E. Norris, and Ami Goulden*

### Introduction: Situating (dis)Ability and Chronic Pain

In Canada, 27 percent of the population identify as living with a (dis)Ability, which constitutes 8 million Canadians (Rabinowitz & Wallace, 2023). Sixty-three percent of working-age Canadians living with a (dis)Ability identified pain as their primary impairment, whereas 46 percent identified mental health (dis)Abilities. Seventy percent of those who identify as living with a (dis)Ability live with two or more (dis)Abilities. Women are more likely than men to identify as (dis)Abled, across all age categories (ibid.). According to Schopflocher, Taenzer and Jovey (2011), women consistently reported higher rates of pain (dis)Abilities, across numerous studies. We need to question why pain is the leading (dis)Ability and why there is a higher representation of women living with pain? Is it related to the stressors on the health care system where people are enduring long wait-times for surgeries, such as knee or hip replacements, where the body's experience of pain is then etched into the body's memory? Or is it in part due to the system's lack of acknowledgment of the pain experience, where the approach to (dis)Ability and pain has been formed around a biomedical expert model of care that discounts the (dis)Abled person's voice and lived experiences?

Throughout history as well as in the modern day, people with (dis)Abilities have experienced oppression and marginalization through every aspect of their lives. Society is entrenched with barriers and inaccessible infrastructures, as evident through the lack of accessible housing and transportation, unreasonable wait-times for health and human services, and complicated and convoluted (dis)Ability policies that make accessing (dis)Ability benefits nearly impossible (MacDonald & Cooper, 2019). Further, societal barriers are created when access to public education ignores (dis)Abled persons' learning needs by negating the implementation

DOI: 10.4324/9781003379591-8

of universal design principles (Wertans & Burch, 2022), or through employment where (dis)Abled persons' potential and abilities are not acknowledged, or accommodations are denied based on the claim of employer's "undue hardship", which can be argued from a number of factors including financial cost and the morale of other employees (Nova Scotia Human Rights Commission, n.d.). The "morale of other employees" seems to pit the (dis)Abled body against the able-bodied, which, in a society based on normative principles and ableist acts, would tend to weigh heavily in favor of the status quo.

Linguistically, within this chapter as an attempt to center lived experiences, persons living with chronic pain will be referred to as "sufferers". The use of the term sufferer repositions (dis)Abled persons living with chronic pain by acknowledging their pain experiences, validating their struggles while witnessing their pain, which has often been brought into question by a biomedical lens that has a psychologizing element of dismissal or minimization of the person's pain, reverting it back to psychological causation, especially for female sufferers (MacDonald, 2008). Further, "(dis)Ability" is written with "dis" in parentheses and a capital "A" in order to:

> emphasize the fact that (dis)Abled persons are more than their difference in abilities … for far too long people with (dis)Abilities have been cast aside, measured against what is perceived to be the "normal" type of body and mind, and denied their agency. This spelling shifts the focus to the talents, personalities, skills and even flaws of the person, rather than the default focus on the (dis)Ability itself, to validate the totality of experience. Further, to navigate the ableist structures in society, persons with (dis)Abilities have had to demonstrate multiple abilities, which have often been overlooked, dismissed, or ignored.
>
> *(MacDonald, Brown, M., & Jones, 2022, p. 286)*

Within this chapter, the terms "(dis)Abled persons" and "people with (dis)Abilities" are both used interchangeably, acknowledging the significance of identity-first language, and appreciating the use of person-first language by some, while emphasizing that people and practitioners alike listen to and follow the preferences and language used by the (dis)Abled person. Later in this chapter, through the case of Sam,[1] we share the experiences of one chronic pain sufferer. Applied to this case are trauma-based practices from a (dis)Ability perspective that emphasize the expertise and voices of chronic pain sufferers encountering the health-care system.

## Ableism

Ableism is not a singular, one-dimensional experience of oppression. It manifests on personal and structural levels, and appears in many forms, including internalized, neoliberal and structural ableism. Ableism is pervasive, and it is often bound to other mechanisms of domination and normalization (Withers, 2012). At the same time, Withers (2012) suggests that "ableism" is a misnomer, in that it implies that people are oppressed because of ability, when they actually experience oppression because of (dis)Ability. Nevertheless, ableist, oppressive processes deeply entrench the marginalization of (dis)Abled people in society as ableism connects to all the challenges faced by (dis)Abled people, since it is secured by notions of whose bodies are important, desired and disposable (Mingus, 2011). This oppression also appears on a personal level through internalized ableism, in which the prejudice and discrimination toward (dis)Abled people shapes their identity and beliefs about themselves (Campbell, 2009). Further, hegemonic notions of the body impact the health and well-being of (dis)Abled people, and their struggles are often the consequence of active marginalization. According to Rauscher and McClintock (1996), ableism manifests when:

> Deeply rooted beliefs about health, productivity, beauty, and the value of human life, perpetuated by the public and private media, combine to create an environment that is hostile to those whose abilities fall outside of the scope of what is currently defined as socially acceptable.
>
> *(p. 198)*

Similarly, Goodley and Lawthom (2019) note, "we already knew that disability relied on its opposite – ability – in order to exist" (p. 234). Indeed, ableism is connected to discrimination and harmful beliefs that uphold notions of healthy and normal in contrast to illness and (dis)Ability. Kafer (2013) points out that ableist assumptions about bodies in turn influence realities of access, affecting both (dis)Abled and non-(dis)Abled people. Kafer (2017) suggests that (dis)Ability may be understood as relational, appearing and arising in the relations between people, policies, beliefs and structures that surround all of us. Indeed, there is a call to address the tendency to see health and (dis)Ability as individualized, depoliticized experiences.

Goodley (2014) describes ableism as the set of practices that produce and promote a typical, individualized, productive, compliant citizen. In turn, this process manifests as neoliberal ableism, a strategy that esteems both this normalized body-mind and abled citizens who are economically prolific and dependent on neoliberal systems of capitalist production (Goodley, 2014). As such, awareness of late-stage capitalism, neoliberalism, as well as the impacts of local, national and international economic realities on the lives of persons with (dis)Abilities is necessary, while staying attentive to the complexities inherent in contemporary times. Indeed, Goodley and Lawthom (2019) note that "neoliberalism and ableism merge together as a deeply inhuman complex" (p. 237). While both neoliberal and structural ableism are distinct phenomena, they are interlinked through their broad harms and traumatic impacts to (dis)Abled people. Structural ableism, as

Dolmage (2017) explains, is the many societal, political and institutional "structures built only for preferred bodies" while excluding those who are not deemed as fitting with "this preferred status" (p. 54). Ableism, in its internalized, neoliberal and structural forms, oppresses (dis)Abled people and perpetuates experiences of trauma in their lives.

## Models of (dis)Ability

Models of (dis)Ability offer explanations on the individual experiences and sociopolitical contexts of (dis)Abled people and communities (Smart, 2004). While there are numerous models of (dis)Ability (Titchkosky et al., 2022), the biomedical model has dominated health care and the social model has presented a counter-perspective (Singh, Murray-Lichtman, & Slayter, 2022).

A biomedical model views (dis)Ability as an individual problem and deficit (Goodley, 2017). This model developed through the nineteenth and twentieth centuries, with a focus on the rehabilitation and remedy of illness (Gough, 2005). The biomedical model aligns (dis)Ability with illness and cure, a categorization based on the pathophysiology of (dis)Abilities and the normalization of specific bodies. Medical professionals hold all power, ranging from diagnosis to determining eligibility for treatment, services and support, with the (dis)Abled person often silenced. Crow (1996) notes that the biomedical model of (dis)Ability holds that "a person's functional limitations (impairments) are the root cause of any disadvantages experienced and these disadvantages can therefore only be rectified by treatment or cure" (p. 208). This biomedical focus on normality signifies illness and (dis)Ability as separate from the realm of human experience and constructed as individual pathology, as abnormal, and as errors to be fixed (Clare, 2017; Fisher & Goodley, 2007). As Greenhalgh (2001) writes, biomedical knowledge is constructed from the formulation of ideas based upon objectification, quantification, pathologization and amelioration. Objectification takes the whole of the (dis)Abled person and splits them into the physical body and the emotional/feeling psyche, with biomedicine claiming expertise over the body. Quantification takes bodily symptoms and turns them into measurable components, where the only parts that count are those that can be quantified. Pathologization exemplifies a disease model of practice, whereby diagnostic labels become the focus with attention given to "fixing" the (dis)Abled body. Amelioration focuses on the treatment, with the aim of returning the (dis)Abled body to a state of normalcy (Titchkosky & Michalko, 2009). The binary split between normalcy and abnormalcy, through a biomedical lens of what constitutes a normal body and a body with impairments, further keeps (dis)Abled persons trapped in internalized, neoliberal and structural webs of ableism where they are constantly being measured against biomedical standards of the ideal body, with the ultimate goal of returning them to as close to a normal state as possible. The compounding traumatic experiences encountered through a biomedical approach brings a (dis)Abled person's reality into question, their identity and lived experiences are denied legitimacy and are replaced by the authoritarian gaze of medical professionals leaving the (dis)Abled person devoid of agency (Greenhalgh, 2001). According to Mackelprang, Salsgiver, and Parrey (2022) the biomedical model – or, as they refer to it, the medical/professional model – is "embedded and institutionalized in the social structures of contemporary Western cultures" (p. 101).

In resistance to the individualization and medicalization of (dis)Ability, (dis)Abled activists and theorists, such as Oliver (1983, 2013), named and developed the social model of (dis)Ability. Within the social model of (dis)Ability, impairment is a "condition or attribute" whereas (dis)Ability is "how society responded to, or failed to respond to, the needs of people with impairments" (Cameron, 2014, p. 137). The impact of living with an impairment are acknowledged in this model, while highlighting the many systemic and structural factors that disregard and exclude (dis)Abled people and communities (Goodley, 2017; Stienstra, 2020). For people (dis)Abled by chronic illnesses and conditions, the social model is insufficient (Wendell, 1996). Environmental changes to a physical building, such as installation of a ramp, while helpful to many (dis)Abled and non-(dis)Abled persons alike, may be missing the actual accommodations needed by a chronic pain sufferer (MacDonald & Friars, 2009; Owen, Hiebert-Murphy, & Ristock, 2018). Oliver (2013) himself noted that the social model of (dis)Ability was not intended to be the only theory and model, encouraging an evolution of the social model as well as building new models.

Models of (dis)Ability bring forward understandings, but alone do not capture the full experiences, spectrum and contexts of (dis)Ability (Kafer, 2013; Titchkosky, Cagulada, & DeWelles, 2022). While (dis)Ability, as Chapman (2022) writes, is "a political and social phenomenon" (p. 433), the biomedical model continues as the dominant model of (dis)Ability today. Further, these models of (dis)Ability do not offer practice approaches when working with specific groups, such as chronic pain sufferers. Comparatively, anti-oppressive theory and practice is a social justice social work approach in working with persons and groups experiencing both individual and structural inequities (Baines & Clark, 2022), including (dis)Abled people and communities (Johnson, Singh, & Slayter, 2022) and, more specifically, chronic pain sufferers (MacDonald, 2008, 2020). Building on anti-oppressive theory and practice (Baines & Sharma, 2022), the social model of (dis)Ability (Oliver, 2013), and the social oppression model of (dis)Ability (Carter, Hanes, & MacDonald, 2017), the Disability Anti-Oppressive Practice (DAOP) model (Hanes, Carter, & MacDonald, 2022) connects the day-to-day lived experiences of (dis)Abled persons to their experiences of oppression, as lived through repeated exposure and assaults of ableism depicted from barriers created through structural, cultural, political, attitudinal and social means. Through this approach, "the aim is to focus on societal access and inclusion, dismantling structural barriers while at the same time working with the (dis)Abled person and their family to address inequities experienced at the individual and familial levels" (Hanes,

Carter, & MacDonald, 2022, p. 247). The DAOP model acknowledges (dis)Abled persons' personal struggles are manifested within structural inequalities through stigmatization, lack of access and inclusion in employment, higher education and society. Practitioners need to be advocates and allies, challenging social policies and societal infrastructures to be accessible and inclusive so that (dis)Abled persons feel heard and a sense of belonging resulting in engagement of full citizenship.

## Situating Trauma-Based Care

In this chapter, we refer to trauma-based care to delineate this approach from trauma-informed care practices that have historically offered little therapeutic value. We have included trauma-informed care considerations and quotations as theoretical and practical approaches referenced by other authors as a means to connect these critical conversations.

Historically, structural ableism and systemic oppressions have prevented (dis)Abled people from having access to adequate supports; while at the same time, trauma-informed approaches have not been at the fore in the development of related services (Hollins & Sinason, 2000). Likewise, Liasidou (2021) notes that "despite their symbiotic relationship, trauma and disability have been historically treated as two distinct experiential entities" (para. 37). In turn, oppressive health care systems and interactions with medical professionals can perpetuate harm, putting (dis)Abled people at risk of retraumatization. Additionally, there is a widely held assumption that when the focus shifts from a biomedical perspective into more socially informed conversations, individuals and institutions are emancipated from power hierarchies, yet all "trauma-informed" work requires a critical gaze (Tseris, 2019). Arguably, most of the "trauma-informed" talk today at best acknowledges the presence of trauma. In large part, notions of "trauma-informed" care within the dominant biomedical neoliberal system is individually and medically focused. Individuals are "responsibilized for their care" within a fiscally constrained system that provides virtually no programmatic care. Trauma itself is decontextualized and depoliticized, whereby individuals are pathologized and often retraumatized (Kinnucan, 2014).

Nair (in Kinnucan, 2014) suggests that sufferers can also make the perfect neoliberal subjects, by minimizing structural harms through individualizing our narratives. Thus, there is a need for critical, collective and intersectional trauma-informed paradigms that specifically situate (dis)Abled experiences within trauma-informed practices (Keesler, 2014; Williamson & Qureshi, 2015).

The notion of best practices for trauma-based care was developed by feminist practitioners in the 1980s. These practices ideally involve the creation of a culture that foregrounds safety, trust, collaboration and empowerment among both service providers and care recipients (Bass & Davis, 1988; Fallot & Harris, 2009; Herman, 1992; Substance Abuse and Mental Health Services (SAMHSA), 2023). While some acknowledge that best practices for trauma-informed care also require a commitment to changing organizational culture, policies and practices, today this is seldom the practice (Harris & Fallot, 2001). Under the pervasive co-influence of dominant biomedical approaches and neoliberal fiscal constraints and the rationalization of social service provision, shifting organizational culture becomes even more critical. There are few trauma-based services, lack of attention to complex trauma and the co-occurrence of trauma, mental health and substance use, lack of trauma-focused training, long wait-lists and one-size-fits-all approaches (Brown, C., Johnstone, & Ross, 2021; Brown, C., Doll, Baines, Johnstone, forthcoming).

Further, trauma-based care involves recognizing the prevalence of trauma and its impact on individuals within the system (including staff), while actively resisting retraumatization, and responding by putting collaborative knowledge into policy and practice (SAMHSA, 2023). While many of these structural interventions have proved helpful to trauma survivors, sufferers still experience trauma from within medical institutions and interactions with medical staff. In fact, "some human service systems aim to adhere to trauma-informed principles while not engaging with the specific experiences of service users" (Tseris, 2019, p. 7). Notably, mainstream trauma-informed approaches have asked (dis)Abled people to build resilience through minimizing risk, bouncing back and buffering themselves against further harm (Runswick-Cole & Goodley, 2013). This narrative aligns closely with a biomedical lens of (dis)Ability, whereas a social constructionist view of resilience views these directives through relational, communal, political and institutional lenses. In their analysis of resiliency within social work literature, Park, Crath and Jeffery (2020) found that the focus on building individual resilience often eclipses the attention from the deep roots of structural oppression. Thus, to work anti-oppressively, researchers and practitioners need to better understand the connections between sufferers' trauma and their unique experiences in the traditional biomedical paradigm, while maintaining a critical and inquisitive stance toward trauma-based approaches. This means *not* mistaking a departure from a biomedical model as an assumed sufferer-informed approach to care.

## Case Study

The accumulation of internalized, neoliberal and structural ableism, and dismissive and harmful encounters with the biomedically based health care system, leads to experiences of trauma for (dis)Abled people. Included in this section is a case to situate the lived experiences of one chronic pain sufferer and highlight practices informed by the DAOP model and sufferer-informed trauma-based approaches.

Sam, a 32-year-old woman, who works in health care, has been diagnosed with reflex sympathetic dystrophy (RSD) after years of hospitalizations and medical procedures attempting to control her pain (MacDonald, 2020). From age 16 to present, Sam has undergone six arthroscopic surgeries on her knee, along with a meniscectomy, a realignment of tendons to straighten the patella, removal of a neuroma, and, finally, a patellectomy. She has been repeatedly hospitalized – for example, the year following the birth of her son her various hospitalizations added up to six months out of the year. As a form of treatment, Sam had numerous sympathetic and epidural blocks, often experiencing complications from uncontrollable vomiting, debilitating migraines and metallic taste, along with the build-up of scar tissue making the blocks difficult to administer and at a greater risk for permanent damage.

Reflex sympathetic dystrophy, often known as chronic regional pain syndrome (CRPS), "is a rare, neuro-inflammatory syndrome characterized by intense chronic pain, swelling, trophic changes, vascular changes, and functional impairment of the limb" (Reflex Sympathetic Dystrophy Syndrome Association (RSDSA), 2021). The predominant symptom is severe and persistent pain disproportionate to the injury.

Sam's uncontrolled pain began following the surgical removal of her kneecap (patellectomy) when she was 27 years old, something that is common for reflex sympathetic dystrophy as it usually follows an injury or surgery to a limb (RSDSA, 2021). There is no objective measure of pain, with the best gauge being a subjective rating of pain with 1 (mild) to 10 (most severe). Sam rated her pain consistently between 8 and 10, often noting it was 10+. Pain was invading all aspects of Sam's life. Caught in a biomedical maze, Sam felt judged and disbelieved, where her experiences and her life's story were dismissed as they were measured up against symptoms defined by the medical establishment. For example, reflex sympathetic dystrophy pain is noted as being a "burning pain", yet Sam described her pain as being "an unfamiliar puzzling pain, of a deep, heavy, invasive character" (MacDonald, 2004, p. 21). Women have historically been judged and pathologized by medicine, especially when "the noxious stimulus does not fit with the degree of pain exhibited" (MacDonald, 2000, p. 52), or the characterization of their pain is outside the diagnostic criteria defined by biomedicine.

Further, as much as Sam wanted to be a mother, her pregnancy was filled with complications. She was hospitalized at three-months' gestation for pain, a lung infection and dehydration. At 34-weeks' gestation she became toxic, was hospitalized, put on bed rest and given an epidural. With Sam's condition continuing to deteriorate, the doctor performed a Caesarian section. Because Sam had an epidural catheter inserted for a week prior to the surgery it was less effective during the C-section resulting in Sam feeling unbearable pain and pressure in her leg. She described it as if her leg was about to explode. A "code 23" (requiring the neonatologist's emergency response) was called immediately following the birth of her son. The neonatologist came running into the operating room with arms stretched out so that nurses could assist with getting the doctor's protective gear secured. The baby was not breathing and needed to be suctioned. For weeks the baby remained in the neonatal unit and Sam remained in hospital for pain control.

Sam's medical journey also included two near-death experiences. First, this occurred when Sam was discharged from hospital with a CADD pump (computerized ambulatory delivery device) for pain medication that was set by the ward nurse at ten times the prescribed dose, so instead of it being set to 4 mg it was set to 40 mg. The second time occurred when she had a massive gastrointestinal bleed that ruptured the day after she traveled across a rural province with no medical facility within miles.

Table 7.1 highlights Sam's experiences of living with chronic pain in column 1, practice implications related to those experiences in column 2, a biomedical critique in column 3 where the authors challenge the dominant biomedical system by unsettling assumptions, and finally, the authors present a sufferer-informed trauma-based approach in column 4.

## Critical Analysis

Reflex sympathetic dystrophy has historically been somewhat of a mystery to medicine with no clear understanding about the symptomology and therefore no clear treatment direction (Bruehl, 2010). Furthermore, given its pathophysiological uncertainty, causation has often been diverted to psychological factors. Sam picked up on this early in her pain journey, with it only intensifying as her condition worsened and treatment attempts failed. As a result, Sam pushed her emotional reactions to living with chronic pain and uncertainty deep beneath the surface. MacDonald (2020) said "the binary split between the emotional and physical experiences of chronic pain is a false divide" (p. 353). Yet, Sam felt she had to keep a lock on her darkest thoughts for if they were to escape, she knew her pain would be labeled psychological and any hope of physiological interventions for pain relief would be lost. Sam's life with pain had created layers of loss and subsequent grief: loss of relationships because she had no energy to maintain them; threat of loss associated with her professional identity and income; and loss of motherhood as she had previously perceived it; just to mention a few. On top of this, Sam felt her identity as a mother was being continually judged, whereby having a (dis)Ability meant she could not be a "good" mother. Hall, Hundley, Collins, & Ireland (2018) found that women with (dis)Abilities during pregnancy, childbirth and postnatal care believed their rights were not respected and they were not treated with dignity; more than 25 percent of the women felt this way throughout the pregnancy process. Furthermore, (dis)Abled women experienced "less choice and control over their experience" (p. 329). Sam internalized these ableist notions, which resulted in significant feelings of self-blame and shame. She felt caught in a biomedical maze, where she desperately hung onto the hope of a medical breakthrough that would reduce her pain, but this came at a cost, for Sam could not afford to share her total pain experience.

One of the most challenging memories that Sam experienced was when she received an overdose of pain medication from the CADD pump that had been programmed by a nurse in the hospital prior to Sam's discharge. What was particularly upsetting was not the threat to her life, but rather when a friend noted if

**TABLE 7.1** (dis)Ability, sufferer experiences and trauma

| Experience | Practice considerations | Biomedical critique | Trauma-based, sufferer-informed approaches |
|---|---|---|---|
| It took 2 to 3 years for Sam to receive a diagnosis and even then, it was questioned. | Increased experiences of isolation and self-doubt. | Physician knowledge is not the only knowledge. Expert knowledge must include the sufferer's self-knowledge. | Sufferers' experiential knowledge is incorporated within clinical practice to develop comprehensive anti-oppressive healing responses. Knowledge from sufferers is integrated within all levels of the organization, from research and practice to feedback opportunities. |
| Sam was experiencing 10+ levels of pain most of the time. Yet, there was no way to measure the intensity of her pain input. | Hopelessness and depression. | RSD pain is rated as more intense than cancer pain or limb amputation (RSDSA, 2021). Yet it is difficult to diagnose especially under the medical gaze devoid of sufferer input. | Treatment is individualized and understands the sufferer's pain and (dis)Ability needs as unique, layered and evolving. Communication between the sufferer and multiple health care providers is expected (e.g., counselor, pain doctor and sufferer). |
| Sam had anesthesiologists refuse her care. She overheard nurses questioning the legitimacy of her pain. | Internalized ableism, questioning one's own identity, meaning, purpose. | Sam felt trapped within a system of health care that was sometimes supportive (e.g., family doctor, obstetrician) yet deeply judgmental by other health care professions (e.g., certain nurses, physicians, etc.). | The organization recognizes that staff, sufferers and families are interconnected; all have meaningful roles within an anti-oppressive, trauma-based approach and move toward the shared understanding that healing occurs in relationships. |

(*Continued*)

**TABLE 7.1** (dis)Ability, sufferer experiences and trauma (*Continued*)

| Experience | Practice considerations | Biomedical critique | Trauma-based, sufferer-informed approaches |
|---|---|---|---|
| Sam felt her right to motherhood was questioned through the glares and stares she received. | Ableist assumptions, inequalities, and gender stereotypes. | Assumptions and stereotypes linked to motherhood (Henderson, Harmon, & Newman, 2016) are well documented in feminist literature, however, Sam had the added judgements of being a (dis)Abled woman (Hall, Hundley, Collins, & Ireland, 2018) who was pregnant and needed to be on pain medication throughout her pregnancy in order to keep her pain and blood pressure out of a critical range | Organizational training programs address the stigmatization of (dis)Abled mothers. Trauma-based care includes (dis)Ability and inclusion education and initiatives for all staff; (dis)Ability motherhood knowledge and experience become well situated within care practices and policies. |
| Sam maintained professional employment throughout all her hospitalizations, using up vacation, sick time, and unemployment sick benefits. | Professional implications, identity crises, financial uncertainty. | Navigating multiple benefits in order to keep paying rent was stressful yet Sam was fortunate than most in that she maintained employment giving her access to sick leave and vacation time, and when these were used up, she was eligible to apply to UI/EI. | COVID-19 pandemic exposed numerous barriers within health care for (dis)Abled persons. When ICU beds were full and respirators were not to be found, the triage system assessed people with (dis)Abilities as having less of a chance of survival than able-bodied people (Hansen, 2020). Acknowledging the devaluation of (dis)Abled persons through all forms of social policy, be it health care, income maintenance or employment, is critical to dismantling ableist structures. |

Sam had died, they would have thought Sam took her own life by reprogramming the CADD pump. The thought of her family dealing with complicated grief created by the question of suicide further shook Sam during a time of overwhelming pain and caregiver judgment.

## Trauma Work with Sufferers

In considering the impact of internalized, neoliberal, structural ableism and of the biomedical model, trauma-based work grounded in the DAOP model and sufferer-informed approaches offer a way to begin practice with chronic pain sufferers. In this chapter, experiences of (dis)Ability, chronic pain and trauma are not separated or individualized, but viewed interconnectedly as well as sociopolitically and structurally. Recognizing that trauma work with sufferers is not universal, we acknowledge the many identities and experiences that chronic pain sufferers hold.

Trauma-based work by practitioners, staff and organizations would do well to respond to sufferers' traumatic disclosures and experiences with validation, while actively engaging in supportive and collaborative service delivery (Klinic Community Health Centre, 2013). Indeed, while there are overall gaps in (dis) Ability specific trauma-based knowledge, sufferers suggest that addressing institutional hierarchies and centering sufferer autonomy are two critical pathways through which one can move forward in challenging the normalization of power and control over (dis)Abled bodies (Hunter, 2021). Moving away from the biomedical model, which negatively labels sufferers as something being wrong with them, may easily be replaced by asking what is happening and what has happened to them (Klinic Community Health Centre, 2013). All too frequently, (dis)Abled people and sufferers have no opportunity to speak about what they are experiencing, and when they do share their experiences, they need to be heard and believed (Klein, Singh, Kynn, & McLean, 2023). Having a voice and having their experiences and input validated consistently by practitioners throughout their accessing of health care services is reflective of the DAOP model and sufferer-informed, trauma-based approaches. Instead of defaulting to an expected list of individualized strategies to cope and striving toward unrealistic measures of resiliency, the practitioner asks what the sufferer needs and hears what works for the sufferer. A practitioner implementing these approaches is asked to truly listen. As C. Brown and MacDonald (2022) explain,

> as practitioners we bear witness, serve as allies and as advocates … it is important to double listen, especially to what is being said, partially said, or not said … it is important to create compassionate and safe spaces where people can speak the unspeakable.
>
> *(p. 127)*

When a sufferer speaks of unimaginable emotional, mental and physical pain, this is heard, believed and validated, thus opening up "the possibility of the story unfolding rather than encouraging it to retreat" (p. 127). The practitioner also listens for combined individual and structural experiences of ableism and trauma, with the latter not always obvious. Shifts in identity and life changes occurring on an individual level may be compounded structurally through inaccessible environments, insufficient accommodations, inadequate financial supports and extensive wait-times to access possible treatments. The sufferer may experience a reduction in their quality of life, wherein their emotional, mental and physical pain worsens, leaving them vulnerable to increased isolation and declining health. Sufferer-informed trauma work emphasizes addressing ableist barriers and structural trauma, in concert with understanding the impact of impairments. Contra-indicated dualisms, such as body versus mind, physiological versus psychological causation, or medical knowledge versus sufferer intuition, are explored through social worker and sufferer engagement for their intertwining complexities and nuances (MacDonald, 2020), aimed at facilitating sufferer centered "agency, power and choice" (Brown, C. & MacDonald, 2022, p. 128).

## Conclusion

In this chapter, we, the authors, explored trauma-based practices as it pertains to people with (dis)Abilities, with the understanding that the (dis)Abled person's struggles are manifested by structural barriers and inaccessible infrastructures. Ableism, by its very nature, creates repeated traumatic experiences, from the presentation of normalcy as the biomedical standard to expert knowledge belonging to professionals. This results in the dismissal of lived experiences and personal choice promoting individualism, which isolates and segregates people with (dis)Abilities, including chronic pain sufferers. Through deconstructing biomedical discourses historical and contemporary displays of ableism are highlighted. Further, practice interventions are situated through the presentation of the Disability Anti-Oppressive Practice Model. The case of Sam, a woman, health service provider and mother, who lived with reflex sympathetic dystrophy, was shared to highlight the importance of critiquing biomedically focused approaches in trauma work. A trauma-based approach works toward breaking down barriers, increasing access to services and social supports, and forming a community of allies and sufferers where safety, voice and control are the founding principles of engagement. Ultimately, we take up trauma-based practices from a (dis)Ability perspective using chronic pain sufferers as the exemplar, hoping that additional connections will be made between working with (dis)Abled persons, their accumulative trauma and trauma-based practices.

## Note

1 This name has been changed to protect confidentiality.

# References

Baines, D., & Clark, N. (2022). Anti-oppressive practice: Roots, theory, tensions. In D. Baines, N. Clark, & B. Bennett (Eds.), *Doing Anti-oppressive social work: Rethinking theory and practice* (4th ed.) (pp. 1–33). Fernwood.

Baines, D., & Sharma, A. (2022). Anti-oppressive practice theory: Building social justice social work. In S.S. Shaikh, B. LeFrançois, & T. Macías (Eds.), *Critical social work praxis* (pp. 118–127). Fernwood.

Bass, E., & Davis, L. (1988). *The courage to heal: A guide for women survivors of child sexual abuse.* Collins Living.

Brown, C., Johnstone, M., & Ross, N. (2021). *Repositioning social work in mental health practice in Nova Scotia.* Nova Scotia College of Social Work, Halifax. https://nscsw.org/mental-health-paper/.

Brown, C., & MacDonald, J. (2022). Critical clinical social work: Working in the context of trauma and (dis)Ability. In D. Baines, N. Clark, & B. Bennett (Eds.), *Doing Anti-oppressive social work: Rethinking theory and practice* (4th ed.) (pp. 118–140). Fernwood.

Bruehl, S. (2010). An update on the pathophysiology of complex regional pain syndrome. *Anesthesiology, 113*(3), 713–725. https://doi.org/10.1097/ALN.0b013e3181e3db38.

Cameron, C. (2014). Social model. In C. Cameron (Ed.), *Disability studies: A student's guide* (pp. 137–140). Sage Publications. https://doi.org/10.4135/9781473957701.

Campbell, F.K. (2009). Disability harms: Exploring internalized ableism. In C.A. Marshall, E. Kendall, M.E. Banks, & R.M.S Gover (Eds.), *Disabilities: Insights from across fields and around the world,* vol. 1 (pp. 19–33). Greenwood.

Carter, I., Hanes, R., & MacDonald, J.E. (2017). Beyond the social model of disability: Engaging in anti-oppressive social work practice. In D. Baines (Ed.), *Doing anti-oppressive practice: Social justice social work* (3rd ed.) (pp. 153–171). Canadian Scholars Press.

Chapman, C. (2022). Disability studies insights for critical social work. In S.S. Shaikh, B. LeFrançois, & T. Macías (Eds.), *Critical social work praxis* (pp. 432–442). Fernwood.

Clare, E. (2017). *Brilliant imperfection: Grappling with cure.* Duke University Press.

Crow, C. (1996). Including all of our lives. In J. Morris (Ed.), *Encounters with strangers.* The Women's Press.

Dolmage, J. (2017). *Academic ableism: Disability and higher education.* University of Michigan Press. https://doi.org/10.3998/mpub.9708722.

Fallot, R.D., & Harris, M. (2009). *Creating cultures of trauma-informed care.* Community Connections, Washington DC.

Fisher, P., & Goodley, D. (2007). The linear medical model of disability: Mothers of disabled babies resist with counter-narratives. *Sociology of Health & Ill*ness, 29, 66–81. https://doi.org/10.1111/j.1467-9566.2007.00518.x.

Goodley, D. (2014). *Dis/ability studies: Theorising disablism and ableism.* Routledge.

Goodley, D. (2017). *Disability studies: An interdisciplinary introduction* (2nd ed.). Sage Publications.

Goodley, D., & Lawthom, R. (2019). Critical disability studies, Brexit and Trump: A time of neoliberal-ableism. *Rethinking History, 23*(2), 233–251. https://doi.org/10.1080/13642529.2019.1607476.

Gough, A. (2005). Body/mind: A chaos narrative of cyborg subjectivities and liminal experiences. *Women's Studies, 34*(3/4), 249–264. https://doi.org/10.1080/00497870590964 147.

Greenhalgh, S. (2001). *Under the medical gaze: Facts and fictions of chronic pain.* University of California Press.

Hall, J., Hundley, V., Collins, B., & Ireland, J. (2018). Dignity and respect during pregnancy and childbirth: A survey of the experience of disabled women. *BMC Pregnancy and Childbirth*, 18(328), 1–13. https://doi.org/10.1186/s12884-018-1950-7.

Hanes, R., Carter, I., & MacDonald, J.E. (2022). Getting to the heart of the matter: A social-oppression model of disability. In D. Baines, N. Clark, & B. Bennett (Eds.), *Doing anti-oppressive social work: Rethinking theory and practice* (4th ed.) (pp. 244–266). Fernwood.

Hansen, N. (April 5, 2020). Who gets medical care during the coronavirus pandemic – and what does that mean for people with disabilities? *CBC News.* https://www.cbc.ca/news/canada/manitoba/manitobans-disability-health-care-coronavirus-1.5520589.

Harris, M.E., & Fallot, R.D. (2001). *Using trauma theory to design service systems.* Jossey-Bass/Wiley.

Henderson, A., Harmon, S., & Newman, H. (2016). The price mothers pay, even when they are not buying it: Mental health consequences of idealized motherhood. *Sex Roles*, 74, 512–526. https://doi.org/10.1007/s11199-015-0534-5.

Herman, J.L. (1992). *Trauma and recovery.* Basic Books/Hachette Book Group.

Hollins, S., & Sinason, V. (2000). Psychotherapy, learning disabilities and trauma: New perspectives. *British Journal of Psychiatry*, 176, 32–36. https//doi.org/10.1192/bjp.176.1.32.

Hunter, M. (2021). *Trauma informed care for survivors with disabilities.* https://traumainformedoregon.org/wp-content/uploads/Trauma-Informed-Care-for-Survivors-With-Disabilities.pdf.

Johnson, L., Singh, R.C.B., & Slayter, E. (2022). A practice model for disability social work: Connecting critical cultural competence, intersectionality, and anti-oppressive practice. In E. Slayter & L. Johnson (Eds.), *Social work practice and the disability community: An intersectional anti-oppressive approach.* Pressbooks.

Kafer, A. (2013). *Feminist, queer, crip.* Indiana University Press.

Kafer, A. (April 6, 2017). Video. *Health rebels: A crip manifesto for social justice.* https://www.youtube.com/watch?v=YqcOUD1pBKw.

Keesler, J.M. (2014). A call for the integration of trauma-informed care among intellectual and developmental disability organizations. *Journal of Policy and Practice in Intellectual Disabilities*, 11(1), 34–42. https://doi.org/10.1111/jppi.12071.

Kinnucan, M. (2014). An interview with Yasmin Nair, part two: The ideal neoliberal subject is the subject of trauma. *Hypocrite Reader.* https://hypocritereader.com/43/yasmin-nair-two.

Klein, L.B., Singh, R.C.B., Kynn, J., & McLean, K.J. (2023). Disabled and/or chronically ill survivors of sexual violence and intimate partner violence. In S.K. Kattari (Ed.), *Exploring sexuality and disability: A guide for academics and health and human service professionals.* Routledge.

Klinic Community Health Care Centre. (2013). *The Trauma Toolkit.* (2nd ed.). https://trauma-informed.ca/wp-content/uploads/2013/10/Trauma-informed_Toolkit.pdf.

Liasidou, A. (2021). Trauma-informed disability politics: Interdisciplinary navigations and implications. *Disability & Society.* https://doi.org/10.1080/09687599.2021.1946679.

MacDonald, J.E. (2000). A deconstructive turn in chronic pain management: A redefined role for social work. *Health & Social Work*, 25(1), 51–58. https://doi.org/10.1093/hsw/25.1.51.

MacDonald, J.E. (2004). One woman's experience of living with chronic pain. *Journal of Social Work in Disability & Rehabilitation*, 3(2), 17–35. https://doi.org/10.1300/J198v03n02_03.

MacDonald, J.E. (2008). Anti-oppressive practices with chronic pain sufferers. *Social Work in Health Care*, 47(2), 135–156. https://doi.org/10.1080/00981380801970285.

MacDonald, J.E. (2020). Counterbalancing life with chronic pain through storying women's experiences of (dis)Ability. In C. Brown & J.E. MacDonald (Eds.), *Critical clinical social work: Counterbalancing for social justice* (pp. 341–365). Canadian Scholars Press.

MacDonald, J.E., Brown, M., & Jones, S. (2022). Social policy across social identities. In B. MacKenzie & B. Wharf (Eds.), *Connecting policy to practice in the human services* (5th ed.) (pp. 272–290). Oxford University Press.

MacDonald, J.E., & Cooper, S. (2019). (dis)Ability policy: A tangled web of complexity. In R. Harding & D. Jeyapal (Eds.), *Canadian social policy for social workers* (pp. 179–200). Oxford University Press.

MacDonald, J.E., & Friars, G. (2009). Structural social work from a (dis)Ability perspective. In S. Hick, H. Peters, & T. Corner (Eds.), *Structural social work in action* (pp. 138–156). Canadian Scholars Press.

Mackelprang, R., Salsgiver, R., & Parrey, R. (2022). *Disability: A diversity model approach in human service practice.* (4th ed.). Oxford University Press.

Mingus, M. (February 12, 2011). Blog post. *Changing the framework: Disability justice. How our communities can move beyond access to wholeness.* https://leavingevidence .wordpress.com/2011/02/12/changing-the-framework- disability-justice/.

Nova Scotia Human Rights Commission. (n.d.). *Duty to accommodate.* https://humanrights .novascotia.ca/duty-accommodate.

Oliver, M. (1983). *Social work with disabled people.* Macmillan.

Oliver, M. (2013). The social model of disability: Thirty years on. *Disability & Society*, 28(7), 1024–1026. https://doi.org/10.1080/09687599.2013.818773.

Owen, M., Hiebert-Murphy, D., & Ristock, J. (2018). Disability, violence, and social change: An introduction. In M. Owen, D. Hiebert-Murphy, & J. Ristock (Eds.), *Not a new problem: Violence in the lives of disabled women* (pp. 1–14). Fernwood.

Park, Y., Crath, R., & Jeffery, D. (2020). Disciplining the risky subject: A discourse analysis of the concept of resilience in social work literature. *Journal of Social Work*, 20(2), 152–172. https://doi.org/10.1177/1468017318792953.

Rabinowitz, T., & Wallace, S. (2023). *New data on disability in Canada, 2022.* Statistics Canada. https://www150.statcan.gc.ca/n1/pub/11-627-m/11-627-m2023063-eng.htm#.

Rauscher, L., & McClintock, J. (1996). Ableism curriculum design. In M. Adams, L.A. Bell, & P. Griffen (Eds.), *Teaching for diversity and social justice* (pp. 198–231). Routledge.

Reflex Sympathetic Dystrophy Syndrome Association (RSDSA). (2021). *Defining CRPS.* https://rsds.org/definition-of-crps/.

Runswick-Cole, K., & Goodley, D. (2013). Resilience: A disability studies and community psychology approach. *Social and Personality Psychology Compass*, 7(2), 67–78. https:// doi.org/10.1111/spc3.12012.

Schopflocher, D., Taenzer, P., & Jovey, R. (2011). The prevalence of chronic pain in Canada. *Pain Research & Management, 16*(6), 445–450. https://doi.org/10.1155/2011/876306.

Singh, R.C.B., Murray-Lichtman, A.J., & Slayter, E. (2022). Mental health and addictions in disability communities. In E. Slayter & L. Johnson (Eds.), *Social work practice and the disability community: An intersectional anti-oppressive approach.* Pressbooks.

Smart, J. (2004). Models of disability: The juxtaposition of biology and social construction. In T. Riggar & D.R. Maki (Eds.), *Handbook of rehabilitation counseling* (pp. 25–49). Springer.

Stienstra, D. (2020). *About Canada: Disability rights* (2nd ed.). Fernwood.

Substance Abuse and Mental Health Services Administration (SAMHSA). (2023). *Practical guide for implementing a trauma-informed approach.* https://store.samhsa .gov/sites/default/files/pep23-06-05-005.pdf.

Titchkosky, T., Cagulada, E., & DeWelles, M. (2022). Introduction. In T. Titchkosky, E. Cagulada, M. DeWelles, & E. Gold (Eds.), *DisAppearing: Encounters in disability studies* (pp. 1–14). Canadian Scholars Press.

Titchkosky, T., & Michalko, R. (2009). *Rethinking normalcy: A disability studies reader.* Canadian Scholars Press.

Tseris, E. (2019). *Trauma, women's mental health, and social justice: Pitfalls and possibilities.* Routledge.

Wertans, E., & Burch, L. (2022). "It's backdoor accessibility": Disabled students' navigation of university campus. *Journal of Disability Studies in Education*, 1–22. https://doi.org /10.1163/25888803-bja10013.

Wendell, S. (1996). *The rejected body: Feminist philosophical reflections on disability.* Routledge.

Williamson, L., & Qureshi, A. (2015). Trauma informed care and disability: The complexity of pervasive experiences. *International Journal of Physical Medicine & Rehabilitation*, (3)2. https://doi.org/10.4172/2329-9096.1000265.

Withers, A.J. (2012). *Disability politics & theory.* Fernwood.

# 8

# BIRTH MATTERS

## Understanding the Impact of Birth Trauma on Women's Well-Being

*Amanda Dupupet and Laura Boileau*

### Introduction

Pregnancy, birth and the postpartum period is a significant and meaningful event in the life of a woman[1] who has the experience. Many women, their families and communities experience birth as a joyful, powerful and beautiful experience. It can conversely be experienced as a terrifying trauma. For some, the birth experience may be both joyful, beautiful, terrifying and disempowering creating a complicated, even confusing, emotional experience.

Women can experience the birth as traumatic due to medical complications that threaten the life of the mother and/or baby, and they can also experience the birth as traumatic due to how they are treated during the experience. For instance, women's experience of how they are treated when a birth is traumatic can include feeling that they have no control, a loss of dignity, a lack of caring, and limited communication between the mother and her care providers (Beck, 2015).

This chapter explores women's experiences of trauma and obstetric violence while giving birth and afterward. First, the chapter offers a definition of birth trauma and its effects. We argue the primary risk factor in developing lasting symptoms of trauma is the way a woman is treated during the perinatal period, which includes pregnancy, birth and after the birth. Symptoms of birth trauma can include feeling numb, angry, anxious, depressed, guilty, humiliated, shame, self-blame, criticism and flashbacks. We then focus on the multiple factors that render birth trauma invisible under the current dominant discourses in both the biomedical model and social constructs of motherhood. Both authors share their own experiences of birth trauma, using them to illustrate the various ways birth trauma can occur and how it is rendered invisible by dominant medical and social discourses. Next, we discuss the obstetric violence movement. Obstetric violence

DOI: 10.4324/9781003379591-9

is a form of birth trauma that consists of emotional, verbal, sexual or physical abuse during pregnancy, birth or in the postpartum experience (Chadwick, 2021; van de Waal, Mayra, Horn, & Chadwick, 2022).

Finally, we address how a collaborative engagement with women can prevent birth trauma as well as help women heal from it. The authors note that they have encountered instances in which health care professionals, including doctors and midwives, unintentionally disempower women and fail to foster collaborative relationships. They observe that individuals from both the medical and midwifery approaches are influenced by prevailing narratives of motherhood, which can further contribute to the underrecognition of birth trauma. The authors emphasize the significance of directing attention toward the relationship between health care professionals and women as a way to prevent or reduce some experiences of birth trauma. For the purposes of this paper, the term "care provider" will refer to any professional supporting the mother through the perinatal period, including medical doctors, nurses and midwives.

In addition, we wish to center women's experiences of birth instead of centering this discussion within the language of post-traumatic stress disorder (PTSD) which is often situated within a psychiatrization, medicalizing, labeling, pathologizing and decontextualizing approach to women's experiences. Birth trauma has remained largely invisible due to a variety of social discourses that influence the perceptions of birth and mothering. Further, in instances of physically traumatic birth, causing physical injury or harm, persistent trauma symptoms may be mitigated through caring and support both through and following the birthing process.

## Birth Trauma

Experiences of traumatic birth are far more prevalent than care providers, families or mothers themselves often realize. According to Alcorn and colleagues (2010), approximately 45 percent of women report they experienced events during the birth of their child as traumatic. Similarly, a recent study in the United States explored the impact of COVID on birth and found 72.3 percent of women studied had significant trauma symptoms post-birth (Diamond & Colaianni, 2022). While women are often seriously impacted by traumatic birth experiences, this often goes unseen. Despite the prevalence of postpartum trauma symptoms, the issue remains largely invisible within the academic literature, among health care professionals and among the wider public (Ayers, Bond, Bertullies, & Wijma, 2016; Dekel, Erin-Dor, Dishy, & Mayopoulos, 2020; Yildiz, Ayers, & Phillips, 2017). The goals of this chapter are to widen the lens for care providers to recognize that birth can be a traumatic event that can cause significant suffering and to highlight that how a woman is treated during birth and afterward can have significant impact on how she perceives and interprets her experience.

Those writing in the field of birth trauma often adopt either the biomedical model or a feminist obstetric violence lens to understand and address the issue.

While research on birth trauma through a biomedical model lens is still in its infancy, those using a feminist lens have been focused on reproductive rights and the treatment of women in birth for decades. The dominant discourse is the biomedical model, which stems from the fields of psychology, psychiatry and health sciences. The biomedical model is mostly centered on diagnostic criteria, prevalence, risk factors and the negative effects birth trauma can have on the infant rather than the overall birth experiences of women (Ayers, Joseph, McKenzie-McHarg, Slade, & Wijma, 2008). The medical model paradigm of birth itself is situated primarily in authoritative knowledge of the body, typically emphasizing the knowledge, authority and expertise of the health professional to the extent of silencing women's voices. The biomedical model maintains a focus on the pathologization of individual women when they do experience significant birthing distress post-birth. Those using only a biomedical lens often neglect to provide an analysis of the limitations of dominant biomedical approaches to birth experiences and how these are shaped by dominant social discourses and practices that influence both how women experience birth and the provision of care in this process. The solutions offered are respectful maternity care, better trauma symptom screening for women and health care providers, and individual therapy when needed (Beck, 2015; Kendall-Tackett, 2014; Olde, van der Hart, Kleber, & van Son, 2006; Yildiz, Ayers, & Phillips, 2017). While the literature from both the medical field and the obstetric violence field address birth trauma, the medical field often precludes reference to the obstetric violence field. This is, at least in part, because the biomedical paradigm does not adequately emphasize the psychosocial, interactive and experiential aspects of care in such a way that acknowledges how women can experience certain forms of care as violent.

The literature on obstetric violence offers a feminist analysis of birth trauma, seeing the experience through the lens of gender-based violence. It is focused on women's experience of mistreatment and advocating for change (Freedman et al., 2018; Sadler et al., 2016). The obstetric violence and reproductive justice movements, particularly in a North American context, emphasize the importance of women having more power and control over their labor and their bodies (Shaw, 2013; van der Waal, Mayra, Horn, & Chadwick, 2022). The obstetric violence movement builds on the work of the women's health movement, which has advocated a move away from the dominant medicalized model of birth, in favour of highlighting the possibility of empowering experiences when women are both well attended and given control over the process. Early work, by, for instance, Ehreinreich and English (1978) examined medical assumptions about medical experts' advice to women. Dreifus (1977) explored the politics of women's health and referred to the medical professions' seizing of women's bodies. More on point, Adrienne Rich (1977) challenged what she called the "theft of childbirth" in her book. Later she extended her analysis with her book *Of Woman Born (2004)*. Whilst in Europe midwives have been central in the birthing process, even with the medicalization of childbirth, in North America the midwifery movement has sought to redress what became an overly medicalized grip on women's reproductive health. While medical knowledge can clearly prevent harm and save lives, medical sociologists and feminist thinkers have been critiquing the medicalization of childbirth for decades, drawing attention to the use of the pacification of women in labor, unnecessary medical interventions such as cesarean sections and episiotomies.

While midwifery care may help support some women in achieving an empowered birth experience with reduced medical procedures, it is important to note that the services of a midwife are not universally available across North America due to limitations on the number of available midwives and the high demand for services. Also, in situations where advanced medical intervention by doctors is required, midwives transfer either some or all aspects of care to an obstetrician and/or other medical specialists. Further, while the tenets of midwifery differ from those of the medical model, globally midwives must often participate in the dominant medical system and when working in hospitals they must comply with the rules and regulations set out by doctors and government officials (Gorham, 1984; van der Waal, Mayra, Horn, & Chadwick, 2022).

Chadwick (2014) argues for the need to create counterstories of birth that allow for an understanding of the complexity of women's experiences. This includes disrupting overly naturalized narratives of birthing, which set women up to feel like failures or that they are not good enough if they required medical assistance. Counter-narratives need to emphasize "the importance of women's agency, their bodily competence and capability as birthgivers and the social and emotional significance of childbirth" (p. 46) and challenge the often inadvertent paradox of continuing to story birth in disembodied, medicalized language. This includes expanding the discursive field to enable telling birthing stories without representing experiences as either "happy" or "difficult and traumatic", which are both tied to notions of being good mothers or women. Similarly, the work of Ussher (1997) demonstrates the importance of challenging the binary divide between the material (corporeal/physical) and the discursive (social, cultural, ideological, political) way of interpreting the world. Women's reproductive body can then be understood as more than the physical, as it is always shaped socially and politically (Cohen Shabot, 2020).

Dominant discourses about birth have the effect of silencing women's stories of trauma and violence, and this lack of support can be retraumatizing. There are many facets of traumatic birth that make it different from other types of trauma. Unlike car collisions, for example, rather than thinking of birth as traumatic, birth is often thought of as primarily a joyfully anticipated event and is viewed as positive by many women and society at large (Ayers, Bond, Bertullies, & Wijma, 2016). Unlike other types of trauma, a woman's experience of birthing itself and the effects of it, are often dismissed by care providers (including obstetricians and midwives), family and friends as the outcome of a healthy baby is viewed as the only thing that matters (Beck, 2004a, 2015). Further, women are often simultaneously dealing with their physical recovery, traumatic experience and sleep deprivation while caring for a new baby, who can be a constant reminder of the trauma (Beck, 2015; Thomas, 2020). While the anniversary of a traumatic event often brings up intense negative emotions, birth trauma is unique as this is also often the child's birthday, a day that most want to celebrate (Beck, 2015). Social pressures, including socially constructed notions of being a "good mother" in the postpartum period, often silence women from speaking of their distress, discomfort and struggles. This can become a self-perpetuating cycle that in effect isolates, retraumatizes and depoliticizes an experience that many women face.

### Definition of Birth Trauma

Beck (2004a), a highly regarded obstetrical nurse researcher in the field of birth trauma, argues that both physiological and psychological events during childbirth can cause trauma symptoms. Physiological events of "actual or threatened serious injury or death to the mother or her infant" can include medical procedures such as use of forceps, vacuum extraction, cesarean section, and NICU (neonatal intensive care unit) stays and psychological experiences such as "intense fear, helplessness, loss of control, and horror" (Beck, 2004a, p. 28). Research has strongly established that common characteristics of a psychologically traumatic birth include women feeling "deprived of caring", "stripped of their dignity", a "terrifying loss of control", "neglected communication" with and between caregivers, and "buried and forgotten" by obstetric staff and midwives (Beck, 2015, p. 4).

In both the biomedical model and the obstetric violence movement there is a growing recognition that the way a woman is treated during labor and delivery can have profound implications for her recovery. Even when a birth is obstetrically uncomplicated and babies arrive at term, trauma symptoms can still be experienced (Dekel, Thiel, Dishy, & Ashenfarb, 2019). The subjective experience of "feeling unassisted, unsupported, uncared for – deprived of a subjectivity that is truly sustained and contained by others – these are clear characteristics of violent and traumatic births" (Cohen Shabot, 2021, p. 6). Some adverse events and medical complications during birth may be unavoidable, but if women feel cared for, communicated with, and treated with respect and dignity, it should be possible to prevent lasting trauma symptoms (Beck, 2015; Garthus-Niegel, von Soest, Vollrath, & Eberhard-Gran, 2013).

Symptoms of Birth Trauma

Common experiences after a traumatic birth can include intense uncontrollable memories, flashbacks or nightmares of the birth (Beck, 2015: Thomas, 2020). Many also experience an intense desire to avoid reminders of the birth. The baby can be a primary reminder of the traumatic experience, but cannot be avoided; mothers may avoid additional reminders such as hospitals, medical staff, pregnant women, other mothers and depictions of birth (Beck, 2011, 2015; Kendall-Tackett, 2014). Some women express feelings of numbness and detachment from everyone, including themselves, and being unable to have any positive feelings (Beck, 2015). Many women also experience a distorted sense of self-blame and guilt or they intensely blame others (Thomas, 2020). Other effects can also include difficulty in concentrating, dissociation, anxiety, panic, hypervigilance, intense anger and insomnia (Thomas, 2020; Beck, 2015). Many of these symptoms are also symptoms of postpartum depression and anxiety. Often health care providers, and mothers themselves, are familiar with "postpartum depression", which has not only been extensively researched, but is also part of everyday conversation. The high degree of similarity in symptoms could lead to a care provider to misinterpret the mother's symptoms as " only postpartum depression" and miss that her current symptoms are actually resulting from a traumatic experience. To render birth trauma more visible and offer appropriate support and treatment, it is important to attend to women's experiences post-birth.

### Lasting Effects of Birth Trauma

Women who perceive the birth as traumatic can experience a variety of short- and long-term effects that, if left unacknowledged and untreated, can worsen over time, leaving some women still feeling impacted decades later (Beck, 2015; Yildiz, Ayers, & Phillips, 2017). In the short term, many women suffer in silence, feeling detached from others, as their dreams of motherhood are shattered by trauma (Beck, 2015). This can be particularly heightened if a woman's care providers, family and community inadvertently reinforce the silencing of her experience by focusing only on the baby (Beck, 2015). The effects of trauma, such as rage, along with the difficulties of adjusting to caring for an infant, also lead to increased strain on relationships at a time when women most need support (Beck, 2004b). Some studies indicate the attachment relationship between the mother and infant can also be impaired due to the effects of trauma, and the distance a woman feels from her child can last for years (Beck, 2015; Dekel, Thiel, Dishy, & Ashenfarb, 2019). The dominant discourses of birth trauma in the biomedical field tend to emphasize the impact on the infant. Not only are women dealing with the effects of trauma, but they are also over-responsibilized, as it is implied that if they do not work to heal themselves it will have lasting consequences for their child. These factors can all increase the risk of suicide, which is one of the leading causes of mortality in the postpartum period (Chin, Wendt, Bennett, & Bhat, 2022).

Longer-term impacts of birth trauma can affect a woman's decision to have future children and impact the experience of future pregnancies and births (Beck, 2015; Garthus-Niegel, von Soest, Vollrath, & Eberhard-Gran, 2013; Thomas, 2020). After multiple losses, Amanda struggled with considering a subsequent pregnancy. Seemingly blind to her experiences of trauma and grief, her doctor was surprised that she was not sure if she wanted to try for another child.

## Influences on the Effects of Trauma

To prevent birth trauma and the possible subsequent effects, practitioners need to identify those at higher risk for the development of trauma symptoms. There are multiple factors that can interact to increase the risk of developing negative effects following birth trauma. Such risks include prior mental health concerns, fear of childbirth, complications in pregnancy and birth, and exposure to prior traumatic events (Andersen, Melvaer, Videbech, Lamont, & Joergensen, 2012; Ayers, Bond, Bertullies, & Wijma, 2016; Chan et al., 2020; Garthus-Niegel, von Soest, Vollrath, & Eberhard-Gran, 2013). Many survivors of sexualized violence report that having vaginal examinations and having the focus of birth on their vaginas feels overwhelming, vulnerable and retraumatizing (Beck, 2004a; Cohen Shabot, 2021; Simkin & Klaus, 2017). Some even describe their labor experiences as "birth rape" (Beck, 2004a; Cohen Shabot, 2021).

Obstetric interventions and physical complications can increase the risk of birth trauma, yet even when a traumatic birth involves a threat of death or serious injury to the mother or infant, it does not necessarily result in the development of trauma symptoms. One study indicated that only a quarter of women whose infants died in childbirth experienced postpartum trauma symptoms (Olde, van der Hart, Kleber, & van Son, 2006). It is the meaning that women make of the experience that determines the development of trauma symptoms. Research indicates the most important influence in the development of trauma symptoms post-birth is women's negative subjective experience of the birth (Beck, 2004a; Garthus-Niegel, von Soest, Vollrath, & Eberhard-Gran, 2013). For women, these experiences include feeling threatened, powerless, dissociated, ignored, abandoned, invisible, unsupported and dissatisfied with their care providers (Ayers, Bond, Bertullies, & Wijma, 2016; Beck 2004a). For Laura, these failures of care increased her perception of physical risk, which greatly increased her distress. Birth is thus much more than just a physiological event. Birth always happens within a social context and is socially constructed, as "we birth with others", and the quality of care (or lack of) being meaningfully held in an embodied connection to others has a significant impact on the development of a healthful adjustment in the postpartum period (Sadler et al., 2016; Cohen Shabot, 2020, p. 10).

## Invisibility of Birth Trauma

### Motherhood Discourse

Women's experience of birth trauma is also rendered invisible by the dominant discourse on motherhood. Women are discouraged from talking about experiences that challenge idealized notions of mothering and birth. The dominant discourse insists that mothers be selfless and take care of others, particularly their newborn baby. Mothers are also expected to be overjoyed by the arrival of their infant, leaving little room for different narratives. When talking about her traumatic birth with family members, Laura was repeatedly told "That's just what we have to go through, it doesn't matter now. At least you have a healthy baby!". Like many other women, it was repeatedly implied that the end of having a healthy baby justified any means (Beck, 2004a). The theme of "at least" also often shows up in the responses of others even when a mother loses a baby during pregnancy. For Amanda, after a third trimester loss, people often responded with comments like, "at least you can have another one" or "at least you have other healthy children". As a result of the minimization of negative experiences and that women comply with social expectations about mothering, women are likely to be reluctant to talk about traumatic experiences and the ongoing impact on them, and they may avoid seeking treatment (Olde, van der Hart, Kleber, & van Son, 2006).

Midwives, nurses, physicians, psychiatrists and other mental health professionals make the same cultural assumptions that birth is supposed to be a joyous event. Laura experienced significant trauma symptoms post-birth and attempted to discuss it with her care providers who kept expressing their confusion "but you don't seem depressed". There seemed to be a complete lack of understanding that she could perceive the birth as traumatic and was suffering as result with intense flashbacks, terror, avoidance and insomnia. Despite ten years of experience as a trauma therapist, until the birth of her first child, Laura also had not considered that birth could be a traumatic event, which in itself reflects the dominant discourse and taken-for-granted reality about birthing.

### Traumatized Health Care Providers

Health care professionals can inadvertently contribute to rendering birth trauma invisible because they are also experiencing trauma symptoms. A study of obstetric staff found that approximately two-thirds of those surveyed experienced situations while providing care to patients that induced lasting feelings of helplessness, fear or horror in the care provider (Slade et al., 2020). A review conducted by Kendall-Tackett and Beck (2022) found that obstetric nurses and midwives also experience symptoms of trauma resulting from caring for their patients. Of note was that, in countries where mothers experience higher rates of trauma symptoms post-birth, they found corresponding higher rates of trauma symptoms in midwives (Kendall-Tackett & Beck, 2022). Care providers experiencing symptoms of trauma such as feeling disconnected and emotionally exhausted, as found in the study by Slade and colleagues (2020), would possibly not be able to consider the emotional impact to the patient that could result from their actions. We know that the care providers themselves, in addition to dealing with life-and-death situations on a day-to-day basis, also struggle to provide care for their patients within often stretched health care systems. Care providers may have entered the profession because they are helpers and care about their patients, but they can often become disillusioned and disconnected by the barriers presented by the system and the traumas that they experience as part of their job.

## *Invisibility in the DSM*

Birth trauma is often rendered invisible because it does not align with the *Diagnostic and Statistical Manual of Mental Disorders* (DSM). Shifting criteria for posttraumatic stress disorder in DSM revisions speaks to the ongoing social and political construction of these diagnoses. Even if a woman is experiencing intense trauma symptoms from all the PTSD categories, health care professionals using the most recent version of the *Diagnostic and Statistical Manual of Mental Disorders* (5th edition, Text Revision) (DSM-5-TR) may only acknowledge the presence of trauma when a person has experienced, witnessed or learned about a close relation experiencing "actual or threatened death, serious injury, or sexual violence" (American Psychiatric Association, 2022, p. 301). A woman, however, can perceive that her life or the life of the baby was at risk, or that she experienced serious injury or sexual violence, even if obstetric staff believe that no such risk was present and her birth was routine.

There are many problems associated with the DSM, as it typically does not fit well with people's experiences. It tends to define human struggles as individual deficits without consideration of social context. It subsequently reinforces pathologizing and medicalizing people's suffering. We need to acknowledge that our current "PTSD knowledge does not address the meaning of a traumatic birth for women" (Beck, 2004a, p. 30). Our concern is that women need to be taken seriously and have their pain, suffering and trauma acknowledged regardless of diagnostic criteria. The invalidation of women's lived experience is too common in birth trauma. Generally, the DSM is reductive, reflecting and upholding dominant discourse (which rarely reflects the experiences or interests of marginalized social groups). Practitioners need to incorporate women's accounts of their experience of childbirth to determine whether or not it resulted in trauma symptoms. In contrast to these formalized guidelines of the biomedical model, the obstetric violence movement strives to make these experiences visible, while situating them in the broader social and systemic contexts in which it occurs.

## Obstetric Violence Movement

Obstetric violence is a form of birth trauma that consists of emotional, verbal, sexual or physical abuse during pregnancy, birth or in the postpartum experience (which can include medical appropriation, non-consensual procedures, overuse or withholding of medical procedures, coercion, neglect, disrespect, bullying or discrimination (Chadwick, 2021; van de Waal, Mayra, Horn, & Chadwick, 2022). These incidents can be active and intentional, passive and unintentional, or related to the actions of individuals or of the broader health system (Bohren et al., 2015).

Building on the prior work of the women's movement, which fought for women to have more freedom, choices, power and control over their own bodies and reproductive rights and to resist the medicalization and psychiatrization of their lives, the obstetric violence movement, which arose in the early 2000s, helped to make birth trauma visible, breaking women's isolation, putting words to their experiences, and understanding the multiple social forces influencing their experience (Boston Women's Health Book Collective & Norsigian, 2011; Chadwick, 2021). The obstetric violence movement is a human rights-based movement that seeks to build cultures of respectful maternity care. It began in Latin and Central America and has spurred global interest in recognizing the dehumanization that can occur as women give birth (Chadwick, 2021; Freedman et al., 2018; World Health Organization (WHO), 2015). As part of this movement, "obstetric violence" was introduced as a legal term in Venezuela to criminalize the abuse and mistreatment of women during childbirth and to recognize it as a form of gender-based violence (D'Gregorio, 2010). The movement has continued to gain momentum globally and several countries have moved to name obstetric violence as an offence in their criminal codes (Chadwick, 2021). The movement has since expanded to recognize how obstetric violence disproportionately affects racialized communities and those with lower socioeconomic status (Chadwick, 2021; van de Waal, Mayra, Horn, & Chadwick, 2022).

The goal of the obstetric violence movement is to disrupt and resist the normalization of oppression and violence during the reproductive period (Chadwick, 2021; van de Waal, Mayra, Horn, & Chadwick, 2022). The obstetric violence movement works to politicize the personal, it gives voice to the mother's experience as important and valid, as well as encouraging outrage at the violation of human rights, and it works to mobilize change. In naming obstetric violence, the movement seeks to help mothers name their experiences and recognize that the problems they experience are influenced by larger social discourses that shape women and their families as well as health care providers' understandings and responses to birth.

The obstetric violence literature points to how a medicalized birth often places the mother as an object rather than the subject of her birth experience (Chadwick, 2021; Cohen Shabot & Korem, 2018; Sadler et al., 2016). The objectification of the mother's body in a medicalized birth renders her invisible, denying her subjective experiences and dehumanizing the birthing process. Obstetric violence can be found in both the overuse of medical technology, such as non-consensual procedures or procedures not medically indicated (for example, the overuse of episiotomies or cesarean sections) and can also be found in the underuse of medical technology where technologies are not available or even withheld (Sadler et al., 2016; Cohen Shabot & Korem, 2018; Shaw, 2013). Even in middle- and high-income countries, where there is greater access to medical technologies, obstetric violence exists in the disparities in access to care and the use of medical technologies between privileged White women and women who are marginalized, such as minorities and those living in poverty, who often experience the underuse of medical technology that might be beneficial (Cohen Shabot, 2021; Cohen Shabot & Korem, 2018; van de Waal, Mayra, Horn, & Chadwick, 2022). This disparity in access to care for marginalized communities is an important issue that requires further attention and research, however it is beyond the scope of this current paper.

When mothers enter into a medicalized birth setting, an expert posture adopted by many medical staff can prevent or interfere with the possibility of working collaboratively with women. Medical professionals are assumed to have the knowledge and power, and the birthing mother is a passive subject to the experience, she often expects to follow the instructions and guidance given by staff in the interest of the safety of both her and her unborn child (Chadwick, 2021; Freedman et al., 2018). During birth, a mother's experiences are often diminished or reduced when she is viewed primarily as a vessel to bring forth the baby, rather than as a human with feelings, rights and intentions (Chadwick, 2021). Due to these cultural norms, the mother may not even be aware that violence during birth is occurring, she may accept certain behaviours during birth as just an unfortunate part of labor and delivery (Freedman et al., 2018; Cohen Shabot, 2021). If women identify misuse of power in the birthing process, such cultural and professional norms contribute to shaming women for voicing their concerns about how they are being treated. Should a mother question her experience during the birth she can be "easily made to feel ashamed of wanting to be respected and cared for as subjects, rather than caring exclusively for the baby's well-being as a good altruistic mother supposedly should" (Cohen Shabot & Korem 2018, p. 2).

## Collaboration with Women

The obstetric violence movement has challenged the unquestioned authority of medical health care workers and the neglect of women's voices. At the same time, within a North American context, many advocate that the solution is to emphasize the importance of women having more power and control over their labor and move away from medicalized birth entirely in favour of midwifery (Shaw, 2013; van der Waal, Mayra, Horn, & Chadwick, 2022). We suggest that the obstetric violence movement's desire to empower women does not have to involve totalizing medicalized birth as unhelpful. For those women who determine they want and need medical health care, the movement needs to empower them to be able to trust medical health care workers who can work collaboratively with them. In situations where women require medical intervention, women need to be able to trust the expertise of the medical professionals. For women who have experienced trauma through abuses of authority in the past, trusting professionals in such a vulnerable setting can be very challenging.

While pregnant, Laura was influenced by the feminist critiques of routine overuse of medical interventions and the dehumanization many women feel in hospital-based obstetrician-attended births and so opted for a home birth under the care of a midwife and a doula. (A doula is a birth professional offering non-medical, emotional, physical and informational support during the perinatal period (see DONA, n.d.) Sudden medical complications required her to be hospitalized and she experienced a series of cascading interventions, resulting in a cesarean section and lengthy hospital stay. Lack of communication and disagreements between medical staff led to Laura feeling increasingly dehumanized, invisible and unsafe. This impacted her ability to trust in the competence of her care providers (medical specialists and midwives) and increased her trauma symptoms for many months after the birth – symptoms that resurfaced in a subsequent pregnancy. She wishes that medical providers would understand and integrate some of the critiques the obstetric violence movement has of their profession, particularly attempting to understand the experience and meaning patients are making, in the hope that women can be cared for collaboratively should they need medical intervention.

Some concepts within the obstetric movement make developing a collaborative model between women and health care professionals difficult. Some authors highlight that defining medical interventions as "violent" infers medical providers are cast as "the abusers" and the birthing women are "the victims" (Sadler et al., 2016; Chadwick, 2021). As this may be how some women experience the situation, concerned obstetric staff need to listen to the ongoing social critiques and those offered by the obstetric violence movement. The way practitioners use their power impacts birthing women. The misuse of power often includes a lack of awareness or acknowledgment of their use of power and control and its impact, which can be true for all types of care providers including medical doctors, nurses and midwives. While in many cases care providers are not intentionally being violent toward birthing women, it still has a traumatic impact. It has been argued that they are caught up in the system "often functioning as an unconscious perpetrator of an existing violent structure" (Cohen Shabot, 2016, p. 9). Of course, even if the effects of interventions are unintentional, these negative effects still need to be mitigated.

The authors also noted that they have encountered instances where even care providers who were committed to empowering women seemed hesitant to provide specific guidance or expertise. Frequently, when advice on how to proceed was sought, care providers responded with phrases like "it is your choice". These responses left the authors with the impression that the care providers were being irresponsible. It appeared that they were misguided in their attempts at empowerment or were possibly reluctant to share their expertise due to concerns about the potential liability if their advice turned out to be incorrect. It seemed that the care providers were hesitant to fully acknowledge and accept the responsibility that came with their influence and power over the birthing process.

Rather than simply relying on the knowledge of women or care providers, collaborative trauma-based interventions need to draw on both. If the relationship is collaborative, women may trust the knowledge of the doctors, midwives and nurses that attend to them during childbirth while still feeling confident to ask questions and make requests rather than collapse and submit. Care providers will also feel confident to give their opinion and make decisions based on their expertise by not abdicating responsibility for all decision making in the hope that women will feel empowered. Olza et al. (2018) showed that women need to feel confident and comfortable when they think they should hand over power and control; and they need to trust in the competence of a care provider with whom they have established a collaborative relationship. At the same time, medical professionals should not exclude women's input in the birth process. Women have important knowledge about what they are comfortable with and can provide information on what they are experiencing that may be critical to positive outcomes.

Some obstetric violence literature simultaneously encourages women to be more involved in the decision-making process during birth while also acknowledging that even when care providers engage mothers in the decision-making process, women may not have the knowledge or expertise in obstetrics to know the correct course of action (Sadler et al., 2016). A care provider (including medical doctors, obstetricians, nurses and midwives) who is committed to a collaborative approach will, however, do their best to provide fully informed care that carefully explains various options, preserves the dignity of the patient and engenders trust. The role of doulas and other support people like partners, family and friends, can also help to support and advocate for the woman in labor. When care providers work collaboratively and are able to recognize the impact of the subjective experience of the mother and attend to her need for respect and communication, as well as manage safety effectively, mothers can feel like an active rather than a passive participant in the experience (Beck, 2015; Sadler et al., 2016). This extends not only to the care providers present in the labor and delivery room, but also to those who help in the postpartum period, including mental health professionals.

## Conclusion

This chapter has sought to make visible how birth trauma can occur or be exacerbated by how a woman is treated throughout pregnancy, birth and the postpartum period. Women often experience birth as traumatic when they are made to feel powerless, out of control, disrespected or degraded during the birth process. Members of the obstetric violence movement have dedicated substantial efforts to shed light on the harmful interventions associated with the medical approach. However, it is important to note that many within this movement have not thoroughly examined their own potential involvement in these practices.

At the same time, obstetric violence and the social silencing and shaming of women who choose to speak out about their traumatic birth experiences contributes to and exacerbates the negative effects of birth trauma. Further, along with addressing the discursive context that contributes to the development of birth trauma, there is a need for practitioners to develop and offer training in trauma-based care, which emphasizes building collaborative relationships with women to both prevent and heal from birth trauma.

## Acknowledgments

We acknowledge the valuable feedback and mentorship we have received on this chapter from Tod Augusta-Scott, Catrina Brown, Brittany Thaxter and Allison Wood

## Note

1 We recognize the need for research, publication, therapy and advocacy for the perinatal experiences of transgender and non-binary folk. While supporting those individuals is within the scope of our clinical practice, this chapter will refer exclusively to "women" as the subject of birth trauma. There are two reasons for this. First, there is a general paucity of research and publications on birth trauma in general, and what does exist has focused only on women. Second, as cisgendered females, this language most closely reflects our respective lived experiences of birth traumas.

## References

Alcorn, K.L., O'Donovan, A., Patrick, J.C., Creedy, D., & Devilly, G.J. (2010). A prospective longitudinal study of the prevalence of post-traumatic stress disorder resulting from childbirth events. *Psychological Medicine*, 40, 1849–1859. doi:10.1017/S0033291709992224.

American Psychiatric Association. (2022). Posttraumatic stress disorder. *Diagnostic and Statistical Manual of Mental Disorders* (5th ed., Text Revision). American Psychiatric Association Publishing.

Andersen, L.B., Melvaer, L.B., Videbech, P., Lamont, R.F., & Joergensen, J.S. (2012). Risk factors for developing post-traumatic stress disorder following childbirth: A systematic review. *Acta Obstetricia et Gynecologica Scandinavica*, 91(11), 1261–1272. https://doi.org/10.1111/j.1600-0412.2012.01476.x.

Ayers, S., Bond, R., Bertullies, S., & Wijma, K. (2016). The aetiology of post-traumatic stress following childbirth. *Psychological Medicine*, 46(6), 1121–2234. doi:10.1017/S0033291715002706.

Ayers, S., Joseph, S., McKenzie-McHarg, K., Slade, P., & Wijma, K. (2008). Post-traumatic stress disorder following childbirth: Current issues and recommendations for future research. *Journal of Psychosomatic Obstetrics & Gynecology*, 29(4), 240–250. https://doi.org/10.1080/01674820802034631.

Beck, C.T. (2004a). Birth trauma: In the eye of the beholder. *Nursing Research*, 53(1), 28–35. https://doi.org/10.1097/00006199-200401000-00005.

Beck, C.T. (2004b). Post-traumatic stress disorder due to childbirth: The aftermath. *Nursing Research*, 53(4), 216–224. https://doi.org/10.1097/00006199-200407000-00004.

Beck, C.T. (2011). A metaethnography of traumatic childbirth and its aftermath: Amplifying causal looping. *Qualitative Health Research*, 21(3), 301–311. https://doi.org/10.1177/1049732310390698.

Beck, C.T. (2015). Middle range theory of traumatic childbirth: The ever-widening ripple effect. *Global Qualitative Nursing Research*, 2, 1–13. https://doi.org/10.1177/2333393615575313.

Bohren, M.A., Vogel, J.P., Hunter, E.C., Lutsiv, O., Makh, S.K., Souza, J.P., Aguiar, C., Coneglian, F.S., Diniz, A.L.A., Tunçalp, O., Javadi, D., Oladapo, O.T., Khosla, R., Hindin, M.J., & Gülmezoglu, A.M. (2015). The mistreatment of women during childbirth in health facilities globally: A mixed-methods systematic review. *PLoS Medicine*, 12(6) . doi:10.1371/journal.pmed.1001847.

Boston Women's Health Book Collective, & Norsigian, J. (2011). *Our bodies, ourselves*. Simon & Schuster.

Chadwick, R. (2014). Bodies talk: On the challenges of hearing childbirth counter-stories. In M. LaFrance & S. McKenzie-Mohr (Eds.), *Women voicing resistance. Discursive and narrative explorations* (pp. 44–63). Routledge.

Chadwick, R. (2021). Breaking the frame: Obstetric violence and epistemic rupture. *Agenda*, 35(3), 104–115. doi:10.1080/10130950.2021.1958554.

Chan, S.J., Ein-Dor, T., Mayopoulos, P.A., Mesa, M.M., Sunda, R.M., McCarthy, B.F., Kaimal, A.J., & Dekel, S. (2020). Risk factors for developing posttraumatic stress disorder following childbirth. *Psychiatry Research*, 290. https://doi.org/10.1016/j.psychres.2020.113090.

Chin, K., Wendt, A., Bennett, I.M., & Bhat, A. (2022). Suicide and maternal mortality. *Current Psychiatry Report*, 24, 239–275. https://doi.org/10.1007/s11920-022-01334-3.

Cohen Shabot, S. (2016). Making loud bodies "feminine": A feminist-phenomenological analysis of obstetric violence. *Human Studies*, 39(2), 231–247. doi:10.1007/s10746-015-9369-x.

Cohen Shabot, S. (2020). We birth with others: Towards a Beauvoirian understanding of obstetric violence. *European Journal of Women's Studies*, 28(2), 1–16. doi:10.1177/1350506820919474.

Cohen Shabot, S. (2021). Why "normal" feels so bad: Violence and vaginal examinations during labour – A (feminist) phenomenology. *Feminist Theory*, 22(3), 443–463. doi:10.1177/1464700120920764

Cohen Shabot, S., & Korem, K. (2018). Domesticating bodies: The role of shame in obstetric violence. *Hypatia*, 33(3), 384–401. doi:10.1111/hypa.12428.

Dekel, S., Erin-Dor, T., Dishy, G.A., & Mayopoulos, P.A. (2020). Beyond postpartum depression: Posttraumatic stress-depressive response following childbirth. *Archives of Women's Mental Health*, 23(4), 557–564. doi:10.1007/s00737-019-01006-x.

Dekel, S., Thiel, F., Dishy, G., & Ashenfarb, A.L. (2019). Is childbirth-induced PTSD associated with low maternal attachment? *Archives of Women's Mental Health*, 22(1), 119–122. https://doi.org/10.1007/s00737-018-0853-y.

D'Gregorio, P. (2010). Obstetric violence: A new legal term introduced in Venezuela. *International Journal of Gynecology and Obstetrics*, 111, 201–202. doi:10.1016/j.ijgo.2010.09.002.

Diamond, R.M., & Colaianni, A. (2022). The impact of perinatal healthcare changes on birth trauma during COVID-19. *Women and Birth*, 35, 503–510. https://doi.org/10.1016/j.wombi.2021.12.003

DONA (International. (n.d.). https://www.dona.org/what-is-a-doula-2/.

Dreifus, C. (1978). (Ed.). *Seizing our bodies. The politics of women's health*. Vintage Books.

Ehrenreich, B., & English, D. (1978). *For her own good. 150 years of the experts' advice to women*. Anchor Books.

Freedman, L.P., Kujawski, S.A., Mbuyita, S., Kuwawenaruwa, A., Kruk, M.E., & Mbaruku, G. (2018). Eye of the beholder? Observation versus self-report in the measurement of disrespect and abuse during facility-based childbirth. *Reproductive Health Matters*, 26(53), 107–122. doi: 10.1080/09688080.2018.1502024.

Garthus-Niegel, S., von Soest, T., Vollrath, M.E., & Eberhard-Gran, M. (2013). The impact of subjective birth experiences on post-traumatic stress symptoms: A longitudinal study. *Archives of Women's Mental Health*, 16(1), 1–10. doi:10.1007/s00737-012-0301-3.

Gorham, D. (1984). Birth and history. *Histoire Sociale – Social History*, XVII(34), 383–394. Retrieved from https://hssh.journals.yorku.ca/index.php/hssh/article/download/38459/34875/45685.

Kendall-Tackett, K. (2014). Childbirth-related posttraumatic stress disorder: Symptoms and impact on breastfeeding. *Clinical Lactation*, 5(2), 56–61.

Kendall-Tackett, K., & Beck, C.T. (2022). Secondary traumatic stress and moral injury in maternity care providers: A narrative and exploratory review. *Frontiers in Global Women's Health*, 3, 3–13. doi:10.3389/fgwh.2022.835811.

Olde, E., van der Hart, O., Kleber, R., & van Son, M. (2006). Posttraumatic stress following childbirth: A review. *Clinical Psychology Review*, 26(1), 1–16. DOI:10.1016/j.cpr.2005.07.002.

Olza, I., Leahy-Warren, P., Benyamini, Y., Kazmierczak, M., Karlsdottir, S.I., Spyridou, A., Crespo-Mirasol, E., Takács, L., Hall, P.J., Murphy, M., Jonsdottir, S.S., Downe, S., & Nieuwenhuijze, M.J. (2018). Women's psychological experiences of physiological childbirth: A meta-synthesis. *British Medical Journal*, 8(10), 1–11. https://doi.org/10.1136/bmjopen-2017-020347.

Rich, A. (1977). The theft of childbirth. *Seizing our bodies: The politics of women's health* (pp. 146–163). Vintage Books.

Rich, A. (2004). *Of woman born: Motherhood as experience and institution.* Virago Press.

Sadler, M., Santos, M.J., Ruiz-Berdún, D., Rojas, G.L., Skoko, E., Gillen, P., & Clausen, J.A. (2016). Moving beyond disrespect and abuse: Addressing the structural dimensions of obstetric violence. *Reproductive Health Matters*, 24(47), 47–55. https://doi.org/10.1016/j.rhm.2016.04.002.

Shaw, J.C.A. (2013). The medicalization of birth and midwifery as resistance. *Health Care for Women International*, 34(6), 522–536. doi:10.1080/07399332.2012.736569.

Simkin, P., & Klaus, P. (2017). *When survivors give birth: Understanding and healing the effects of early sexual abuse on childbearing women* (9th ed.). Classic Day Publishing.

Slade, P., Balling, K., Sheen, K., Goodfellow, L., Rymer, J., Spiby, H., & Weeks, A. (2020). Work-related post-traumatic stress symptoms in obstetricians and gynecologists: Findings from INDIGO, a mixed methods study with a cross-sectional survey and in-depth interviews. *BJOG: An International Journal of Obstetrics and Gynecology*, 127(5), 600–608. https://doi.org/10.1111/1471-0528.16076.

Thomas, K. (2020). *Birth trauma: A guide for you, your friends and family to coping with post-traumatic stress disorder following birth* (2nd ed.). Nell James Publishers.

Ussher, J. (1997). *Body talk. The material and discursive regulation of sexuality, madness and reproduction.* Routledge.

van der Waal, R., Mayra, K., Horn, A., & Chadwick, R. (2022). Obstetric violence: An intersectional refraction through abolition feminism. *Feminist Anthropology*, 1–24. https://doi.org/10.1002/fea2.12097.

World Health Organization (WHO). (2015). The prevention and elimination of disrespect and abuse during facility-based childbirth. WHO statement. Retrieved from https://apps.who.int/iris/bitstream/handle/10665/134588/WHO_RHR_14.23_eng.pdf%3Bjsessionid=CCAC68126815369075482A729017F62E?sequence=1.

Yildiz, P.D., Ayers, S., & Phillips, L. (2017). The prevalence of posttraumatic stress disorder in pregnancy and after birth: A systematic review and meta-analysis. *Journal of Affective Disorders*, 208, 634–645. https://doi.org/10.1016/j.jad.2016.10.009.

# 9

# THE TRAUMA OF YOUTH HOMELESSNESS

## Youth on the Street

*Jeff Karabanow, Andrea Titterness, Jean Hughes, Haorui Wu and Samantha Good*

## Introduction

Homelessness is a complex social problem, especially when we acknowledge the trauma associated with homelessness and youth. Homeless populations often suffer from deep and frequently unaddressed traumatic life experiences that intersect with systemic structural inequities (Wu & Karabanow, 2020) – including the influence of gender, age, sexual orientation, race and ethnicity – that lead to homelessness and also make it difficult to exit the street. In this chapter, we will focus on the role that trauma plays in propelling youth into homelessness and how young people experiencing street life continue to experience trauma as part of their lived experiences which together make it difficult to be able to exit the street.

> I've been on and off [the street], like, I've been in and out of institutions, group homes, sugar daddies, the streets, garbage dumpsters, forty below nights ... (Noam, 22, Toronto).
>
> *(Karabanow, 2004a, p. 40)*

According to many of street youth who took part in Canadian studies (Karabanow, 2004a, 2004b, 2008, 2010; Karabanow et al., 2007; Karabanow, Kidd, Frederick, & Hughes, 2018), life on the street was viewed as a *safer* environment than the one they had come from, indicating that living on the streets can be perceived as a better option than continuing to experience trauma at home:

DOI: 10.4324/9781003379591-10

I always thought that being on the street was at least better … less dangerous than staying with my dad. I wasn't beat up every day on the street … (Chris, 18, Montreal).

*(Karabanow, 2006, p. 54)*

That was the whole reason I would never try to live back home: in the last day/ night that I slept there, my dad grabbed me by my throat and put me up against the wall 'cause I was thinking about leaving. So that was his answer 'cause my dad's very short tempered and high fused. … I would rather stay on the street than move back there (Lisa, age 24, Halifax).

*(Karabanow, 2008, p. 775)*

… I didn't want to live with my dad. He was an asshole, he used to beat me around and shit … (Don, 17, Halifax).

*(Karabanow, 2006, p. 54)*

However, the trauma experienced at home will continue to be manifested in, and to shape, the lives of homeless youth. We will begin by talking about youth's experiences of trauma preceding street life, followed by a discussion of the trauma they commonly experience while living on the streets. Youth participants' voices from Karabanow's research are peppered throughout the discussion. Despite the efforts youth often make to escape trauma and violence and to cope and survive outside their families, the subsequent trauma of living on the street often compounds existing trauma and further retraumatizes them. Although, formal child and youth welfare solutions to this dilemma are failing to provide many youth with the care and support they need (Bender, Yang, Ferguson, & Thompson, 2015; Karabanow 2004a; Zlotnick, 2009), we will end with a brief discussion of what appears to help youth exit street life and the need for clear future directions in addressing these problems.

## Trauma Preceding Street Life

Trauma refers to an enduring emotional response to a distressing event and is a risk factor and precursor to homelessness in both youth and adult populations (McManus & Thompson, 2008). Although homeless youth are not a homogenous group, consistently high rates of abuse and neglect strongly suggest that childhood trauma – commonly known as adverse childhood experiences (Centers for Disease Control and Prevention, 2013) – is at least one mechanism contributing to early homelessness (Davies & Allen, 2017), and youth who end up on the street often have shared experiences as survivors of trauma (ibid.; Karabanow, 2008; Karabanow et al., 2007; McManus & Thompson, 2008). Family poverty and/ or disfunction, sexual, physical and/or emotional abuse in the home, and negative child welfare involvement are the three most common influences on street life (Karabanow, 2004b, 2006, 2008; Karabanow et al., 2007; Karabanow, Kidd, Frederick, & Hughes, 2018).

According to van der Kolk (2014), "People's income, family structure, housing, employment, and educational opportunities affect not only their risk of developing traumatic stress but also their access to effective help to address it" (p. 350). Economic instability in the family of origin can contribute to homelessness in youths, which can manifest as a lack of access to affordable housing (Damron, 2015). As one youth noted: "'I grew up in a really, really rough neighborhood ... it's the five buildings that you can basically call a "crack lot." There was a lot of drugs, a lot of alcohol, a lot of violence' (Chris, 18, Montreal)" (Karabanow, 2004a, p. 29). Such precarious housing situations can then disrupt an individual's access to, and utilization of, education (Kull, Morton, Patel, Curry, & Carreon, 2019; Toolis & Hammack, 2015), including high rates of absenteeism, poor grades, difficulty with peers and dropping out (Jones, Bowen, & Ball, 2018). The negative downstream effects of disrupted education can persist into adulthood (Baker-Collins, 2013), attesting to the importance of programs and initiatives that advocate for stable schooling for youth experiencing homelessness (Julianelle, 2008), including adopting a trauma- and violence-informed approach to education (Jones, Bowen, & Ball, 2018). While family poverty can promote homelessness in youth, homelessness often cannot be isolated from an abusive and traumatic home environment, something that will be discussed below.

Childhood physical and sexual abuse is a common experience among unhoused youth (Green et al., 2012). A study of 329 homeless youth found that 48% reported some form of prior intra-familial abuse (Ryan, Kilmer, Cauce, Watanabe, & Hoyt, 2000), including situations in which a caregiver cannot intervene when a youth is being abused because the caregiver is afraid or has also recently been abused (Tyler, 2006). Unhoused youth have often experienced two or more forms of childhood abuse (Bender, Brown, S.M., Thompson, Ferguson, & Langenderfer, 2015).

While several studies did not distinguish between males and females, several studies indicate that unhoused female youth are more likely than males to have experienced sexual abuse prior to living on the streets (Cauce et al., 2000; Gwadz, Nish, Leonard, & Strauss, 2007; Rew, Taylor-Seehafer, & Fitzgerald, 2001), and are more likely than males to experience sexual abuse while living on the streets (Tyler, Hoyt, & Whitbeck, 2000). There are also gender disparities in relation to experiencing maltreatment, with more males experiencing physical neglect and physical violence than females, but emotional abuse and sexual abuse are more prevalent in females (Coates & McKenzie-Mohr, 2011; Gwadz, Nish, Leonard, & Strauss, 2007).

Unhoused youth report greater rates of abuse and/or maltreatment than stably housed youth (Wolfe, Toro, & McCaskill, 1999) and are more likely to experience more traumatic events prior to, and after entering, life on the streets (Coates & McKenzie-Mohr, 2011). These findings indicate that homeless youth are carrying a burden of traumatic events, which can be compounded by living on the streets.

While living on the streets is understandably dangerous, it is important that we understand how living at home is often experienced as emotionally, physically and/or sexually dangerous, as is subsequent foster care for many (Karabanow, 2004a). Contact with family can mitigate some of the effects of sexual violence (Kidd et al., 2021), but with homeless youth reporting greater levels of abuse and/ or maltreatment in their family of origin compared to stably housed youth (Wolfe, Toro, & McCaskill, 1999), home might not be the safest option. As one Toronto youth noted: "'If home was good and if it was safe, I'd be back there in a minute …' (George, 18)" (Karabanow, 2006, p. 54).

Many youth live in foster homes prior to entering life on the streets and report higher rates of physical and sexual violence after becoming homeless compared to homeless youth who did not live in foster care (Bender, Yang, Ferguson, & Thompson, 2015). Further, homeless youth with a history of foster care also spent more months living on the streets than homeless youth without a history of foster care, were less likely to have a high school diploma or General Education Diploma (GED), had higher rates of depression, post-traumatic stress disorder (PTSD) and substance-use disorder than non-foster-care youth (ibid.). While multifactorial in nature, factors associated with foster care that might contribute to elevated rates of homelessness for youth include aging out of the system without proper support in place and the lack of housing and educational stability during their time in foster care (Kurzawski, 2021; Zlotnick, 2009).

Interestingly, homeless youth attribute the age at which they exited welfare care to be the greatest predictor of homelessness, along with the lack of an important personal relationship (Serge et al., 2002). Overall, the child welfare system, though well-intentioned, may inadvertently reinforce a traumatic and chaotic upbringing, thus contributing to a greater likelihood of youth homeless-ness and further traumatization. As one Halifax 19-year-old noted: "'… it was hard moving from one [foster] family to another family to another family … I have no kind of relation, nothing to them … it was hard' (Trevor)" (Karabanow, 2004a, p. 33).

## Trauma on the Streets: Homelessness as Trauma

There is no doubt that past experiences of trauma can play a role in whether someone ends up homeless; however, homelessness is not only a consequence of trauma, but is a form of psychological, emotional and social trauma itself (Goodman Saxe, & Harvey, 1991). Indeed, high rates of victimization have been found among homeless young people both before (92 percent) and after (75 per-cent) leaving home (Wright, Milligan, Bender, & DePrince, 2022). It is often an immeasurable struggle for young people as they attempt to survive on the streets – seeking out shelter, food, clothing, money and safe environments (Karabanow, 2004a). Homelessness comes with a greater risk of physical violence, alongside severely limited resources, and the use of coping strategies for survival such as substance use, risky sexual behaviour and sex work (Coates & McKenzie-Mohr, 2011; Karabanow, Kidd, Frederick, & Hughes, 2018). Youth interviewed in Halifax have recounted many forms of hardships they face on the street:

> You hardly get any sleep when you are sleeping on the streets, cause the pavement was hard, it was cold out, there was traffic noise ... the police bother you all the time (Luke, 16).
>
> *(Karabanow, 2006, p. 67)*

> I've had people just go off on rants, like "fuck you, you stupid worthless piece of shit, blah, blah, blah, get a fucking job, why don't you just go fucking die," and like, try to spit on me. I've been kicked and stuff ... I've had people throw stuff at me out of cars and shit. Like just, people get pissed off, man (Fatima, 19).
>
> *(Karabanow, Hughes, Ticknor, & Kidd, 2010, p. 50)*

> I am always stressed and depressed, that what it means to be on the street ... street kids get into drugs to deal with their lives ... I get high to forget that I really don't have anything to look forward to ... (Nina, 20).
>
> *(Karabanow et al., 2007, p. 6)*

> Some nights you're stuck sleeping on the sidewalk almost freezing to death you know? That really sucks. When you're on the street there are a lot of people trying to get you doing drugs and stuff and that's no good. And, uh, a lot of times the cops are – right –prejudiced against street people, so I get beat up by the cops here and there (Wesley, 16).
>
> *(Ibid., p. 10)*

> I've sat on the streets and bawled my eyes out panhandling. [Be]cause you get to the point where you don't want to be there and you're so hungry ... and people walk by and no one gives you anything except dirty looks and mean comments ... (Benjamin, 17).
>
> *(Karabanow, Hughes, Ticknor, & Kidd, 2010, p. 52)*

These daily struggles to cope, aligned with feeling vulnerable, marginalized, devalued and alienated, foster a sense of disempowerment, hopelessness and injustice, combined with unfulfilled basic needs (Karabanow, 2004a; Karabanow et al., 2007). Street communities can be surrogate families for many young people:

> ... We all look out for each other. Like if someone's giving us a hard time we stick up for each other and it's like the main community outside of being homeless ... like we have a community within the homeless community who we look

out for each other and we talk to each other and if we need a place to stay then there may be a building that has a heater there that's warm and we look out for each other when a new person comes out on the street and we try to help them out as much as we can ... (Frank, 21, Halifax).

*(Karabanow, 2006, p. 65)*

While street communities can be supportive and caring settings, there is also much evidence that "street tribes" can also be exploitative, violent and dehumanizing (Karabanow, 2006). Along with threats to their own safety, people who are homeless may be exposed to violence at a higher rate, such as being a witness to a mugging or stabbing (Fitzpatrick, La Gory, & Ritchey, 2003). Additionally, homeless women and Two-Spirit, Lesbian, Gay, Bisexual, Transgender, Queer, Intersex, and Asexual (2SLGBTQIA+) populations, in particular, face various forms of trauma (sexual, physical and emotional) both before and during life on the street (Beijer, Scheffel Birath, DeMartinis, & af Klinteberg, 2018; Hamilton, Poza, & Washington, 2011).

I used to live in a small rural community ... they're very closed minded, homophobic, racist people and ... the community long with my family were not very supportive [when I came out as gay] ... and my father kicked me out and I had nowhere to go (Mike 16, Toronto).

*(Karabanow, 2004a, p. 32)*

Indeed, a Canadian national survey found young women, 2SLGBTQIA+, and Indigenous youth experienced heightened adversity (Gaetz, O'Grady, Kidd, & Schwan, 2016). The authors also highlighted the necessity of considering the impact of exposure to violence when assessing the risk and distress of these populations. In so many ways, being homeless involves living one's private world (e.g., the need to go to the bathroom or to sleep) within public spaces) a very alienating, traumatic and overwhelming experience (Karabanow, 2006). As noted by one of Karabanow's Canadian youth study participants:

When you do that [public work], there's no privacy in your life at all, you know. Like people will, like I used to be followed to see where I was going after I would leave a corner, to see what I was spending my money on and stuff. And like, it's that sort of like violation ... It's like it's none of your business and there's just no privacy on the street and you know, like yeah, I always used to think like man, it's bad that I'm standing out here crying but it's like, if I had an apartment or a room, I would go there and cry ... So it's like, there's nothing, just yeah ... I cried because I just had no shelter and privacy or nothing (Lisa 17, Halifax).

*(Karabanow 2006, p. 58)*

In all, trauma can be both the cause and effect of homelessness, possibly perpetuating a negative cycle that contributes to individuals remaining homeless. Street youth who were interviewed often referred to mental health issues that began before their life on the street but are further exacerbated by the experience of homelessness. One Halifax youth stated: "I've had a lot of emotional problems growing up, and being on the street just seems to make them worse. I don't really ever feel happy ... I'm always worried about things ... like where will I be in two days? Where will I wake up tomorrow, stuff like that?" (Karabanow et al., 2007, p. 13).

Homelessness must also be understood as a housing, income, gendered and racial problem, threatening the just foundation of our society (Karabanow, Bozcam, Hughes, & Wu, 2021). As countries face overwhelming housing market challenges, coupled with inadequate income support mechanisms and increased acknowledgment of historical and current racial discriminatory system structures, and set alongside gender-based violence (Wu, Karabanow, & Hoddinott, 2022), we are witnessing higher numbers of people living in shelters, on the street, in park encampments and/or surviving in precariously housed situations (such as "couch surfing").

Tight housing markets (e.g., high levels of rent and low rental housing vacancy rates) have had a devastating effect on the homelessness crisis, leading many to argue that homelessness is a direct result of economic, structural and systematic inequities (Andermann et al., 2021; Olivet, Dones, & Richard, 2019; Olivet et al., 2021). Gender-based violence also contributes to homelessness, which disproportionately affects more women than men (Andermann et al., 2021). Additionally, the heterogenous nature of the homeless population suggests that interventions need to be tailored to specific groups of homeless individuals (e.g., homeless women or homeless youth) (ibid.), adding to not only the complexity of the etiology of homelessness, but also to the complexity of its solution (Karabanow, Wu, Doll, Leviten-Reid, & Hughes, 2023).

Young people on the street tend to live in very excluded domains, due to their age, income, vulnerabilities, lack of education and employment, difficulty in navigating systems (e.g., housing and income assistance and other social services) and lack of social, human and material capital (Karabanow, 2008). According to Noble (2012), unemployment rates among homeless youth in Canada were as high as 73 percent ten years ago. Factors that contribute to unemployment more recently include mental health, housing stability and substance use (Slesnick, Zhang, & Yilmazer, 2018). In a mixed-methods study on employment and homelessness, it was found that trauma experienced as a result of living on the streets impaired employment-seeking and employment-sustaining, perhaps out of fear of discrimination, poor coping with mental health, and/or substance-abuse issues (Ferguson, Bender, Thompson, Maccio, & Pollio, 2012).

Among homeless youth, initial sources of income reflect doing what they can to survive. These include activities such as prostitution, stealing, or selling personal items, while less desperate endeavours such as government assistance are more predominant over time (Slesnick, Zhang, & Yilmazer, 2018). Homeless youth who engage in prostitution are at increased risk of developing health complications and mental health issues (Srivastava et al., 2019; Yates, MacKenzie, Pennbridge, & Swofford 1991). Juvenile entry into prostitution is linked to sexual and emotional abuse experienced prior to entering life on the streets (Stoltz et al., 2007) and is also associated with ongoing high levels of trauma (Roe-Sepowitz et al., 2012). At the same time, some homeless youth have been found to engage in protective factors while engaged in survival sex (Greenfield, Alessi, Manning, Dato, & Dank, 2020). Taken together, these studies suggest that trauma experienced prior to life on the streets can influence the employment activities in which street youth engage, including employment that is potentially traumatizing, thus perpetuating the cycle of retraumatization.

Homelessness is also a racialized problem, with deep racial disparities in homelessness and its related systems (e.g., criminal legal, child welfare, education and health) particularly for Black and Indigenous people. Most racialized people experience homelessness at higher rates than White people, largely due to long-standing historical and structural racism, ongoing oppression and inequity (Olivet, Dones, & Richard, 2019; Olivet et al., 2021). In particular, youth who identify as female and as a racial minority and as a sexual minority (e.g., 2SLGBQIA+) are more likely to engage in couch-surfing rather than staying in a shelter (with unknown safety) (Petry, Hill, Milburn, & Rice, 2022). Furthermore, intergenerational trauma in Indigenous and Black communities (which have been gravely impacted by colonial practices that have destroyed communities, families, traditions, rituals and languages) have resulted unsurprisingly in deep levels of mental, emotional, physical and spiritual suffering (Menzies, 2006; Milburn et al., 2010). Therefore, youth homelessness needs to not only be seen through a trauma- and violence-informed lens, but also through one that takes into account gender-based differences in experience alongside those marginalized by race, sexual orientation and gender identity.

As previously noted, homelessness also increases the risk of further victimization and retraumatization. Within societies worldwide, people experiencing homelessness are often marginalized, isolated, stigmatized, blamed and discriminated against. Homeless youth are highly vulnerable to violence and victimization, and retraumatization becomes a distinct possibility. Almost all homeless youth have experienced at least one traumatic event since becoming homeless in addition to the ongoing traumatic nature of homelessness itself (Gwadz, Nish, Leonard, & Strauss, 2007). Youth who leave home environments to escape traumatic experiences may find that whilst one form of trauma (such as family violence and bullying) decreases, other forms of trauma may increase (Bender, Yang, Ferguson, & Thompson, 2015; Coates & McKenzie-Mohr, 2011). Coates and McKenzie-Mohr (2011) reported that, on average, street youth faced approximately 11 to 12 types of traumatic events, half of which would occur before and half of which would occur after becoming homeless. Female youth experienced increased levels of physical violence and consistent levels of sexual violence before and after becoming homeless, while male youth had a decreased incidence of sexual violence after entering street life, but physical violence remained consistent (Coates & McKenzie-Mohr, 2011). Again, these studies demonstrate that homeless youth are likely to have experienced trauma prior to becoming homeless and are likely to be retraumatized once they are homeless.

Homelessness poses dire consequences for physical, spiritual, psychological, emotional and social health and well-being. People experiencing homelessness are at increased risk of trauma, mental health challenges and substance-use problems (Fazel, Geddes, & Kushel, 2014; Karabanow et al., 2007). Severe mental health problems are associated with traumatic experiences and are prevalent in the long-term adult homeless population (Caton et al., 2005). Significant research has established a relationship between experiences of violence, abuse, trauma and mental health struggles; and, for some, entry to street life. A recent review shows that while mental health problems have been associated with an increased risk of becoming homeless, homelessness can directly produce, or exacerbate, the mental health struggles (Ridley, Rao, Schilbach, & Patel, 2020). The challenges of homelessness are also detrimental to physical health, with the life expectancy of people living in shelters being 8 to 13 years less than the general population (Hwang, Wilkins, Tjepkema, O'Campo, & Dunn, 2009). People may become caught in a cycle, whereby traumatic experiences lead to poor mental health and subsequent efforts using poor coping mechanisms (which can produce their own dangers, such as substance use and risky behaviors) that in turn may affect an individual's ability to achieve, or maintain, stable housing. Without timely and efficient interventions, such as supportive housing and mental health services, people are often left in dangerous circumstances with a higher risk of experiencing further traumatic events, triggering long-term, compounded, negative influences on their health and well-being. The significant stress of just surviving day-to-day living has an understandable impact on mental and physical health. This struggle is not about an individual's deficit but, arguably, the inhumane and unjust conditions that an individual is expected to deal with. The next section explores ways forward.

## A Way Forward: Intervening with Trauma and Homelessness

Clearly, the vast majority of people experiencing homelessness have faced traumatic events, such as being exposed to violence, experiencing losses, and often dealing with severed significant familial relationships. While some may argue that the deep interaction of trauma and homelessness suggests we will not be able to combat homelessness without first addressing the underlying traumas (Hopper, Bassuk, & Olivet, 2010), this position does not adequately acknowledge that the experience of *being without a home* itself is traumatic (as it involves a lack of stability, a loss of safety and identity, and the disconnection from one's community at large) (Karabanow, 2004a, 2008; Kidd, 2003). Importantly, unacceptable experiences of violence and trauma in childhood and youth intersecting with poverty, sexism, racism and homophobia were indeed very often the reason why youth entered street life to begin with. And while these intersecting layers need to be addressed, the immediate crisis response at the level of basic human needs with the assistance of government intervention must first prioritize the development and provision of safe housing and living conditions to remedy the immediate trauma associated with lack of safe and secure housing. Healing from trauma cannot begin without this.

Being unhoused means one cannot obtain the basic needs for survival – as such, sustainable, affordable and appropriate housing – a solution to which is a key foundation for stability and healing (Karabanow, 2004a; Karabanow, Kidd, Frederick, & Hughes, 2018; Kidd, 2003). Shelter systems continue to be the most common and predominant response to homelessness. However, they are band-aid emergency offerings and are not a long-term solution. Shelters can be violent, dangerous, crowded and crisis-filled environments, and they can be overwhelming and triggering for victims of trauma. These environments may be especially intimidating for people who are marginalized or vulnerable such as girls, women, and/or 2SLGBTQIA+ and individuals of different diversity (e.g., Indigenous, African) (Flock & Benjamin, 2019; Johnsen, Cloke, & May, 2005).

To address the factors associated with shelter systems, supportive housing initiatives are a promising response to homelessness. Supportive housing programs pair housing assistance with support services for people with physical, mental or developmental disabilities and/or substance-use issues (Rog et al., 2014). Supportive housing strives to meet people where they are, providing people with shelter as well as access to a variety of supports, treatments and services. However, homelessness is increasingly exacerbated by late capitalist neoliberal constrained fiscal policies and the virtual dissolution of the welfare state and social programming. System-wide infrastructure failures occurring at the municipal, state and federal government levels and whose catastrophic impacts on population health and the response to the COVID-19 pandemic are the consequence of the decades-long devolution of government and neglect of investment in public infrastructure, including public and social housing and a modern public health and mental health system (Allegrante & Sleet, 2021). We need to continue to advocate for more and better services for those on the street, especially as, since the pandemic, the myriad of both public and non-profit organizations are strained, overwhelmed, stressed and under-supported.

Secure housing alone, however, is not sufficient to repair trauma related to being homeless. The early life trauma people experienced initially that led them to living on the streets and developing mental health and substance-use problems needs to be addressed. Supports that provide empathic care and a sense of belonging in order to begin to reverse feelings of marginalization, disempowerment and hopelessness need to be embedded within living arrangements. Homeless people often exist within ruptured community bonds and limited healthy social support to cope with the impact of trauma. As such, we need to build "cultures of hope" (Karabanow, 2004a) that provide both basic needs and meaningful care. A social justice/anti-oppressive response that provides housing stability and a sense of belonging begins with a trauma- and violence-informed care foundation. Speaking eloquently about a particular anti-oppressive service, one young Montreal girl notes: "When I'm here, I feel like a human being; when I leave, I feel like a street kid" (Karabanow, 2004a, p. 1). When one is focused on daily protection and survival, it can be difficult to imagine the steps to building stability and community. Therefore, providing stable housing and promoting a sense of community are important ingredients to begin repairing and healing trauma (Karabanow, Kidd, Frederick, & Hughes, 2018).

Indeed the Government of Canada (2018) has acknowledged the critical importance of trauma and violence approaches (TVIA) (Ponic, Varcoe, & Smutylo, 2016), articulating four central integrated principles that emphasize the following goals: (1) Understand trauma and violence and their impacts on people's lives and behaviours; (2) Create emotionally and physically safe environments; (3) Foster opportunities for choice, collaboration and connection; (4) Provide a strengths-based and capacity-building approach to build client coping and resilience capacities (Wathen, Schmitt, & MacGregor. 2023, p. 262). These goals, however, will need to be followed up with clear action plans that are seen in government budgets designated for program development, training and evaluation in the complex area of trauma and violence work.

In addition to the procurement of stable, community-based, supportive housing, attention also needs to be paid to how the traditional conceptualization of trauma imposes unnecessary restrictions on prevention of trauma and healing. The medicalized construction of trauma and diagnoses (such as post-traumatic stress disorder) can be stigmatizing and deflect attention from the structural elements of trauma (Coates & McKenzie-Mohr, 2011). By trying to diagnose and treat people's coping mechanisms for homelessness (e.g., substance use, mental illness) we pathologize the individual and at the same time ignore the larger social inequalities at play. Coates and McKenzie-Mohr (2011) state:

> The study of trauma has been strongly influenced by the domains of psychiatry and psychology, and within these realms the concept has most often been individualized, medicalized, universalized and decontextualized. As long as the construction of trauma is understood merely as an individual phenomenon, attention is not paid to potential social and political roots of a problem, forms of oppression, and experiences of families and communities.
>
> *(pp. 85–86)*

By shifting the focus of trauma to incorporate how systemic factors contribute to the initial experience and maintenance of trauma, affected individuals will no longer be identified as agents to their situation, *but as individuals caught in unhealthy societal structures.* Social changes are required to minimize homelessness and assist individuals. This shift helps identify actionable steps that societies can take to repair and prevent trauma instead of placing the onus of change on the traumatized individual. Indeed, the research of Wenzel and colleagues (2019) examined the effects of permanent housing for people who were homeless and found that housing may offer respite from everyday discrimination, but the persistence of discrimination and particularly racism in society requires structural solutions addressing implicit bias and systemic inequities. In this way, the collective support that can be offered in diverse forms in the community setting that can be established to help homeless individuals who have experienced trauma to heal (Wenzel, Rhoades, LaMotte-Kerr, & Duan, 2019). In addition, Wathen, Schmitt, and MacGregor (2023) argue:

> given increased attention to structural issues, from racism to poverty, and their impact on every aspect of people's lives, it is increasingly obvious that we must not only implement interventions that approach TVIC [trauma- and violence-informed care] from a structural stance, but also that we develop more nuanced and rigorous ways to assess these efforts
>
> *(p. 273)*

Utilizing a trauma- and violence-informed approach to care when working with homeless individuals is a way in which the reconceptualization of trauma can promote more effective care. Trauma- and violence-informed care is ideally a comprehensive approach that acknowledges the impact of trauma and the specific context of trauma in an individual's life (Hopper, Bassuk, Olivet, 2010; Wathen, Schmitt, & MacGregor, 2023). Trauma- and violence-informed care needs to emphasize safety and security when addressing traumatic experiences, while avoiding blame and retraumatization Since victims of trauma often feel unsafe, and homelessness comes with a myriad of risks and dangers, working on building safety is a key aspect of trauma- and violence-informed care. "The greatest need of any traumatized individual is to feel safe, and this often requires attention to various practical dimensions" (Wilson, Friedman, & Lindy, 2001, p. 247). Clear roles and boundaries, mutual respect, awareness of triggers, privacy/confidentiality, and cultural and diversity competency are some of the ways to cultivate a safe environment (Hopper, Bassuk, Olivet, 2010). Additionally, taking a user-informed approach to the design and evaluation of the services provides those who utilize such services an opportunity to rebuild a sense of control and empowerment in their lives (Hopper, Bassuk, Olivet, 2010; Karabanow 2004a). As experiences of trauma and violence may differ by demographic variables (e.g., gender, sexual orientation and race), the overall social and cultural context of an individual's life should be integrated into trauma- and violence-informed service frameworks (Karabanow 2004a; McManus & Thompson, 2008).

There is very limited research on interventions such as dialectical behavior therapy, cognitive behavior therapy and solution-focused and strength/empowerment-based approaches with trauma among street youth (Karabanow & Clement, 2004; Kidd, 2003, 2004, 2006; McManus & Thompson, 2008). Further, most of these models tend to focus on the individual deficit and pathology with very little, if any, attention to the social context of an individual's life and the meanings those individuals make of their experiences. Therapeutic services that do exist tend to be associated with institutional settings such as hospitals and government services and promote a short-term, one-size-fits-all approach that aligns with the institution's fiscal policy of programming (Brown, C., 2021; Brown C., Johnstone, & Ross, 2021; Brown, C., Johnstone, Ross, & Doll, 2022). By themselves, such therapeutic services are not nearly adequate to address the complexity of trauma experiences often associated with homelessness. There are extensive waiting lists for most services and greater training and resources should be made available to staff. As for the homeless populations, utilizing therapeutic services through a private practice is not an option. Community-based programming that is attuned to the complex experiences of homelessness and trauma is needed – such as trauma- and violence-informed approaches (Wathen, Schmitt, & MacGregor, 2023). Approaches will need to address the pain and suffering that homeless youth have experienced and what this has taught them about themselves and the world. Additionally, the issue of family violence and abuse needs more attention at all levels and the overall failure of the subsequent involvement of child welfare and foster families among those youth who live on the streets.

We believe that an integrative and outreach-based model that speaks to deep client-based engagement and that grounding support "where young people are" are necessary in this work (McManus & Thompson, 2008). Further, prioritizing the voices of homeless youth means being responsive to their needs; respectful, knowledgeable and considerate of their situations; non-judgmental and accepting of differences; participatory and democratic; supportive throughout the long-term involvement; and non-bureaucratic and action-oriented (Karabanow, 2004a; Kidd, 2003; Gaetz, 2004). This view is client-centered and collaborative and will need to be integrated for those who would benefit from therapeutic strategies that can attend to the complex relationship between mental health struggles related to experiences of trauma and homelessness. A holistic, non-medicalized approach needs to be consistent throughout the work, with the youth's explanations of trauma- and violence-based, anti-oppressive, structurally aware interventions as being helpful. This parallels Karabanow's perspective on interventions that employ social development (providing basic needs in safe, as well as collective and empowering spaces), active participation (allowing young people to actively engage and co-author interventions), awareness of structural elements (understanding of individual, community and structural influence on their situations), consciousness-raising (exploring their collective and structural experiences) and social action (advocating for change)

(Karabanow 2004a). Together, this approach can provide young people with meaningful support along with empowered and hopeful avenues to move forward and begin the healing process. This foundation will go a long way, with government support and financing, and the development of programming that allows for community-based, congruent co-occurring therapeutic trauma and violence interventions.

## Conclusion

Over the years, the street youth literature has highlighted both the "push" (e.g., poverty, family problems, abuse and school problems) and "pull" (e.g., independence, freedom and drug/alcohol use) aspects of how, and why, youth become homeless. Much of this debate revolves around individual pathology and structural forces. Social justice/anti-oppressive/trauma-informed, as well as trauma- and violence- based, interventions adopt the latter vision, believing that political, economic, environmental and social forces propel the individual to street life. Understanding the "whole" person entails a holistic perspective of how individual experiences exist within the discourses and structures of society. For example, acknowledging that most youth exist on the street due to a lack of affordable, safe and appropriate housing as well as adequate support following experiences of family violence and problems. There is now greater acknowledgement that trauma and violence are pervasive realities that permeate throughout the lives of homeless youth, both preceding and during their experiences of homelessness. Trauma- and violence-informed interventions that seek to provide stability and support while providing for basic needs (e.g., shelter, food and clothing) in a pragmatic and immediate fashion, while fostering the strengths of participants through community building, is the direction in which we need to move. These elements function to create a safe and caring environment where participants can build empowered and supportive communities. In other words, when taken together, these elements forge a "culture of hope" for an otherwise vulnerable, marginalized and, too often, forgotten population.

## References

Allegrante, J.P., & Sleet, D.A. (2021). Investing in public health infrastructure to address the complexities of homelessness. *International Journal of Environmental Research and Public Health*, 18(16), 8887, 1–8. https://doi.org/10.3390/ijerph18168887.

Andermann, A., Mott, S., Mathew, C.M., Kendall, C., Mendonca, O., Harriott, D., McLellan, A., Riddle, A., Saad, A., Iqbal, W., Magwood, O., & Pottie, K. (2021). Evidence-informed interventions and best practices for supporting women experiencing or at risk of homelessness: A scoping review with gender and equity analysis. *Health Promote Chronic Disease Prevention Canada*, 41(1), 1–13. doi: 10.24095/hpcdp.41.1.01.

Baker-Collins, S. (2013). Childhood stress and mobility among rural homeless youth. In S. Gaetz, B.O'Grady, K. Bucci eri, J. Karabanow, & A. Marsolais (Eds.), *Youth homelessness in Canada: Implications for policy and practice.* Canadian Observatory on Homelessness Press.

Beijer, U., Scheffel Birath, C., DeMartinis, V., & af Klinteberg, B. (2018). Facets of male violence against women with substance abuse problems: Women with a residence and homeless women. *Journal of Interpersonal Violence*, 33(9), 1391–1411. https://doi.org/10.1177/0886260515618211.

Bender, K., Brown, S.M., Thompson, S.J., Ferguson, K.M., & Langenderfer, L. (2015). Multiple victimizations before and after leaving home associated with PTSD, depression, and substance use disorder among homeless youth. *Child Maltreatment*, 20(2), 115–124.

Bender, K., Yang, J., Ferguson, K., & Thompson, S. (2015). Experiences and needs of homeless youth with a history of foster care. *Children and Youth Services Review*, 55, 222–231.

Brown, C. (2021). Critical clinical social work and the neoliberal constraints on social justice in mental health. Special Issue on Social Justice. *Research on Social Work Practice*, 1–9. doi: 0.1177/1049731520984531.

Brown, C., Johnstone, M., & Ross, N. (2021). *Repositioning social work practice in mental health in Nova Scotia.* Report. Nova Scotia College of Social Work.

Brown, C., Johnstone, M., Ross, N., & Doll, K. (2022). Challenging the constraints of neoliberalism and biomedicalism: Repositioning social work in mental health. *Qualitative Health Research*, 32(5), 771–787. https://doi.org/10.1177/10497323211069681.

Caton, C.L., Dominguez, B., Schanzer, B., Hasin, D.S., Shrout, P.E., Felix, A., et al. (2005). Risk factors for long-term homelessness: Findings from a longitudinal study of first-time homeless single adults. *American Journal of Public Health*, 95(10), 1753–1759. http://dx.doi.org/10.2105/AJPH.2005.063321.

Cauce, A.M., Paradise, M., Ginzler, J.A., Embry, L., Morgan, C.J., Lohr, Y., & Theofelis, J. (2000). The characteristics and mental health of homeless adolescents: Age and gender differences. *Journal of Emotional and Behavioral Disorders*, 8(4), 230–239. https://doi.org/10.1177/106342660000800403.

Centers for Disease Control and Prevention. (2013). *Adverse childhood experiences (ACE) study.* Retrieved from http://www.cdc.gov/ace/about.htm.

Coates, J., & McKenzie-Mohr, S. (2011). Out of the frying pan, into the fire: Trauma in the lives of homeless youth prior to and during homelessness. *The Journal of Sociology & Social Welfare*, 37(4), 65–96.

Damron, N. (2015). *No place to call Home: Child & youth homelessness in the United States.* Poverty Fact Sheet. Institute for Research on Poverty.

Davies, B.R., & Allen, N.B. (2017). Trauma and homelessness in youth: Psychopathology and intervention. *Clinical Psychology Review*, 54, 17–28.

Fazel, S., Geddes, J.R., & Kushel, M. (2014). The health of homeless people in high-income countries: Descriptive epidemiology, health consequences, and clinical and policy recommendations. *The Lancet*, 384(9953), 1529–1540. https://doi.org/10.1016/S0140-6736(14)61132-6.

Ferguson, K.M., Bender, K., Thompson, S.J., Maccio, E.M., & Pollio, D. (2012). Employment status and income generation among homeless young adults: Results from a five-city, mixed-methods study. *Youth & Society*, 44(3), 385–407.

Fitzpatrick, K.M., La Gory, M.E., & Ritchey, F.J. (2003). Factors associated with health-compromising behavior among the homeless. *Journal of Health Care for the Poor and Underserved*, 14(1), 70–86. doi:10.1353/hpu.2010.0829.

Flock, I., & Benjamin, E. (2019). *Best practices in addressing homelessness*. University of British Columbia Housing Research Collaborative. https://housingresearchcoll aborative.scarp.ubc.ca.

Gaetz S. (2004). Safe streets for whom? Homeless youth, social exclusion, and criminal victimization. *Canadian Journal of Criminology and Criminal Justice*, 46, 423–455.

Gaetz, S., O'Grady, B., Kidd, S., & Schwan, K. (2016). Without a home: The national youth homelessness survey. Canadian Observatory on Homelessness Press.

Goodman, L., Saxe, L., & Harvey, M. (1991). Homelessness as psychological trauma: Broadening perspectives. *American Psychologist*, 46, 1219–1225.

Government of Canada (2018). *Trauma and violence-informed approaches to policy and practice*. https://www.canada.ca/en/public-health/services/publications/health-risks -safety/trauma-violence-informed-approaches-policy-practice.html.

Green, H.D., Tucker, J.S., Wenzel, S.L., Golinelli, D., Kennedy, D.P., Ryan, G.W., & Zhou, A.J. (2012). Association of childhood abuse with homeless women's social networks. *Child Abuse Neglect*, 36(1), 21–31. doi: 10.1016/j.chiabu.2011.07.005.

Greenfield, B., Alessi, E.J., Manning, D., Dato, C., & Dank, M. (2020). Learning to endure: A qualitative examination of the protective factors of homeless transgender and gender expansive youth engaged in survival sex. *International Journal of Transgender Health*, 22(3), 316–329. https://doi.org/10.1080/26895269.2020.1838387.

Gwadz, M.V., Nish, D., Leonard, N.R., & Strauss, S.M. (2007). Gender differences in traumatic events and rates of post-traumatic stress disorder among homeless youth. *Journal of Adolescence*, 30(1), 117–129.

Hamilton, A.B., Poza, I., & Washington, D.L. (2011). "Homelessness and trauma go hand-in-hand": Pathways to homelessness among women veterans. *Women's Health Issues*, 21(4), 12–16. http://dx.doi.org/10.1016/j.whi.2011.04.005.

Hopper, E.K., Bassuk, E.L., & Olivet, J. (2010). Shelter from the storm: Trauma-informed care in homelessness services settings, *The Open Health Services and Policy Journal*, 3(1), 80–100.

Hwang, S.W., Wilkins, R., Tjepkema, M., O'Campo, P.J., & Dunn, J.R. (2009). Mortality among residents of shelters, rooming houses, and hotels in Canada: 11 year follow-up study. *BMJ* (Online), 339(7729), 1068. https://doi.org/10.1136/bmj.b4036.

Johnsen, S., Cloke, P., & May, J. (2005). Day centres for homeless people: Apaces of care or fear? *Social & Cultural Geography*, 6(6), 787–811.

Jones, A.S., Bowen, E., & Ball, A. (2018). "School definitely failed me, the system failed me": Identifying opportunities to impact educational outcomes for homeless and child welfare-involved youth. *Children and Youth Services Review*, 91, 66–76.

Julianelle, P. (2008). Using what we know: Supporting the education of unaccompanied homeless youth. *Seattle Journal for Social Justice*, 7, 477.

Karabanow, J. (2004a). *Being young and homeless: Understanding how youth enter and exit street life*. Peter Lang Publishing.

Karabanow, J. (2004b). Making organizations work: Exploring characteristics of anti-oppressive organizational structures in street youth shelters. *Journal of Social Work*, 4(1), 47–60.

Karabanow, J. (2006). Becoming a street youth: Uncovering the stages to street life. *Journal of Human Behavior in the Social Environment*, 13(2), 49–72.

Karabanow, J. (2008). Getting off the street: Exploring young people's street exits. *American Behavioral Scientist*, 51(6), 772–788.

Karabanow, J. (2010). Street kids as delinquents, menaces and criminals. Another example of the criminalization of poverty. In D. Crocker & V.M. Johnson (Eds.), *Poverty, regulation and social exclusion* (pp. 138–147). Fernwood.

Karabanow, J., Bozcam, E.S., Hughes, J., & Wu, H. (2021). Lessons learned: COVID-19 and individuals experiencing homelessness in global context. *International Journal on Homelessness*, 2(1), 160–174. https://doi.org/10.5206/ijoh.2022.1.13798.

Karabanow J., & Clement P. (2004). Interventions with street youth: A commentary on the practice-based research literature. *Brief Treatment & Crisis Intervention*, 4, 93–108.

Karabanow, J., Hopkins, S., Kisely, S., Parker, J., Hughes, J., Gahagan, J., & Campbell, L.A. (2007). Can you be healthy on the street? Exploring the health experiences of Halifax street youth. *Canadian Journal of Urban Research*, 16(1), 12–32.

Karabanow, J., Hughes, J., Ticknor, J., & Kidd, S. (2010). The economics of being young and poor: How homeless youth survive in neo-liberal times. *Journal of Sociology and & Social Welfare*, 37, 39–64.

Karabanow, J., Kidd, S., Frederick, T., & Hughes, J. (2018). *Homeless youth and the search for stability*. Wilfrid Laurier University Press.

Karabanow, J., Wu, H., Doll, K., Leviten-Reid, C., & Hughes, J. (2023). Promoting emergency response for homeless service agencies: Field-based recommendations from two municipalities in Nova Scotia, Canada. *Natural Hazards Review*, 24(2), 06023001. https://doi.org/10.1061/NHREFO.NHENG-1498.

Kidd, S.A. (2003). Street youth: Coping and interventions. *Child & Adolescent Social Work Journal*, 20, 235–261.

Kidd, S.A. (2004). "The walls were closing in and we were trapped": A qualitative analysis of street youth suicide. *Youth and Society*, 36, 30–55.

Kidd, S.A. (2006). Factors precipitating suicidality among homeless youth: A quantitative follow-up. *Youth & Society*, 37, 393–422.

Kidd, S.A., Gaetz, S., O'Grady, B., Schwan, K., Zhao, H., Lopes, K., & Wang, W. (2021). The second national Canadian homeless youth survey: Mental health and addiction findings / La deuxième enquête nationale auprès des jeunes sans abri: Résultats en matière de santé mentale et de toxicomanie. *The Canadian Journal of Psychiatry*, 66(10), 897–905.

Kull, M.A., Morton, M.H., Patel, S., Curry, S., & Carreon, E. (2019). *Missed opportunities: Education among youth experiencing homelessness in America*. Chapin Hall at the University of Chicago.

Kurzawski, J. (March 31, 2021). *The link between foster care, homelessness, and criminalization*. Homeless Hub. https://www.homelesshub.ca/blog/link-between-foster-care-homelessness-and-criminalization.

McManus, H.H., & Thompson, S.J. (2008). Trauma among unaccompanied homeless youth: The integration of street culture into a model of intervention. *Journal of Aggression, Maltreatment & Trauma*, 16(1), 92–109. https://doi.org/10.1080/10926770801920818.

Menzies, P. (2006). Intergenerational trauma and homeless aboriginal men. *Canadian Review of Social Policy*, 58, 1–24. https://www.proquest.com/scholarly-journals/intergenerational-trauma-homeless-aboriginal-men/docview/222289446/se-2.

Milburn, N.G., Batterham, P., Ayala, G., Rice, E., Solorio, R., Desmond, K., Lord, L., Iribarren, J., & Rotheram-Borus, M.J. (2010). Discrimination and mental health problems among homeless minority young people. *Public Health Reports*, 125(1), 61–67. https://doi.org/10.1177/003335491012500109.

Noble, A. (2012). *It's everybody's business: Engaging the private sector.* Retrieved from: https://raisingtheroof.org/wp-content/uploads/2020/12/RtR_PS_FullReport_EN_web_01-13.pdf.

Olivet, J., Dones, M., & Richard, M. (2019). The intersection of homelessness, racism, and mental illness. In M.M. Medlock, D. Shtasel, Nhi-Ha T. Trinh, & D.R. Williams (Eds.), *Racism and psychiatry* (pp. 55–69). Humana Press.

Olivet, J., Wilkey, C., Richard, M., Dones, M., Tripp, J., Beit-Arie, M., ... & Cannon, R. (2021). Racial inequity and homelessness: Findings from the SPARC Study. *The ANNALS of the American Academy of Political and Social Science*, 693(1), 82–100.

Petry, L., Hill, C., Milburn, N., & Rice, E. (2022). Who is couch-surfing and who is on the streets? Disparities among racial and sexual minority youth in experiences of homelessness. *Journal of Adolescent Health*, 70(5), 743–750.

Ponic, P., Varcoe, C., & Smutylo, T. (2016). *Victims of Crime Research Digest No. 9.* Department of Justice, Government of Canada, Ottawa.

Rew, L., Taylor-Seehafer, M., & Fitzgerald, M.L. (2001). Sexual abuse, alcohol and other drug use, and suicidal behaviors in homeless adolescents. *Issues in Comprehensive Pediatric Nursing*, 24(4), 225–240.

Ridley, M., Rao, G., Schilbach, F., & Patel, V. (2020). Poverty and mental illness: Causal evidence. *Working Paper*, 1–26.

Roe-Sepowitz, D.E. (2012). Juvenile entry into prostitution: The role of emotional abuse. *Violence Against Women*, 18(5), 562–579.

Rog, D.J., Marshall, T., Dougherty, R.H., George, P., Daniels, A.S., Ghose, S.S., & Delphin-Rittmon, M.E. (2014). Permanent supportive housing: Assessing the evidence. *Psychiatric Services*, 65(3), 287–294.

Ryan, K.D., Kilmer, R.P., Cauce, A.M., Watanabe, H., & Hoyt, D.R. (2000). Psychological consequences of child maltreatment in homeless adolescents: Untangling the unique effects of maltreatment and family environment. *Child Abuse & Neglect*, 24(3), 333–352.

Serge, L., Eberle, M., Goldberg, M., Sullivan, S., & Dudding, P. (2002). Pilot study: The child welfare system and homelessness among Canadian youth. *National Homelessness Initiative.*

Slesnick, N., Zhang, J., & Yilmazer, T. (2018). Employment and other income sources among homeless youth. *The Journal of Primary Prevention*, 39(3), 247–262.

Srivastava, A., Rusow, J.A., Holguin, M., Semborski, S., Onasch-Vera, L., Wilson, N., & Rice, E. (2019). Exchange and survival sex, dating apps, gender identity, and sexual orientation among homeless youth in Los Angeles. *The Journal of Primary Prevention*, 40(5), 561–568.

Stoltz, J.A.M., Shannon, K., Kerr, T., Zhang, R., Montaner, J.S., & Wood, E. (2007). Associations between childhood maltreatment and sex work in a cohort of drug-using youth. *Social Science & Medicine*, 65(6), 1214–1221.

Toolis, E.E., & Hammack, P.L. (2015). The lived experience of homeless youth: A narrative approach. *Qualitative Psychology*, 2(1), 50.

Tyler, K.A. (2006). A qualitative study of early family histories and transitions of homeless youth. *Journal of Interpersonal Violence*, 21(10), 1385–1393. https://doi.org/10.1177/0886260506291650.

Tyler, K.A., Hoyt, D.R., & Whitbeck, L.B. (2000). The effects of early sexual abuse on later sexual victimization among female homeless and runaway adolescents. *Journal of Interpersonal Violence*, 15(3), 235–250. https://doi.org/10.1177/088626000015003001.

van der Kolk, B. (2014). *The body keeps the score.* Penguin Books.

Wathen, C.N., Schmitt, B., & MacGregor, J.C.D. (2023). Measuring trauma- (and violence-) informed care: A scoping review. *Trauma, Violence & Abuse*, 24(1), 261–277. https://doi.org/10.1177/15248380211029399.

Wenzel, S.L., Rhoades, H., LaMotte-Kerr, W., & Duan, L. (2019). Everyday discrimination among formerly homeless persons in permanent supportive housing. *Journal of Social Distress and the Homeless*, 28(2), 169–175. https://doi.org/10.1080/10530789.2019.1630959.

Wilson, J.P., Friedman, M.J., & Lindy, J.D. (Eds.) (2001). *Treating psychological trauma and PTSD*. Guilford Press.

Wolfe, S.M., Toro, P.A., & McCaskill, P.A. (1999). A comparison of homeless and matched housed adolescents on family environment variables. *Journal of Research on Adolescence*, 9(1), 53–66.

Wright, N.M., Milligan, T., Bender, K., & DePrince, A.P. (2022). Revictimization patterns among unhoused youth. *Journal of Interpersonal Violence*, 37(19–20), NP17227–NP17247. https://doi.org/10.1177/08862605211028302.

Wu, H., & Karabanow, J. (2020). COVID-19 and beyond: Social work interventions for supporting homeless population. *International Social Work*, 63(6), 790–794. https://doi.org/10.1177/0020872820949625.

Wu, H., Karabanow, J., & Hoddinott, T. (2022). Building emergency response capacity: Social workers' engagement in supporting homeless communities during COVID-19 in Halifax, Nova Scotia, Canada. *International Journal of Environmental Research and Public Health*, 19, 12713. https://doi.org/10.3390/ijerph191912713.

Yates, G.L., MacKenzie, R.G., Pennbridge, J., & Swofford, A. (1991). A risk profile comparison of homeless youth involved in prostitution and homeless youth not involved. *Journal of Adolescent Health*, 12(7), 545–548.

Zlotnick, C. (2009). What research tells us about the intersecting streams of homelessness and foster care. *American Journal of Orthopsychiatry*, 79(3), 319–325.

# 10

# FROM GENERATION TO GENERATION

## The Legacy of Trauma

*Nachshon Siritsky*

### Introduction

Intergenerational trauma is both historic and ongoing, pointing to the importance of decolonization and a social justice focus in the healing process. Mental health struggles often co-exist with social inequities and challenges that reflect the legacy of trauma of prior generations. In this chapter, I argue that current approaches to mental health fail when dealing with intergenerational trauma, largely because they fail to address the ongoing trauma people experience through oppression, discrimination and racism. Intergenerational trauma is amplified by neoliberal economic and social welfare state policies, which increasingly cut back social support and services and which reinforce social inequities, thus reinforcing and worsening intergenerational trauma (Morrow & Weisser, 2012). Furthermore, without an intersectional approach to this issue that acknowledges the root cause of so many of these issues, namely the role of colonization in instigating and perpetuating this trauma, it will continue to haunt generations to come.

### A Personal Reflection

This chapter is grounded in the lived experience of someone with intergenerational trauma and varied intersectional identities that all impact one another. The illusion of scientific objectivity is often increasingly reflected in evidence-based claims that center discussion of trauma in the body, biochemical medicine and neuroscience. Current discursive practices of decolonization emphasize the importance of speaking from a personal perspective as an important step in providing a more comprehensive understanding of the issues that impact so many of us who have been harmed by colonial and oppressive systems. The failure to acknowledge how the

DOI: 10.4324/9781003379591-11

past continues to influence the present is, in itself, a form of violence that functions as an abdication of responsibility and a form of erasure of the violence that created it. This chapter contributes to the necessary foundation for the reconciliations, reparations and amends that must take place before any healing from trauma can happen.

Speaking one's truth from a first-person perspective is, in itself, a destabilizing act of resistance. As someone who identifies as transgender non-binary, it has taken years of unlearning to be able to come out publicly as myself. As a second-generation holocaust survivor, whose father was hidden, similarly to Anne Frank, in order to stay safe, I was raised to believe that I should hide who I am in a world with transphobia and anti-Semitism. I often felt like I needed to choose which part of me to share, because the world "was not ready to handle" both aspects of me simultaneously. It was only through my experiences working with Indigenous communities and elders, as well as beginning to read about and reflect upon the profound impact of intergenerational trauma and the need for a decolonizing stance to ensure intergenerational healing, that I came to understand the interconnectedness of all of the intersectional injustices that I had both experienced and witnessed.

Overt and covert messages from individuals, organizations and governments reinforced the belief that I could somehow choose between my identities and decide which one the world could handle, while compartmentalizing the rest of myself. This fragmentation is central to the colonial belief system, and my trauma made it difficult for me to recognize or question these assumptions or fully understand their consequences. The truth is that hiding myself was actually what caused me psychological harm, but I did not realize it at the time. It was only through the act of transitioning publicly that I have come to understand the power of authenticity as a revolutionary action. Messages such as those I received are transmitted not only consciously, but unconsciously, not only through words but through stories, attitudes, reactions and in countless other ways. These individual and social messages are reinforced through policies, laws and the distribution of resources. For me, additional traumas amplified these messages and encouraged me to lock the closet door where I sought refuge. It took deep unconscious and somatic work, in addition to the many structural pieces of gender-affirming care that I was finally able to access after moving to a country where my existence was less overtly threatened, to begin to come out as me.

Understanding the influence of intergenerational trauma, as contextualized within a larger colonial framework, is crucial to beginning to understand the deepest and most powerful antecedents to the illusion of the present. In fact, true critical analysis cannot examine the structural influences upon anyone's lives without also reflecting upon the intergenerational patterns and dynamics at play, and the ways these patterns are replicated across the intersectional power and privilege and across the globe. While this chapter seeks to reflect the broad diversity of experiences impacted by this topic, it is nevertheless rooted in my personal experiences, although mitigated by the other influences that have shaped this book.

## Intergenerational Trauma

The term intergenerational trauma emerged in Canada through Dr. Vivian Rakoff's documentation of disproportionately high rates of psychological distress among second-generation holocaust survivors (DeAngelis, 2019). In the 1960s, clinicians studied the intergenerational transmission of trauma, finding that the children of holocaust survivors felt secondary traumatic stress, chronic depression, anxiety, guilt, self-criticism, insomnia, nightmares, mistrustfulness, difficulty regulating aggression and difficulty expressing emotions (Matz, Vogel, Mattar, & Montenegro, 2015). Accordingly, "the parent's trauma is an ongoing part of the children's day to day mental lives" (p. 186).

In this holocaust research, participants described their parents' trauma as having produced a negative effect on their professional and private lives. One participant, Amy, described it as, "Being maimed with bitterness, a really angry view of the world and feeling powerless, feeling like a victim". Robert and Kevin both felt a pervasive sense that they had to be vigilant throughout their lives with regard to when and to whom they disclosed that they were Jewish. This remains a common experience among many Jews: indeed, some choose to assimilate to avoid facing potential violence, racism and discrimination, while others continue to be conscious of who they disclose being Jewish to in order to reduce danger. The privilege of invisibility comes at a price: hiding brings its own experience of shame and anxiety. For example, Debbie described learning from her parents that it was dangerous if people knew she was Jewish. This left her feeling she must remain hidden in both her private and professional life. According to Debbie, "[T]his thing that when fear would inspire a desire to be invisible, or need to be invisible, and that on some level things I was taught about in my family about how being seen is dangerous. This push pull about the longing to be seen, and the fear to be seen" (Matz, Vogel, Mattar, & Montenegro, 2015, p. 19).

Overall, research found that there were often negative psychological impacts of familial holocaust legacies on survivors' children's lives, which included feelings of anger, fear and uncertainty. The children experienced their legacy experiences of the holocaust as a "burdensome responsibility", "put upon them" by their families, and from which they often wished to be freed (ibid.).

Intergenerational or transgenerational trauma is often experienced as "orphaned" trauma – the echo of a trauma that pre-existed us. This is the lived experience of those who grew up in homes or communities that were shaped by trauma that happened before they were born. Frequently, those old traumas continue to be activated and/or reinforced by contemporary injustices. Making sense of the legacy of grief and trauma that one did not oneself experience can be very difficult. Feelings like guilt and shame can be induced as a result of the emotions that are present but unnamed. As a coping mechanism, many children believe that the distress they observe is somehow their fault, or their responsibility to fix – a belief that can amplify trauma-related symptoms (Clark, 1995). This is often what leads many to the helping professions, which in turn opens them up to the influence of vicarious trauma and can contribute to a number of other issues. In the case of the children of holocaust survivors, for example, they often worry that, if they cause trouble or are too demanding, they may exacerbate the pain of their parents. They also report living with the burden and weight of their parents' or relatives' experiences (Matz, Vogel, Mattar, & Montenegro, 2015).

While the initial intergenerational research focused on holocaust survivors and their children, scholars began to apply these same concepts to others, such as communities of African descent and Indigenous communities. The theoretical framework of intersectionality asserts that all those who have been historically marginalized and oppressed have their own unique experiences, which can sometimes cause a sense of alienation from the larger whole, which is experienced as tonally privileged. However, an analysis of power and privilege reveals that intersectional experience is part of a larger whole, and that this sense of alienation and exclusion perpetuates the status quo, by causing diverse communities to compete against one another for scarce resources or to turn to lateral violence among themselves. When we focus on how we are different from one another, and the ways in which our experiences are often not validated or recognized, we miss out on the healing and revolutionary potential that is possible when we come together to advocate for systemic changes to address the structural inequities and, indeed, hatred that have been in place for generations.

An intergenerational trauma lens can also elucidate the experiences of communities and individuals who have experienced significant violence (such as civil war, genocide, war-related migration, mass violence, political instability, or domestic violence, or have been forced to become refugees, or have parents with significant mental health problems) – who all shared similar ongoing reactions to intergenerational trauma.

## Lack of Culturally Responsive Support

The colonial project is maintained through the establishment of false silos between individuals, communities and disciplines of knowledge, which prevent the collective dismantling of oppressive systems. While an intersectional lens is crucial to understanding the need for culturally responsive support, any discussion on intergenerational trauma within a Canadian context must specifically address the racist foundations of Canadian policy. The Doctrine of Discovery (the profound impact of intergenerational trauma and the need for a decolonizing stance to ensure intergenerational healing), and the theological construct of *Terra nullius* (which defines as "empty and ownerless" any land that is inhabited by people who are not Christian) are examples of the use of religious rhetoric to justify the murder, exploitation and oppression of Black and Indigenous communities. Together, the impact of historical and current racism and gender discrimination are evident in the lived experiences of people of African and Indigenous backgrounds.

Intergenerational trauma and systemic injustice continue to haunt these communities to this day on every single level, including the psychosocial determinants of health that are often the focus of current government policies. Population health perspectives in Canada emphasize the need to take steps to become culturally responsive, particularly regarding the Indigenous population. This is necessary but nevertheless profoundly inadequate to counter the systemic extermination of generations of Indigenous communities, and the racism that is embedded into every part of the system. The Truth and Reconciliation Commission's findings are only the beginning of the reckoning that must take place (see Truth and Reconciliation Commission, various years).

Marginalized and oppressed groups, such as individuals of African descent, Indigenous communities, Two-Spirit, Lesbian, Gay, Bisexual, Transgender, Queer, Intersex, and Asexual (2SLGBTQIA+) and refugees continue to experience significant and systemic barriers for accessing services, which is exacerbated by a lack of cultural/social appropriateness and an absence of trauma-informed practices. In particular, there is a lack of appropriate mental health services and long-term funding for mental health that acknowledges intergenerational trauma. Smaller and remote communities such as those in rural parts of the country, along with the often-isolated Indigenous communities in the Northern parts of Canada, often have very little, if any, access to mental health care and within marginalized communities, stigma and discrimination are a significant barrier.

Most planning and funding of initiatives to address mental health and addictions challenges fail to acknowledge or address the deeper systemic root causes of the symptoms that they claim to target or treat. Trauma, anxiety, depression and substance-use problems are commonly interrelated, but a failure to acknowledge the intergenerational legacy that caused these actually perpetuates the stigma that continues to harm these communities to this very day. Research that examines the prevalence of such coping behaviors can be misused and inadvertently contribute to the prejudice that magnifies the traumas that continue to influence these communities. For example, when people feel anxious or depressed, dominant biomedical approaches to mental health asserts a diagnosis and treatment plan that includes medicating the symptoms, in order to help people "function" within the system. This serves to preserve existing social relations of power and privilege, which positions those suffering as unwitting accomplices in exchange for survival.

Many of those experiencing the effects of intergenerational trauma are pathologized, stigmatized and medicated. This is exacerbated by the lived experiences of those who grew up in the shadows of intergenerational trauma, who were born not understanding why the adults in their world were so distressed, and who often developed coping strategies to make sense of their lived experiences. It is not uncommon for a child to blame themselves for their parents' discontent. For those children who were born into systemic and intergenerational trauma, the degree of blame that they often internalized was proportional to the degree of trauma that they sensed present around them. Therefore, many of those born into family systems with intergenerational trauma, will internalize the doubt, shame and self-recrimination around them. This makes them particularly receptive to internalizing the blaming messages of a pathologizing biomedical approach that places responsibility for illness upon the shoulders of the individual, rather than acknowledging the systemic and historic factors that led to the situation.

In our current system, symptoms and struggles are typically seen as individual pathology, viewed through a deficit and biological lens, rather than understanding how they are often produced by intergenerational trauma and systematic oppression. Consequently, the social and political context is not acknowledged, and this maintains the status quo.

In contrast, some research and writing on trauma and violence points to the need for intergenerational healing within families and communities. A growing body of research recommends engaging with communities to learn from those with lived experience what can be most impactful to support intergenerational healing and foster new structural and cultural norms that mirror the values and aspirations community members have for themselves and their children (Porter, Martin, & Anda, 2017; Ross & Bookchin, 2020). It is imperative that intergenerational trauma among African Canadian and Indigenous communities be addressed in a far more comprehensive and systematic manner. It is not enough to add a "diversity division" to an existing biomedical system that was designed to promote colonial values, and that is resourced and managed in such a way as to perpetuate the status quo, for doing so ensures the perpetuation of intergenerational legacies of inequity.

In a recent Nova Scotia study, it was reported that social workers are concerned that mental health professionals, including some practicing social workers, do not always recognize the intergenerational trauma among African and Indigenous Nova Scotians and are often ill-equipped to respond effectively (Brown, C., Johnstone, & Ross, 2021, p. 134). This report indicates that there is very little community-based work or commitment to providing culturally and socially appropriate services, for example, to African Nova Scotians, Indigenous communities, and 2SLGBTQIA+ communities (ibid.). The failure of the system to provide education or resources to address these observed disparities and systemic injustices contributes to the profound burnout and moral distress of social workers and other health care providers. As practitioners learn to recognize these injustices, this distress grows. But because of the intersectional silos that prevent a comprehensive overhaul of the system, most health care workers experiencing moral distress find themselves being pathologized and treated as individuals who are "burned out" and need to go on leave. Consequently, the system's status quo remains, despite a growing vacancy rate as social workers and other health care workers seek to work in the private sector.

Sadly, this exodus of health care professionals will likely only continue to grow, due to their frustration with the system's failure to own and address these intergenerational and systemic issues. Despite their training, the limitations of the mental health care system, for example, does not allow these health care professionals to offer the type of comprehensive care and support they know are needed. People's struggles are too often decontextualized, treated as individual pathology and medicalized. The growing privatization of the health care system as a solution to a lack of public services will however only perpetuate social injustice and inequity by ensuring that those who do not have money will have difficulty accessing the resources and support they need to survive, let alone thrive.

## Dominant Capitalist Neoliberalism and Biomedical Service Provision

Today, mental health services are problematically rooted in capitalist neoliberalism and biomedicalism that emphasize fictional notions of objectivity, science and evidence-based practice (Bullen, Deane, Meissel, & Bhatnager, 2020). The dominant ideological world view that guides mental health care ignores the social and historical context of people's lives and thus does not adopt critical or culturally appropriate services. As a result, "evidence-based" programs often highlight the privilege of certain knowledge and knowers over others. The salience of a Western Eurocentric and colonial approach to work in the social service field results in a failure to recognize and meet the needs of marginalized groups (ibid.). As the current dominant approach to health and mental health is shaped by an entrenched neoliberal political economic policy, meeting the needs of those who have experienced intergenerational trauma will require a seismic change of understanding and commitment to change (Martin, 2012; Waitzkin, 2020).

Colonization is far from over. Intergenerational trauma continues to be manufactured by our current economic policies. Colonization is perpetuated by the pathologization and criminalization of those who continue to be oppressed and discriminated against in a system that works against them. Furthermore, social work as a profession, particularly child welfare, has been used to perpetuate violence on those it is meant to help (Needham, 2022). The Canadian Association of Social Workers has apologized for its role in perpetuating the harms of colonization by its support of policies that were clearly intended to dispossess Indigenous people from their land (Canadian Association of Social Workers (CASW), 2019). When social work has sought to speak out against the mechanisms by which capitalism, biomedicalism and colonization perpetuate harm upon so many people, they are often silenced by organizational policies and practices.

Social workers working in the mental health system overwhelmingly express a deep frustration and sense of moral distress, according to the recent report commissioned by the Nova Scotia College of Social Workers (Brown, C., Johnstone & Ross, 2021). Those social work voices, committed to social justice, have very little influence or autonomy within the hierarchy of mainstream organizations. Under the fiscal constraints of neoliberalism, social workers are often disturbed by the long wait-lists, one-size-fits-all, very short-term organization of service provision, with a focus on efficiency rather than care. This deliberate approach, shaped by cutbacks, does not allow for the development of relationships, or the development of appropriate support for marginalized communities, and does not allow the provision of adequate care, far less the capacity to being to address intergenerational trauma (Brown, C., Johnstone & Ross, 2021; LaMarre, Smoliak, Cool, Kinavey, & Hardt, 2019).

## Ongoing Systemic Violence and Adversity: Well-being Inequities

No less than the many military public statues that fill community parks and public spaces, police violence is a graphic and public reminder of the ways that the colonial apparatus continues to dominate and control the narrative. Media reports and movies reinforce stereotypes of criminality, and also eclipse the countless micro-aggressions that perpetuate the intergenerational trauma that strikes deep at the psyche of communities ravaged by colonial brutality for centuries. The witnessing and experiencing of police violence has been identified as a source of profound harm by multiple generations of African Nova Scotian/African Canadians and Indigenous Canadians (Lee & Robinson, 2019). This has a "spill-over effect" on Black people's mental health. The recent violent murders of George Floyd and Breonna Taylor by police in the United States has been highlighted by the Black Lives Matter movement. Black men struggling with mental health problems have also been notably at high risk of being shot and killed by police, which only exacerbates the problem. Waldron argues,

> … the racial terrorism of anti-Black police violence is a deeply felt wound in Black communities that extends beyond the individuals who directly experience it and that this type of collective trauma must be understood as an urgent public health crisis.
>
> *(Waldron, 2021, p. 29)*

Among Indigenous people, depression, anxiety, post-traumatic stress disorder and substance-use problems are related to stressful/traumatic experiences and, according to Bombay, Matheson and Anisman (2009) "shared collective experiences of trauma experienced by First Nations peoples, coupled with related collective memories, and persistent sociocultural disadvantages, have acted to increase vulnerability to the transmission and expression of intergenerational trauma effects" (p. 6). Intergenerational trauma creates social, structural and historical causes of adversity in Indigenous communities (Boksa, Joober, & Kirmayer, 2015) and are reflected in current mental health and substance-use issues and experiences. Like intergenerational trauma, the concept of historical trauma "takes the perspective that the consequences of numerous and sustained attacks against a group may accumulate over generations and interact with proximal stressors to undermine collective well-being" (Bombay, Matheson, & Anisman, 2014, p. 320).

Bombay argues that this cumulative historical trauma is responsible for well-being inequities. The colonization of Indigenous people evidenced, for example, by the Indian Act (first introduced in 1876), the Indian Residential Schools (which operated in Canada between the 1870s and the 1990s), the Sixties Scoop (which coincided with the residential schools as a government strategy to remove Indigenous children from their homes and communities), child welfare practices and ongoing systemic racism has produced intergenerational trauma. Similar to the experiences of other marginalized and oppressed groups, there are significant barriers for Indigenous people accessing services, which is exacerbated by a lack of cultural appropriateness. While biomedically based approaches increasingly dominate mental health care, Khan (2008) notes that Indigenous people have a holistic view of mental wellness, as did many other cultures that were colonized. Consequently, dominant biomedical Western European models tend not be useful frameworks and arguably, despite their hegemonic authority, are limiting for most. For Indigenous people, wellness involves a balance with family, community and the larger environment. According to Khan (2008) effective approaches to treatment involve "identifying the strengths of families and communities and developing programs that build on these strengths" (p. 7 ).

In the Nova Scotia study (Brown, C., Johnstone, & Ross, 2021) mentioned above, one service provider described the mental distress resulting from intergenerational trauma and the impact of this on parenting and family functioning:

> Attachment wounds is a huge one that I see over and over again with almost every mom I see through Child Protective Services. Definitely there's so much intergenerational trauma in a huge percentage of my clients … Definitely those clients that grew up in poverty and how that's affected them, the opportunities that they had or didn't have, most of them didn't have and how that, and then also the communities that they grew up in and what they weren't exposed to and what they were exposed to, that then further marginalized them and set them on a course that made it really difficult for them to thrive. – Lori, provider.
>
> *(p. 135)*

The effects of colonial policies and practices on individual and community well-being must be addressed when understanding the overrepresentation of poverty, homelessness, incarceration, experiences of violence, substance use, depression, anxiety and suicidality among Indigenous people. Collective historical and current trauma, loss and grief, are reflected in these issues (Boksa, Joober, & Kirmayer, 2015). According to Kirmayer, Brass, & Tait (2000),

> However, framing the problem purely in terms of mental health issues may deflect attention from the large scale, and, to some extent, continuing assault on the identity and continuity of whole peoples. To these organized efforts to

destroy Aboriginal cultures are added the corrosive effects of poverty and economic marginalization.

*(p. 15)*

Research has further established that Indigenous people are overrepresented among homeless populations, and the prevalence of Indigenous homelessness appears to be increasing in Canadian cities. Bingham et al. (2019) explored gender differences among Indigenous Canadians experiencing homelessness and mental illness and investigated mental health, substance use and service use among Indigenous people who met criteria for homelessness and mental "illness". Women had significantly higher rates of trauma, suicidality, substance dependence and experiences of violence compared to men.

Bingham and colleagues (2019) found that Indigenous women were six times more likely than Indigenous men to be victims of forced sexual violence, and were significantly more likely to experience post-traumatic stress and suicidality. Indigenous women continue to experience multiple forms of violence, social exclusion and marginalization (Bingham et al., 2019; Brennan, 2009). This is consistent with the widely documented violence against Indigenous women, girls and Two-Spirit individuals in Canada and reflects the ways that intersectional oppression amplifies trauma.

The report on the Missing and Murdered Indigenous Women, Girls and Two-Spirit Individuals (Angelino, Burns, LaForme, & Giroux, 2023) shows the unique intersectionality of race, gender and sexuality that colonial intergenerational trauma created and perpetuates. This is maintained and amplified by the commodification of sexuality and the ubiquity of human trafficking. The failure to examine intergenerational trauma from an intersectional lens leads to the failures of the system to take responsibility and address this as part of the larger Truth and Reconciliation effort (Truth & Reconciliation Commission of Canada, 2015). This report enables this problem to be seen as separate, which, in turn, ensures that the deeper issues are not addressed. For instance, when providing housing and support, services need to be culturally appropriate and reflect trauma-based care that acknowledges the experiences of Indigenous women (Martin, 2012; Palmater, 2016; Porter, Martin, & Anda, 2017). When non-cisgendered males become homeless they are impacted even further by violent victimization, post-traumatic stress and suicidality, and this is synergistically exacerbated for those who identify as Indigenous or are visibly "other" due to their race.

Elias and colleagues (2012) conducted a study on the effect of intergenerational trauma related to the negative experiences of residential schools and found that experiences of trauma and suicidality were related to intergenerational trauma among survivors and their children. It is clear that the colonization of Indigenous people and the intergenerational trauma Indigenous people have experienced have been significant determinants of health and mental health. Indigenous people experience major depression at twice the national average (Khan, 2008). Suicide rates are twice the national average and increasing among youth (ibid.). The stark reality of Indigenous suicide rates tells a powerful story of the pain and suffering that intergenerational trauma and ongoing oppression has caused (Bodnar, 2014).

Adopting culturally aware and decolonizing approaches is not consistent with biomedically based diagnostic approaches that center in individual pathology without addressing the larger sociocultural and socioeconomic context. Often the effects of trauma are pathologized, whereby the interpretation of symptoms are separated from their source. Intergenerational trauma can be the cause of many mental health challenges, and, specifically, the intergenerational trauma that has been unacknowledged, misunderstood and reinforced by social injustices (Bortolon & Brand, 2021). It is imperative to develop community-based and community-led programming in dialogue and consultation with Indigenous and Black populations: these should be trauma-informed and informed by the ancestral values and teachings of these communities, rather than reflect Euro-Western approaches. It is especially vital that consultations be done in a way that is trauma-informed and grounded in the intersectional experiences and perspectives of Indigenous women, girls and Two-Spirit individuals, all of whom are at a higher risk of the intergenerational traumas noted above. And yet, consultations are often perceived as excuses for action. Therefore, it is imperative that, at the same time, larger restorative justice initiatives begin and ongoing social inequities are addressed.

## Intergenerational Trauma and the Importance of a Hermeneutic Lens

A hermeneutic lens is critical because it emphasizes the need to unpack how meaning is socially shaped. This lens emphasizes exploring and valuing the meaning-making process. Often, the stories that we tell ourselves, to try to make sense of symptoms or experiences, can instead contribute to further mental health challenges, due to the misattribution of causality and the internalization of shame and blame. This is evident in the child that grows up not understanding why their parent or guardian is behaving in a certain way, and therefore assumes that it is their (the child's) fault. This interpretation is too often reinforced with the biomedicalized focus of the health care system, which pathologizes and interprets every symptom as an individual problem. Without an intergenerational or systemic lens, feelings or behaviors that seem to have no direct cause can seem "crazy". For this reason, a better understanding of the role of trauma is needed – especially those traumas that are poorly understood, because as in the case of intergenerational traumas, the traumas happened before the person was born.

When trauma is collective and spans multiple generations or is ongoing, as is the case for oppressions that are connected to colonization, then the outcomes of intergenerational trauma become far more complex. According to Ngameni et al. (2022), these become the collective efforts to create meaning and ensure safety that become transmitted and socially reinforced. Menakem (2020) notes: "Trauma in a person, decontextualized over time, looks like personality. Trauma in a family, decontextualized over time, looks like family traits. Trauma in a people, decontextualized over time, looks like culture."

To speak about intergenerational trauma is to speak about a footprint. The concept implies that something pre-existed us and continues to haunt us. Devgan (2018) described growing up with intergenerational trauma as if one is living in a haunted house, somehow always intruding on a secret, learning the language of shame and fear viscerally.

Young (2018) calls for the transformation of our legacies from burdens into gifts. This is essential to breaking the intergenerational pattern of transmission, where shame and blame can lead to self-sabotaging behaviors, as we internalize social stigma. Instead of turning the finger on oneself, healing involves recognizing the systemic and transgenerational impacts upon every individual experience. This is the way that the master's tools *can* dismantle the master's house (Lorde, 1984).

Many who work in the field of trauma or intergenerational trauma are interested in this topic because they are impacted by their own lived experiences. However, the neoliberal biomedical professional practice encourages the illusion of neutrality, and autobiographical elements are rarely acknowledged. Often efforts to seem skilled or knowledgeable leads to pathologizing, labeling and medicating (Beazley, 2021). Such distancing behaviors complicate the field of discussion, because much of what has been written on the topic is impacted by that which is not acknowledged. This is further reinforced by the neoliberal biomedical "scientific" need to preserve the illusion of objectivity. The biomedical and pharmaceutical approach to mental health serves a regulatory function, by redirecting attention away to the larger systemic and structural social justice issues that are at the root of mental health distress (Brown, C., Johnstone, & Ross, 2021).

When people feel anxious or depressed, or begin to have a sense that things are terribly wrong, science asserts a diagnosis and treatment plan that includes medicating the symptoms in order to help people "function" within the system. When those experiencing symptoms of intergenerational trauma are pathologized, stigmatized and medicated, the focus remains on individual deficit, rather than to both acknowledge and challenge the larger social context.

Perhaps, the best visual of what intergenerational healing can be seen in the popular cartoon of the generations trying to stop the trauma, from one parent to the next: the great-grandparent is seen cursing, the grandparent is seen trying to stop the pattern by being silent, while the next generation is trying to say positive affirmations to their offspring. This cartoon has many iterations across the internet, in part because it conveys deep truths that resonate for many of us. Specifically, in the cartoon we can see a great-grandparent saying "I hate you" and the grandparent that is silent, while the parent has put up a shield and says "I love you" to the child that is the inheritor of the healed legacy of intergenerational trauma.

Instead of simply repeating the pattern, we can recognize these as moments where we can suddenly see clearly. Such revelatory moments are liminal opportunities for healing (Bond, 2021). The most important first step is to understand that complex feelings are actually part of a legacy of violence that was passed down, through the internalization of wounds, beliefs and behaviors. When we realize this, then we are freed (Boisen, 1936).

However, these insights must be accompanied by systemic solutions that address the structural issues related to the intergenerational trauma that are still causing harm. For example, the intergenerational trauma caused by colonization or the conditions of self that are related to post-traumatic familial slavery can never be healed simply by naming the issues or by providing a diagnostic label. Deeper systemic justice is also desperately needed: the righting of historic wrongs through reconciliation and reparations, as well as the fixing of ongoing systemic injustices and the unlearning of pervasive racism, prejudice and discrimination. We live in systems that reflect the brokenness that leads to the harms that are carried and transmitted to the next generation (Yellow Bird, 2020).

And yet, just as importantly, it is imperative that the symptoms of intergenerational trauma are recognized and named for what they are, because the failure to do so silences rather than amplifies its effects and also serves as a form of silent collusion. The systemic abdication of responsibility and historic ongoing blaming of the victim perpetuates the stigma at the root of orphaned trauma. This, in turn, too often results in those suffering seeking solace through self-medication or acting out their frustrations. The focus cannot be on individuals through labeling, diagnosing and providing pharmaceutical treatment within a mainstream individualized biomedical lens, but instead on culturally appropriate community-based support and overall social restructuring that can redress the underlying intergenerational and historical causes, alongside ongoing support and services.

There are parallels between intergenerational trauma (from the generation that survived the trauma) and transgenerational trauma (from the first generation following the trauma to subsequent generations), as well as the similarities between the experiences of diverse intergenerational traumatic experiences. When trauma is decontextualized over time, people tell harmful internalized stories about themselves that are too often blaming and shaming.

When we stop blaming ourselves for traumas that pre-existed our birth, but that have continued to impact us, then we can begin to focus our efforts on what needs to happen at a systemic level to create the kind of structural changes that can support our healing journey. Foundationally, the healing of intergenerational trauma cannot only happen on an individual level because the wounds are reinforced by larger systems that reinforce pervasive intergenerational traumas.

## Critical Social Justice

Systemic approaches with intersectional solutions are desperately needed in order to address the deeper social injustices that underly many of the intergenerational traumas that are the legacy of colonization. Intergenerational trauma is a critical social justice issue that requires a collective reframing for intergenerational healing to occur. We need to encourage society's collective understanding of the pervasive intergenerational impact of colonization and racism. By pathologizing mental health symptoms, rather than recognizing them as the consequence of systemic injustices, the status quo is preserved, and individuals are responsibilized (Clarke & Yellow Bird, 2021).

There is, too often, an inadequate understanding of the ways in which all those who experience mental health challenges are in fact experiencing the legacy of trauma caused by prior generations, amplified by the ways that systemic racism, queerphobia, paternalism and colonialism remain central to current governmental policies and the mainstream health care system. The larger structural issues of colonialism and its systemic injustices are rarely acknowledged, yet these issues must be addressed for healing to be possible.

The effects of intergenerational trauma among people of African descent need to be recognized and addressed in a way that is not decontextualized and pathologized. It is important to clearly identify the historical source of the trauma – slavery. Multigenerational trauma co-exists with ongoing oppression, and institutionalized racism today only deepens both the oppression and the effects of trauma. Under neoliberalism and ongoing fiscal constraints, we see less and less trauma-based support available. Those that exist have waiting-lists and tend to be short term and standardized, with one-size-fits-all approaches. It is difficult to offer or advocate for whole-person care that emphasizes the social determinants of health and mental health when there are next to no services available and even fewer that address diversity and intergenerational trauma (Brown, C., Johnstone, & Ross, 2021; Carey & Hodgson, 2018).

Intergenerational trauma continues to be reproduced by our current economic policies. Colonization is perpetuated by the pathologization and criminalization of those who seek to dissent, with prisons often serving as colonial nation states' largest psychiatric service providers, yet without any actual therapeutic support (Butler, Nicholls, Samji, Fabian, & Lavergne, 2022). In both the United States and Canada, the overrepresentation of Black, Indigenous and people of color (BIPOC) individuals in the criminal justice system is but one example of the ways in which intergenerational trauma is transmitted and perpetrated. Rather than addressing the systemic injustices, such policies of individual blaming perpetuate the disproportionate number of children who are placed into "care", so often ensuring the continued presence of intergenerational trauma. Systemic changes are not adequately addressed, and existing relations of power are simply reproduced (Needham, 2022).

Education, science and justice policies entrench these dynamics into community culture and the stigma associated with mental health struggles often results in people not seeking help (Aziz, 2007; Žižek, 1997). Movies, television, books, laws, policies, academic practices … these all reinforce these unconscious values, reminding us that being "different" is shameful (Tremain, 2006). History and pop culture both overflow with examples of how difference is punished. For those of us whose families experienced intergenerational trauma, these messages reinforce the earlier ones received. We learn shame, silence and complicity as the key to survival (Naidu, 2021). Colonization's reliance upon religion, education and other social systems further reinforces these messages (Redvers, Guzmán, & Parkes, 2023).

To the extent that much of its goal has been the control and exploitation of the land and its peoples, the truest threat to colonial world order is the perspective of Spirit, which affirms that our uniqueness is a gift (Dueck & Marossy, 2021). While there are many understandings of the Spirit, Indigenous ways of knowing and being stand in direct conflict with colonial and false claims of objective knowledge. Shame has a crucial role in the ways in which colonial religion functions: trauma begets shame and becomes the glue by which trauma is passed down from one generation to the next, in particular, in the case of complex trauma. In many ways, the issue of intergenerational trauma and healing is a spiritual one.

Religion has often been weaponized as a tool to promote and sanctify the colonial quest. Central to this process has been the harnessing of shame as a way to create loyalty and obedience. Shame has a crucial role in the ways in which colonial religion functions, and it also becomes the glue by which trauma is passed down from one generation to the next (Clark, Classen, Fourt, & Shetty, 2014). Shame is an overarching construct that perpetuates trauma and is maintained through traumatic reactions such as the "F" responses that can lead to "fight", "flight", "fawn", "freeze" or "flop" and manifest in a variety of symptoms that are reinforced socially (Schwartz, 2017).

Wordlessly, those of us who grew up surrounded by intergenerational trauma learned what was safe and what was not safe. These messages are then introjected by the next generation of children growing up in environments that either do – or do not – align with the social norms of that era. This ensures the enduring dominance of certain groups over others, perpetuating the systemic injustice that itself perpetuates the transmission of generational patterns (Tremain, 2006). Intergenerational trauma perpetuates existing social inequities that look different for different communities, and are amplified by those who have multiple intersectional experiences of oppression and are more visibly "other" in our colonized and colonizing world.

Today, much of trauma work is based on somatic therapy, including eye movement desensitization and reprocessing (EMDR) and the neuro-experiential integrative model, brainspotting (BSP). While such therapies may help individuals cope with the intensity of emotions related to their distress, they do little to address the root causes that maintain the systemic traumas that contribute to the distress. Unfortunately, these models all center on the individual and are not integrated into the cultural framework of the individual or their experiences of intergenerational trauma (Langford, 2021). If anything, they become formulaic techniques offering questionable promises. To the extent that many intergenerational wounds are interwoven with acts of violence to one's people or community, it is essential that healing approaches integrate the cultural or spiritual beliefs of the individual. It is critical that approaches foster hope and possibility, and they are offered in communities by communities.

Wells-Wilbon (2021) notes that a significant form of intergenerational and transgenerational violence has been the attack on African and Indigenous communities' spiritual beliefs, through the ways that colonization has weaponized religion and become integrated into dominant narratives, which, in turn, help to perpetuate "othering" practices. Indeed, current colonial approaches to health perpetuates the false distinction between physical, mental, spiritual and social well-being. Yellow Bird (2020) has written extensively about the ways in which colonization seeps into the psyche through the internalization of colonial values through multiple methods, noting the trauma of Christian colonizing beliefs that outlawed Indigenous spiritual and communal practices. Religion has been a primary strategy for colonization, and therefore spirituality must be used cautiously when integrated into clinical intervention and only after determining whether this is something a client wants or does not want. It is therefore essential to complete a thorough assessment prior to the integration of spiritual practices into the therapeutic context, lest these bring up trauma from adverse religious experiences (Koenig, Al-Zaben, & VanderWeele, 2020).

## Conclusion

For those of us who grew up in the shadows of intergenerational trauma, we learned how to survive by the ways that we absorbed the wounds and unwritten rules of those who raised the ones who raised us and all of the generations that preceded us. Like trying to decipher hieroglyphs, the process of healing often involves recognizing and naming the symptoms that distress us for what they are, critically reflecting on how traumatic meanings emerged, engaging in ceremonies or behaviors that allow us make sense of them, and challenging their ongoing power in our lives. When we are liberated from the power and impact of our pain, suffering and loss we can be freer to embody an alternative, a more authentic and preferred, sense of who we are. Healing from the impact of intergenerational trauma can transform trauma into roadmaps for healing and new beginnings. But none of this is possible without larger systemic efforts to ensure reconciliation, reparations and restorative justice that become actualized through changes in policy, funding and practices, as well as through the integration of these new ways of understanding the social and historical context that has shaped so much current suffering and inequity

## References

Angelino, A.C., Burns, J., LaForme, C., & Giroux, R. (2023). Missing and murdered Indigenous women, girls, and Two Spirit people: A paediatric health crisis. *The Lancet Child & Adolescent Health*, S2352–4642.

Aziz, C. (2007). Transnational activist coalition politics and the de/colonization of pedagogies of mobilization: Learning from anti-neoliberal Indigenous movement articulations. *International Education*, 37(1).

Beazley, A. (2021) Normativity, marginality, and deviance in a psychiatric placement: A parallel process. *Transactional Analysis Journal*, 51(1), 91–105, doi: 10.1080/03621537.2020.1853355.

Bingham, B., Moniruzzaman, A., Patterson, J., Sareen, I., Distasio, J., O'Neil, J., & Somers, J. (2019). Gender differences among Indigenous Canadians experiencing homelessness and mental illness. *BMC Psychology*, 7, 57. https://doi.org/10.1186/s40359-019-0331-y.

Bodnar, A. (2014). Perspectives on Aboriginal suicide: Movement toward healing. In P. Menzies & F. Lavallee (Eds.), *Journey to healing: Aboriginal people with addiction and mental health issues: What health, social service and justice workers need to know* (pp. 285–299). Centre for Addiction and Mental Health.

Boisen, A. (1936). *The exploration of the inner world: A study of mental disorder and religious experience*. Harper and Brothers.

Boksa, P., Joober, R., & Kirmayer, LJ. (2015). Mental wellness in Canada's Aboriginal communities: Striving toward reconciliation. *Journal of Psychiatry & Neuroscience*, 40(6), 363–365. doi: 10.1503/jpn.150309.

Bombay, A., Matheson, K., & Anisman, H. (2009). Intergenerational trauma: Convergence of multiple processes among First Nations peoples in Canada. *International Journal of Indigenous Health*, 5(3), 6–47.

Bombay, A., Matheson, K., & Anisman, H. (2014). The intergenerational effects of Indian Residential Schools: Implications for the concept of historical trauma. *Transcultural Psychiatry*, 51(3), 320–338. doi: 10.1177/1363461513503380.

Bond, A.J. (2021). *Discomfortable: What is shame and how can we break its hold?* North Atlantic Books.

Bortolon, C., & Brand, R.M. (2021). Psychosis, trauma and dissociation: Evolving perspectives on severe psychopathology. *European Journal of Psychotraumatology*, 30(12), 1. doi: 10.1080/20008198.2021.1893985.

Brennan, S. (2009). *Violent victimization of Aboriginal women in the Canadian provinces*. Retrieved from http://www.statcan.gc.ca/pub/85-002-x/2011001/article/11439-eng.htm.

Brown, C., Johnstone, M., & Ross, N. (2021). *Repositioning social work in mental health practice in Nova Scotia*. Retrieved February 5, 2023: https://nscsw.org/mental-health -paper/.

Bullen, P., Deane, K., Meissel, K., & Bhatnager, S. (2020). What constitutes globalised evidence? Cultural tensions and critical reflections of the evidence-based movement in New Zealand. *International Journal of Psychology*, 55(1), 16–25.

Butler, A., Nicholls, T., Samji, H., Fabian, S., & Lavergne, M.R. (2022). Prevalence of mental health needs, substance use, and co-occurring disorders among people admitted to prison. *Psychiatric Services*, 73(7), 737–744. https://doi.org/10.1176/appi .ps.202000927.

Carey, L.B., & Hodgson, T.J. (2018). Chaplaincy, spiritual care and moral injury: Considerations regarding screening and treatment. *Frontiers in Psychiatry*, 9, 619. https://doi.org/10.3389/fpsyt.2018.00619.

Canadian Association of Social Workers (CASW). (2019). *Statement of Apology and Commitment to Reconciliation.* Retrieved February 5, 2023: https://www.casw-acts.ca/files/attachements/Statement_of_Apology_and_Reconciliation_FINAL_2021.pdf.

Clark, F.C. (1995). Anger and its disavowal in shame-based people. *Transactional Analysis Journal*, 25(2), 129–132. https://doi.org/10.1177/036215379502500205.

Clark, C., Classen, C.C., Fourt, A., Shetty, M. (2014). *Treating the trauma survivor: An essential guide to trauma-informed care.* Routledge.

Clarke, K., & Yellow Bird, M. (2021). *Decolonizing pathways to integrative healing in social work.* Routledge.

DeAngelis, T. (2019) The legacy of trauma. *Monitor on Psychology*, 50(2), 36. Retrieved February 10, 2023. https://www.apa.org/monitor/2019/02/legacytrauma#:~:text=One%20of%20the%20first%20articles,14.

Devgan, S. (2018). A haunted generation remembers. *Contexts*, 17(4), 36–41. https://doi.org/10.1177/1536504218812867.

Dueck, A., & Marossy, M. (2021). Prolegomena for the development of indigenous psychologies of spirituality: Colonization, decolonization, and indigeneity. In: A. Dueck (Ed.), *Indigenous Psychology of Spirituality.* Palgrave Studies in Indigenous Psychology. Palgrave Macmillan. https://doi.org/10.1007/978-3-030-50869-2_2.

Elias, B., Mignone, J., Hall, M., Hong, S.P., Hart, L., & Sareen, J. (2012). Trauma and suicide behaviour histories among a Canadian Indigenous population: An empirical exploration of the potential role of Canada's residential school system. *Social Science & Medicine*, 74, 1560–1569. doi:10.1016/j.socscimed.2012.01.026.

Khan, S. (2008). Aboriginal mental health: The statistical reality. "Aboriginal People" issue of *Visions Journal*, 5(1), 6–7.

Kirmayer, L.J., Brass, G.M., & Tait, C.L.(2000). The mental health of Aboriginal peoples: Transformations of identity and community. *The Canadian Journal of Psychiatry.* 45(7), 607–616. doi:10.1177/070674370004500702.

Koenig, H., Al-Zaben, F., & VanderWeele, T. (2020). Religion and psychiatry: Recent developments in research. *BJPsych Advances*, 26(5), 262–272. doi:10.1192/bja.2019.81.

LaMarre, A., Smoliak, O., Cool, C., Kinavey, H. & Hardt, L. (2019) The normal, improving, and productive self: Unpacking neoliberal governmentality in therapeutic interactions. *Journal of Constructivist Psychology*, 32(3), 236–253. doi:10.1080/10720537.2018.1477080.

Langford, P. (2021). Somatic experiencing, EMDR and brainspotting: An African-centered critique. In R. Wells-Wilbonn &Anthony Estreet (Eds.), *Trauma and mental health social work with urban populations: African centered clinical interventions* (pp. 40–51). Routledge.

Lee Smith, J.R., & Robinson, M.A. (2019). "That's my number one fear in life. It's the police": Examining young black men's exposures to trauma and loss resulting from police violence and police killings. *Journal of Black Psychology*, 45(3) 143–184. doi:i1.o0.r1g1/107.171/0770/90509759789481491986655152.

Lorde, A. (1984) The master's tools will never dismantle the master's house. In *Sister outsider: Essays and speeches* (pp. 110–114). Crossing Press.

Martin, D. (2012). Two-eyed seeing: A framework for understanding Indigenous and non-Indigenous approaches to Indigenous health research. *The Canadian Journal of Nursing Research*, 44(2), 20–42.

Matz, D., Vogel, E.B., Mattar, S., & Montenegro, H. (2015). Interrupting intergenerational trauma: Children of Holocaust survivors and the Third Reich. *Journal of Phenomenological Psychology*, 46, 185–205.

Menakem, R. (2020) Notice the rage, notice the silence. *On Being with Krista Tippett*. Retrieved August 15, 2023: https://onbeing.org/programs/resmaa-menakem-notice-the -rage-notice-the-silence/.

Morrow, M., & Weisser, J. (2012). Towards a social justice framework for mental health recovery. *Studies in Social Justice*, 6(1), 27–43.

Naidu, T. (2021) Modern medicine is a colonial artifact: Introducing decoloniality to medical education research. *Academic Medicine 96* (11S), S9–S12. doi: 10.1097/ ACM.0000000000004339.

Needham, F. (2022). The bond is broken: Data shows the number of Indigenous kids in foster care is going up. Statistics Canada. *APTN News*. Retrieved February 10, 2023: https://www.aptnnews.ca/national-news/statistics-canada-indigenous-people-housing -issues-child-welfare/#:~:text=More%20than%20three%20per%20cent,years%20of %20age%20and%20younger.

Ngameni, E., Moro, M., Kokou-Kpolou, C.K., Radjack, R., Dozio, E., & El Husseini, M. (2022). An examination of the impact of psychosocial factors on mother-to-child trauma transmission in post-migration contexts using interpretative phenomenological analysis. *Child Care in Practice*, 1–16. https://doi.org/10.1080/13575279.2022.2071220.

Palmater, P. (2016). Shining light on the dark places: Addressing police racism and sexualized violence against indigenous women and girls in the national inquiry. *CJWL/ RFD*, 28(2), 253–284.

Porter, L., Martin, K., & Anda, R. (2017). Culture matters: Direct service programs cannot solve widespread, complex, intergenerational social problems. Culture change can. *Academic Pediatrics*, 17(7), S22–S23.

Redvers, N., Guzmán, C., & Parkes, M. (2023). Towards an educational praxis for planetary health: A call for transformative, inclusive, and integrative approaches for learning and relearning in the Anthropocene. *The Lancet Planetary Health*, 7(1), 77–85. Ahead of print: https://doi.org/10.1016/S2542-5196(22)00332-1.

Ross, N., & Bookchin, S. (2020). Perils of conversation: #MeToo and opportunities for peacebuilding. *Gender in Management: An International Journal*, 35, 391–404.

Schwartz A. (2017). *The complex PTSD workbook: A mind-body approach to regaining emotional control and becoming whole*. Althea Press.

Tremain, S. (2006). On the government of disability: Foucault, power, and the subject of impairment. In L. Davis (Ed.), *The Disability Studies Reader* (2nd ed.) (pp. 185–196). Routledge.

Truth and Reconciliation Commission of Canada. (2015). *Canada's Residential Schools: The Final Report of the Truth and Reconciliation Commission of Canada* (Vol. 1). McGill-Queen's Press.

Truth and Reconciliation Commission of Canada. (Various years). Reports. Retrieved from: https://nctr.ca/records/reports/.

Waitzkin, H. (2020). Moving beyond capitalism for our health. *International Journal of Health Services*, 50(4):458–462. doi:10.1177/0020731420922827.

Waldron, I.RG. (2021). The wounds that do not heal: Black expendability and the traumatizing aftereffects of anti-Black police violence. *Equality, Diversity and Inclusion: An International Journal*, 40(1), 29–40. doi: 10.1108/EDI-06-2020-0175.

Wells-Wilbon, R. (2021). Reclaiming our right to wholeness and wellness. In R. Wells-Wilbon & A. Estreet (Eds.), *Trauma and Mental Health Social Work with Urban Populations: African Centered Clinical Interventions*. Routledge.

Yellow Bird, M. (2020) Decolonizing from the inside out. *ReRooted* Episode 22. Video. Retrieved February 6, 2023: https://youtu.be/lEyS4wlyDvc.

Young, D. (2018). *Black therapists rock: A glimpse through the eyes of experts.* Black Therapists Rock in.

Žižek, S. (1997) Cogito, madness and religion: Derrida, Foucault and then Lacan. Retrieved February 5, 2023: https://www.stephenhicks.org/wp-content/uploads/2019/04/ZizekS -Cogito-Madness.pdf.

# 11

# INTERGENERATIONAL TRAUMA

Rising Above the Intersectional Impact of
Racism and Gender on the Health and
Well-Being of African Nova Scotian Women

*Barb Hamilton-Hinch and Catrina Brown*

## Introduction

The impact of intergenerational and historical trauma across systematically oppressed populations in Canada, including people of African ancestry, continues to impact women's health and well-being. In this chapter we draw on research that examined the lived experiences of racism and gender-based discrimination among women of African ancestry living in Nova Scotia and the factors that contributed to their survival, success, health and well-being. These women spoke about gender-based racism (James et al., 2010). This study adds to existing research where women gave spoken about gender-based racism (Essed, 1991; Fraser & Reddick, 1997). Together these studies explore the implications of gendered racism on their health, the health of their families and their community. In this chapter, we focus on Hamilton-Hinch's Nova Scotia study, which demonstrates through the voices of African Nova Scotia women the theme of "silence" that emerged, consisting both of "being silenced" by others or by pervasive racism/sexism and also the intentional "silencing of oneself" as self-protection.[1] Suggestions for addressing health inequalities while simultaneously confronting racism and gender-based racism, for system-level change are offered.

The intersectionality of race and gender are central determinants of the well-being of women of color (Crenshaw, 1991). The unique challenges Black women experience due to these factors have been examined in a number of Canadian studies (Beagan & Etowa, 2011; Beagan, Etowa, & Bernard, 2012; Enang, 1999; Este & Bernard, 2006; Etowa, 2005; Etowa, Keddy, Egbeyemi, & Eghan, 2007; Etowa, Thomas, Oyinsan, & Clow, 2007; Etowa, Wiens, Bernard, & Clow, 2007; Etowa, Beagan, Eghan, & Bernard, 2017; Waldron, 2012, 2019, 2020). The Racism Violence Health study (James et al., 2010) examined the experiences of racism and its effects

DOI: 10.4324/9781003379591-12

on the well-being of individuals, families, and communities in the African Canadian diaspora. Inherent within these African Canadian studies, but not yet fully explored, are experiences that told the story of how Black women living in Nova Scotia have survived and succeeded in the face of racism and gender discrimination.

Barb Hamilton-Hinch (the first author of this chapter) identifies as an eighth-generation African Nova Scotian woman. She is from the African Nova Scotian communities of Beechville (father), and Cherry Brook (mother), and grew up as the youngest of six children. She knows the sacrifices many women make in order to survive. When Barb was a child, her mother cleaned homes for white families. She eventually elevated herself to a manager of a hotel restaurant and, later, an insurance broker. She recalls the weight of racism her mother would bring home. As a daughter, sister, mother and aunt, Barb has lived the pain and power of silence. She personally found the women's experiences shared in the study to be very powerful. The forced silence of people living with the effects of racism is never *not* there. This work is very personal to Barb, as it elevates the voices of some women, and exposes the intergenerational trauma of racism that continues to exist today.

Silence can mean hiding who one is, or parts of oneself. Catrina Brown (the second author of this chapter) recalls how her mother told her she was Jewish when she was 14 years old. Until then, Catrina sensed there was something not spoken, something hidden, something secret in her mother's life. Her mother had been hiding that she was Jewish. While growing up in Scotland, which had been bombed many times during World War Two, she was often woken in the middle of the might to find safety in a bomb shelter. As she was Jewish, she knew she faced significant danger. Long after, she continued to feel that being Jewish was dangerous and she wanted to protect both herself and her children from hatred, from anti-Semitism. This is not an uncommon Jewish story. Much goes unspoken, hidden and is carefully rendered silent. Silence is linked to a sense of fear and vulnerability, of protection, survival, safety and caution against risk. Silence is often forced from a history of subjugation and domination.

Both authors of this chapter have historical stories of subjugation and erasure through slavery and genocide that reverberate in the present. These historical stories have needed to be spoken for the millions who have been brutalized, dehumanized and murdered. Silence is often related to oppression, to the danger of speech – of terrible consequences. Yet even when spoken, there are echoes of silence. Many continue to be brutalized, oppressed, and silenced. In the research of African Nova Scotian women in this chapter, there are the sounds of silence. The women describe forced and subordinated silence, and silence as power, control and survival.

## Intergenerational Trauma

Historical and present-day realities of the impact of racism and gender-based discrimination continue to be evident in the lived experiences of people of African descent (Bernard & Smith, 2018; hooks, 2000, 2003; Jones, 2008; Waldron, 2020, 2021; West, Donovan, & Daniel, 2016). Both race and gender are socially and politically constructed determinants of health, which are reflected in the differential impact of social value and power, and the continued discrimination and prejudice experienced by racialized women relative to non-racialized women (Juster & Lupien, 2012; Lorde, 1984). Today, people of African descent living in Canada and the United States experience high rates of incarceration, unemployment, and difficulty in accessing advanced education and equitable health care (Codjoe, 2001; James, 2012; African and Canadian Legal Clinic, 2015; Wortley & Owusu-Bempah, 2011).

In the context of Nova Scotia, the largest of the four Atlantic Canadian provinces, African Nova Scotians have a significantly higher rate of unemployment, are less likely to attend university and have double the prevalence of low income than the rest of Nova Scotians (Office of African Nova Scotian Affairs, 2014). Inequities in access to advanced education, employment and equitable health care as well as other key social determinants of health, all serve to impact the personal and social development and integration of individuals of African ancestry (Raphael, 2004, 2009; World Health Organization (WHO), 2001). Racism has similarly impacted the health of people of African Nova Scotian ancestry who experience increased rates of anxiety, depression and high blood pressure as compared with individuals of European descent (Etowa, 2005; James et al., 2010; World Health Organization, 2014). It has also been noted that individuals of African descent do not see themselves represented in a variety of health care settings, which in turn can produce barriers for navigating and accessing such systems and contributes to the ongoing development of historical trauma (McGibbon & Etowa, 2009).

Historical trauma in relation to race examines the trauma of enslavement and the everyday experiences of racism as factors contributing to poor health outcomes among people of African descent (Beagan & Etowa, 2009, 2011, 2012; Collins, 1990, 2000a; Crawford, 2007; DeGruy, 2005; Dobbins & Skillings, 2000; Edmonds, 2001; Essed, 1991; Etowa, Keddy, Egbeyemi, & Eghan, 2007; Etowa, Thomas, Oyinsan, & Clow, 2007; Gee, Walsemann & Brondolo, 2012; hooks, 2003; James et al., 2010; Jones & Shorter-Gooden, 2003; Jackson & Naidoo, 2012; Lynam & Cowley, 2007; Veenstra, 2009; Wallace & Bell, 1999; Waldron, 2020; Wells-Wilbon, 2021; Williams & Williams-Morris, 2010).

Research that examines the marginalization of Black women indicates they are more likely to live in poverty and experience homelessness and disparities in health than their White counterparts (Utsey et al., 2007; Williams & Sternthal, 2010; Office of African Nova Scotian Affairs, 2014). In relation to Nova Scotia, previous research has examined Black nurses in the health care system (Etowa, 2005), the childbirth experiences of African Nova Scotian women (Enang, 1999), older African Nova Scotian women and the menopause (Etowa et al., 2005), and racism, violence and the health of African Canadians in Halifax, Calgary and Toronto (James et al., 2010) and has indicated widespread racism.

Despite the consequences of racism, many women of African Nova Scotian descent have been defined as leaders and role models in African Nova Scotian and Canadian communities and beyond. These include Rose Fortune, the first Black policewoman in Nova Scotia; Viola Desmond, a Black hairdresser who refused to be removed from the "white section" of a movie theatre to the "Blacks-only section"; Daurene Lewis, the first Black female mayor in Canada; Portia White, who broke the color barrier to become the first Black Canadian concert singer to achieve international fame; the Honorable Mayanne Francis, who became the first Black female Lieutenant Governor in Canada; and Corrine Sparks, who became the first Black female judge in Canada. These women reveal the ability to survive and succeed in a deeply racist society.

## Racism Violence and Health Project: The Voices of Black Nova Scotian Women

The Racism Violence Health study defined health as "a state of complete physical, mental and social well-being and not merely the absences of disease or infirmity" (World Health Organization, 1948, p. 100). This definition encompasses the impact of racism and gender-based discrimination on the overall well-being of individuals and has not been changed since 1948. The Racism Violence Health study showed that racism was endemic and significantly affected African Canadians in all facets of their lives (James et al., 2010). While this study examined these factors at the Canadian national level, we will focus in this chapter on Hamilton-Hinch's earlier examination (2016) of Black Nova Scotian women leaders and their lived experiences of discrimination together with the factors that may contribute to their survival, success, health and well-being. Specifically, Hamilton-Hinch's (2016) study explored the lived experiences of racism, and gender discrimination among 20 leaders of African descent from the original Racism Violence Health interviewees. Aspects of their stories are shared here with the use of pseudonyms.

As the original research was focused on racism, the women did not explicitly talk about gender in the study. Women talked about feeling invisible, unable to speak or afraid to challenge racist actions or comments. They felt silenced. Nonetheless, gender-based experiences such as the "strong Black women's syndrome" or those related to being the primary care provider of children, family and community, were central to their stories. Black feminist thought emphasizes the intersection of sexism and racism and the women reported on their experiences of gendered racism. Black women's intersectional experiences of racism and sexism are often reflected in the experiences of feeling invisible and unheard.

The women's accounts of their experiences produced counterstories. Counterstories are a form of discursive resistance that enables "telling the stories of those [individuals] whose experiences are not often told" (Yosso & Solórzano, 2005, p. 26). The women's voices challenged narratives often told about Black women that helped to create counterstories. Within the women's experiences were stories of the oppressions they experienced and the tools they used and developed to improve their future including "Being Silenced", "Becoming Aware of and Using Silence", "Surviving Discrimination" and emphasizing now was the "Time for Change". The results illustrate the commonalities of racism and gender-based discrimination among the women (Hamilton-Hinch, 2016).

## Being Silenced

In describing their lived experiences of racism, many women shared the ways they survived at the same time as they often talked about feeling invisible and being unable to speak. Several women, while talking about their lived experiences of racism as a child, shared how they were either silenced by others because of discrimination, silenced by loved ones in a protective way or chose to silence themselves for their own protection. The theme of "silence" therefore consisted of both "being silenced" by others or pervasive racism/sexism and intentional "silencing of oneself" as self-protection. In their conversations about being silenced, the women described not being able to speak because of the discriminatory attitudes and behaviors toward them. Specifically, they spoke of the numbness that descended on them in the course of being silenced and how this contributed to their resistance to discriminatory attitudes and behaviors. In addition, they talked about how they were assaulted by forced silence psychologically, emotionally and physically. Their voices were muzzled, their responses were stifled, and their presence made invisible or ignored. Some women reported losing the ability to speak out, because of fear, lack of confidence, or the difficulty and danger of putting into words what they were experiencing. Bernadette describes her experience of keeping silent in the following way:

> So you know I feel sometimes, down and out, depressed, you know, and inadequate, and doubtful about myself, especially if I am in a group of mostly white people. I don't know how to act sometimes. I get scared not knowing what to say because I think if I say something, it will offend them because I'm not, you know, I'm not being like – I'm not trying – I'm not conformed to their own ideology of what I should be in society. [Bernadette]
>
> *(Hamilton-Hinch, 2016)*

Several women spoke of fear of losing their jobs or being punished (being passed over for promotions or unfair evaluations) and as such, they would continue to experience discrimination. Being silent was the only way to guarantee survival in the context of some of the women's experiences. However, Bettina explains the importance of challenging discrimination that leads to silencing and helping people to name it:

> Help people name when it's institutional racism. Help them name when somebody is personally attacking them because of their race or because of their gender

or sexual orientation. Give it some language. And that's a huge level of account-ability. Don't be silent, you know, help people create – healing occurs when people are able to create safe spaces. And there has to be safe spaces for people to talk about this and in talking about it [racism] that means naming it. [Bettina]

*(ibid.)*

Stories of being fired from a job, being let go or being abused in the workplace reminded some of the women of their own vulnerability and that of their children. Many spoke of feeling pressured to present an image of pride and keep-ing it together, so as not to permit being ascribed to Black stereotypes such as being uneducated and angry. The pressure to avoid stereotypes often manifested in silence and was described as painful, confusing and frustrating. The effects of being silenced can leave a person feeling numb. Bettina states:

I think it's because we've numbed. It's like, there it is again, but you don't rec-ognize it anymore. You begin to expect the worst and accept the worst, which makes it difficult to move beyond the racism. You are blocked. [Bettina]

*(ibid.)*

This reference "to being numbed" or shutting down was seen as a protective response to stress. The participants experienced the inability to speak or move. They stood in shock and disbelief about what they were hearing. Some of the women became bed-ridden but did not know how to name why they felt depressed or suicidal. The daily exposure to discrimination made it difficult to name or deal with. In some cases, women described being on autopilot and moving monotonously through their day doing only what was expected of them. As Ninika points out:

If I was to go to my doctor and say that, you know, I'm stressed because of incidences of racism. You know, I might be diagnosed as having poor coping styles opposed to – and that may be for a lack of understanding what it is that I'm truly experiencing because that person doesn't experience racism … it may be perceived as more of a psychological disorder. [Ninika]

*(ibid.)*

It was felt that a diagnosis of a psychological disorder by a physician with no experience of racism, may simply contribute to being silenced. Experiencing these conditions on a daily basis can cause an individual to become debilitated, as indi-cated in Bettina's reflection of her experience of working with individuals who faced racism, whereby she describes racism as "trauma":

[…] When I think – and I think as someone in the mental health profession and the only way I can describe it is if you are constantly being traumatized – it's post-traumatic stress disorder. [Bettina]

*(ibid.)*

Many of the women described chronic pain, depression, anxiety, suicidal thoughts, drug and alcohol abuse, cardiovascular disease, eating 'disorders', type 2 diabetes, hypertension and other health conditions they believed were associated with their exposure to racism. As Bettina states:

> You can't be safe if you're always on guard. And that hypervigilance only leads to mental health issues of depression, anxiety, high blood pressure. Pure mental health issues and pure physical health issues that get manifested in other diseases. [Bettina]
>
> *(ibid.)*

Many children are taught at a young age the old expression: *"children are to be seen and not heard"*. In certain circumstances this can be considered a form of voluntary silencing. Women in Hamilton-Hinch's (2016) study recognized that in some instances this was done to keep the children safe from discrimination. One woman in the study reflected on her experience of being silenced as a child by her parents, while being taught to act a certain way when she went into town. She expressed the level of comfort she had when living in an all-Black community and going to an all-Black school. She acknowledged having teachers of European descent but reflects on the expectations her parents placed on her when she was in town in the company of White people. The children were expected to be quiet and to look perfectly well kept.

Many young Black children are taught early on what is expected of them in the presence of White adults. It is a form of silencing. Particularly for Black women who were often subjected to domestic work and childcare in the homes of White middle- to upper-class families and expected to be seen but not heard. Camia explains:

> ... but in a sense of the way that you're expected to act, you know, because you're now in the company of White people. That generation, my parent's generation, like they went into town, like, "Hush, be quiet, wipe that stuff off your face." You have to, like you know, you have to look like perfect little beings. [Camia]
>
> *(ibid.)*

Women in Hamilton-Hinch's (2016) study indicated they and others would not go into town unless their hair was combed, their make-up applied and their clothing neatly pressed, suggesting pressure to present an image of dignity and to avoid stereotypes of Black women, including being unkempt, dirty, uneducated and a welfare mother. Further, being silenced reaches as far as being conscious of not drawing attention to yourself, of becoming invisible.

## Becoming Aware of and Using Silence

Many women spoke of how, upon becoming aware of having been silenced, they learned self-silencing as a tool for surviving discrimination, particularly when they were offended and expected to provide a response. They were at least to some extent able to mitigate being silenced in reaction to the actions or attitudes of others through their own deliberate use of silence as a means of silencing their oppressor. This was particularly useful when discriminatory comments or "jokes" were being heard. In other words, rather than responding to their oppressor, the women remained silent and did not verbally or physically respond. The women became aware that oppressors were attempting to silence them and chose to use silencing as a protective tool after arriving at the "aha" moment or the moment in which they gained insight. This often frustrated and silenced their oppressor, as the oppressor did not know how to respond.

Many of the women interviewed recounted how reflection on discriminatory experiences, and their physical and behavioral reactions to those experiences (instant reaction, sweating of the palms, clenching of the jaw, a body twitch, nausea, being completely debilitated) led to becoming aware of the power of silencing. The women began to reflect on and develop an awareness of what had caused their silence, their "illness" (depression, anxiety, compromised mental health, high blood pressure), their inability to respond by sharing the exchanges of the internal and external happenings of their body with family, friends, community members and even physicians. Ava describes the power of silencing:

> ... Sometimes I say nothing, but I do that purposely because sometimes it comes back and it will – that person's going to learn more when they're smacked in the face themselves – when they do it to themselves – than when I do it ... And then they become all apologetic about what they said. And I let them talk because that's their confession to you. Hey, I'm not going to say, "Well, don't worry about it blah, blah, blah. I'm glad that you recognize that. And thank you for bringing it to my attention." ... So that's my opportunity for educating at that time. [Ava]
>
> *(Hamilton-Hinch, 2016)*

Ava suggests that it is important to recognize and know your own strengths of silencing. Through the use of counterstories shared with each other, other women of African descent can see how women have often silenced themselves as a tool to survive the pain of discrimination and move forward.

## Surviving Discrimination

The African Nova Scotian women described their lived experiences of racism, how it impacted their lives and how they survived discrimination. Despite the challenges, hardships and negative experiences women endured, their stories portrayed the ability to press on. When exploring how women persevered *the church, family and community* were commonly described as positive influences on surviving. Through their stories women illustrated how these influences supported their survival in the face of racial discrimination, and how they helped to contribute to positive mental health. The women often described historic memories, those gained through stories of ancestors' tenacious spirits and strategies for survival, which helped them to cope in the face of discrimination. Hearing and retelling these stories became a part of the women as they continued to share them with the next generation. The stories not only became a part of them, but in many cases influenced their socialization (Mogadime, 2008). These women illustrated how, when stories are told and retold over long periods of time, they get "into the bones and under the skin" (Schatzki & Natter, 1996, pp. 4–5). Beverly states:

> It's like we have a [historical] memory and, when we realize it, we come to terms with what happened to us, it strengthens us, you know. It's like you find it doesn't break you down, it gives you this internal fortitude. [Beverly]
>
> *(Hamilton-Hinch, 2016)*

Knowing your history helps to define who you are, and memory represents a protective armor passed on by people's ancestors. The women spoke of the resilience of their ancestors and their ability to survive in spite of their circumstances, passing on this history and connection to their ancestors to the next generation, acknowledging the fortitude of people of African ancestry. This memory, referred to by participant Beverly, has propelled her to fight against racism.

Similarly, through oral traditions, women reported learning ways of being and acting and the "social codes" expected of them as matriarchs. They were responsible for caring for the family and community regardless of the toll it sometimes took on their health. Ninika states:

> I think Black women have gotten to a point, because we're taking care of everybody else's wellness emotionally and physically that we put ourselves on the backburner. It's such an easy thing to do. And we burn ourselves out and don't even realize we're burnt. [Ninika]
>
> *(ibid.)*

Not unlike women who face the gendered role expectation of caregiving, many women reflected on how they would forget to take care of themselves in order to take care of others. By itself, this research cannot indicate whether the gender-based expectations of Black women are different from those of women who do not also face oppression based on race. However, the expectation of women is evident in research by Bryson and colleagues (2014), Dickens and Chavez (2018) and Wharton and Erickson (1995), which examines the role and expectations of women who work and care for others.

Feminist policy research in particular has shown that women's care-giving role often means women taking care of others at the expense of themselves (Gaunt, 2013; Maxwell, 2012; Thomas, Hacker, & Hoxha, 2011) regardless of race.

However, specific differences and similarities between and among women across a range of intersectional needs further exploration.

Social institutions such as the church, family and community were seen by many women as a place for refuge and engendering strength. Women indicated how the church is the backbone of most African Nova Scotian communities. The church is often the first teacher about racism, equality and social justice. In addition, the women talked about the church as being more than just an institution and how stories told in the spirituals, sung by the choir, helped heal. Camia explains that community and congregation members go to church:

> ... with a heavy heart ... and get healed by the choir as much as by the sermon. Music as a form of release and a form of renewal has been documented through time immemorial as having the capacity to transform your whole spirit. [Camia]
>
> *(Hamilton-Hinch, 2016)*

The family unit was also often described by women as an integral part of the African Nova Scotian community and a source of support. Many reflected on how they depended on their family and extended family such as the church and community for informal counselling. For some women, the church provided another source of support and understanding, similar to that which they received from their immediate family. Shiona shares how important the Black community is for her:

> The Black community, for me, is a sense of support, a sense of, community. It gives me a sense of community, it gives me a sense of belonging, of sanity [laugh], family. And it's a sort of place of refuge and a place where I can totally be by myself and be comfortable.
>
> *(ibid.)*

## Taking Action for Change

The women indicated the importance of being active in advocating for change. Being silenced, becoming aware of the physical and emotional symptoms of having been silenced, and using silencing of others as a protective and educational practice, led to a gradual remaking of some of the women and, through them, their communities. Taking action for change refers to a transformation, a new way of looking at the self – a re-imagining of the self and the community. Taking action for change against racism and gendered racism was highlighted by the women.

The women often described the need to be educated about remaking the self and community when describing taking control of their lives and taking control of the community as a community. Doing so would mean not being silenced and numbed by the oppressive and racist actions of others. One of the ways Dencil sees it as being possible to heal from this "cancer" of racism is "to come together again as Black people, people as a whole, to help our young people get the proper education". Ava expresses the importance of knowing who we are as Black women, in order for the next generation to move on:

[W]e have to re-establish ourselves … it goes back to a knowing and, I think a firm foundation again. And if we understand who we are, then what they say – will it really matter? Because you can't keep me in a box. You see, you tried to keep me in a box 400 years ago, and I still stand, and I really wish our people – if I had any message, that would be the message to our people – we are free. Only we keep ourselves in bondage by thinking, – by using our past and bringing it into the present. But we need to leave it back there, if only to learn to push us forward, not to keep reliving, because then the ones that want to keep us there, they don't have to do any work 'cause we're doing it for them. That's not who we are – [that's] who they say we are. [Ava]

*(Hamilton-Hinch, 2016)*

Camia and other women in the study think about ways to move forward:

And I think we don't believe that we can learn our way out of it and take the indigenous knowledge and reinvent ourselves to survive this next leg. And then we're lost. That's what we have to do. We have to re-believe in ourselves. [Camia]

*(ibid.)*

Some of the women carefully selected their paths of education and employment in order to help remake themselves and to re-imagine the Black community and Black people in general. The women in this research made a conscious choice to become role models for the continued advancement of future generations. In addition, they acknowledged the role they played in preparing the next generation of Black women. Bettina talks about her sense of responsibility as part of being a Black woman:

But I also think Black women who are in positions, you know, I'm a participant in the Black middle class. I have a responsibility to make sure I bring along the next person. When you work in an institution like this, bringing one along is hard work, you know, and you're always identifying the places if you're mindful of your race politic and your community politic to say to my supervisor or to my director, "We need to do more in the Black community about this". Consistently keeping race on the agenda of institutions is exhausting, emotionally hard work, that is you are politically aware and you are using your privilege as a Black middle-class person or a person in a place of privilege, it's exhausting. [Bettina]

*(ibid.)*

As the women shared their strong concern for upcoming generations, some spoke specifically about their own professional and educational choices. Their chosen professions in education, social work, health and law have given them a position where they can provide direct or indirect support to young people, particularly young people of African descent. For example, Samantha advocates for the African Nova Scotian community "to exercise as many rights as we can".

Bettina talks about the need to make the health care system more accountable to the African Nova Scotian community:

> I work in the health care field, and deal with issues around lack of research, which is about racism, and it's construction about how issues around health and wellness that affect the Black community – high diabetes, heart disease, sickle cell, anything that has a strong common denominator where even though we're only maybe 7–10% of the population, where 100% of that 10% of the population are suffering from these diseases and all we're getting is a menial treatment which are treatments that could be preventative based. And I think the health care system needs to be responsive to that. [Bettina]
>
> *(ibid.)*

The women also expressed the desire to see a different future for their community and their children, where they can celebrate the past, the present and the future and where they can contribute and not be judged or excluded because of the color of their skin, their sex, gender identity, income or education.

### Rising Above Stories of Survival

It is important to understand how people, in spite of historical and generational trauma, move themselves and their communities forward. Hamilton-Hinch's (2016) study tells a story of surviving racial and gender-based discrimination from the perspective of recognized women leaders of African ancestry living in Nova Scotia in 2016. Equally evident was the impact that racism and gender-based discrimination had on their overall health. Certainly, a history of African Nova Scotians emerges from the stories that are told and retold. Women demonstrated how they survived by drawing on the experiences and strength of their ancestors, their families, the church and themselves. Within the context of this work, understanding the themes among Black Nova Scotian women of "surviving discrimination" and "taking action for change" builds upon an awareness of surviving and colonization, the effects of being silenced, and using silence oneself.

The impact of colonization has often silenced people of African ancestry, which then constrains them from defending themselves or others when experiencing discrimination (Dotson, 2011; Spivak, 1998). Dotson (2011) refers to the notion of silencing in two ways: testimonial quieting and testimonial smothering. The women in the current study (Hamilton-Hinch, 2016) experienced both types of silencing. The invalidation of people's knowledge is a form of "testimonial quieting" and epistemic injustice (Collins, 2000a, 2000b; Dotson, 2011; Fricker, 2010). Regardless of their academic, political and social positions, the women in the study described often feeling invisible, believing that their opinions, thoughts or knowledge were not respected, valued or considered relevant. In contrast, Dotson's research (2011), suggests that "testimonial smothering" occurs when populations that have been marginalized do not speak or respond in situations that resemble microaggression. Rather than confront racism and sexism in the workplace, for instance, many of the women described how they remained silent in order to retain their jobs. In other words, they felt speaking out threatened their livelihood, which impacted both themselves and their families. Some women talked about how difficult it was to be a woman and experience sexism while also experiencing the impact of racism in their lives. One woman told the story of how a White man she trained was given a promotion over her and there was nothing she could do. Narratives and other bodies of work on the experiences of Black women leaders across North America reveal similar stories of their silencing in the face of discrimination, affecting their journeys toward achieving greater equity (see, for example, Angelou, 1969; Rice, 2010; Wright Myers, 2002).

Some of the women in Hamilton-Hinch's (2016) study were explicit about how they remained silent in order to avoid conflict and disapproval and to protect themselves and others. Indeed, remaining silent is often a form of survival. The women did not want to be seen as the "angry Black woman" and wanted to protect their positions for themselves and for other Black people. They did not want to give their employer a reason to dismiss them. For many, being silenced, whether involuntarily or voluntarily, manifests itself in depression, stress, anxiety, high blood pressure, poor mental health and other debilitating conditions (Etowa, 2005; James et al., 2010). There are many health consequences of being silent. The stress of surviving, not speaking up, remaking self and the community were described as having a long-term effect on the women's mental and physical health. As we have documented, research indicates that racism can have a direct negative effect on the health and well-being of people of African ancestry because of the historical trauma of being of African descent. However, as some women became more aware of how and why they were silent or being silenced it created an awareness and an awakening that led them to take action for change. Many of the women sought employment and education that empowered them with the tools to help, protect and support other people of African descent.

Most women described becoming aware of their body's responses to feeling silenced and of their silence as a reaction to, and protection against, the racism that was either occurring or anticipated. As they talked to other women who shared similar experiences and responses, a consciousness-raising emerged. The stories they told and retold began to take on new meanings. The women began to use silence in new ways. They discovered silence was a potential tool for personal agency and resistance against discrimination.

Henry (1993, 2015) argued that the complexity of Black women's lives as leaders is rarely examined in relation to resistance and power. This research demonstrates Black Nova Scotian women's use of silence is an expression of agency and power. Indeed, the women in the study stepped beyond being voluntarily silenced. They knowingly used silence as a way to avoid responding to the kinds of remarks that did not warrant the dignity of a response. This method of resisting racism can make the perpetrator aware of their actions.

Through their awareness of racism, the use of silence as agency and resistance and through the power of formal and informal education the women have established themselves as leaders in many professions. Through their survival, and indeed their thriving, the women see themselves as contributing to the next generation of leaders and helping to change the trajectory of career paths often reserved for people of African ancestry.

The original Racism Violence Health study (James et al., 2010) did not set out to intentionally focus on the intersectionality of gender and race (Enang, 1999; Etowa et al., 2005; Henry, 1993, 2015; Mogadime, 2008). However, despite this, we gained insight on the influences that gender had on women's responses to racism and discrimination and their combined impact on women's overall health and well-being through the African Nova Scotian women interviewed. Comparisons of men's and women's interviews would further our understanding of how gender influences responses to racism.

## Conclusion

The lived experiences of discrimination and racism and their impact on the well-being of African Nova Scotian women are explored in this chapter. The women's stories connect the impact of discrimination based on race and gender on their health and well-being. The women credit their power and strength to their ancestors, the church, family and community for making it possible for them to push through tough times. They stand on the shoulders of those who came before them. Their fears and anxieties about racism for themselves, their families and their communities were evident, as was the toll it continues to take on their well-being. The women's stories stressed that their experiences of silence ultimately, perpetuates the systems of gendered racial discrimination.

These experiences suggest the need for the development and enactment of health-related social policies to improve health outcomes that address the race- and gender-related challenges experienced by these women. Canadian statistical and epidemiological information needs to be collected in order to allow for an intersectional analysis of how race, sex, gender and class impact the health and well-being of Black women.

In order to ensure social polices increase awareness of and challenge the impact of discrimination on well-being they should include: (1) mandatory and ongoing training for employers, policymakers and leaders on the impact of discrimination; (2) recruitment of employees across all sectors who reflect the racial diversity of the population; and (3) addressing how professionals deliver services to clients from racially and ethnically diverse populations (Davis-Murdoch, 2005; Etowa, 2007; Seeleman, Suurmond, & Stronks, 2009). This could help to minimize the sense of invisibility experienced by racialized populations (Bernard, 2000, 2001, 2002; Enang, 1999; Etowa, Keddy, Egbeyemi, & Eghan, 2007; Etowa, Thomas, Oyinsan, & Clow, 2007; Krieger, 2003; McGibbon & Etowa, 2009; Sharif, Dar, & Amaratunga, 2000). Many of the women indicated they do not seek professional health care and would rather speak to a family member, friend or their pastor, suggesting the need for an increase of racialized counseling professionals with a specialization in intersectional analysis of health and well-being.

The emotional labor of silence is evident in the stories of the women. The inter-generational trauma of gendered-racism and the resilience of the women is unmistakable in their stories. Yet, there is no place of reprieve from the pain caused by racism, from the pain of being silent or being made to be silent as a form of protection or resistance. The lived experiences of the Black women in this chapter, their strength, resistance, faith and struggle of survival needs to be elevated and shared. Through their stories, the recognition and impact of gendered racism in their lives have been explored: the question remains, what is the next step for societal change?

## Note

1 This chapter reports on Hamilton-Hinch's (2016) secondary data analysis of gender-based racism among Nova Scotian women from the national Racism Violence Health study (James et al., 2010). Of the 120 interviews in the national study, 20 were with Nova Scotian women of African/Black ancestry. It is these women's voices that we draw on here. The semi-structured interviews included open-ended discussion questions that examined these women's experiences of racism as violence.

## References

African and Canadian Legal Clinic. (June, 2015). Civil and political wrongs: The growing gap between international civil and political rights and African Canadian life. *A report on the Canadian Government's compliance with the International Covenant on Civil and Political Rights.* Report presented to the United Nation Human Rights Commission.

Angelou, M. (1969). *I know why the caged bird sings.* Random House.

Beagan, B.L., & Etowa, J.B. (2009). The impact of everyday racism on the occupations of African Canadian women. *Canadian Journal Occupational Therapy, 76*(4), 285–293.

Beagan, B.L., & Etowa, J.B. (2011). The meanings and functions of occupations related to spirituality for African Nova Scotian women. *Journal of Occupational Science, 18*(3), 277–290.

Beagan, B.L., Etowa, J.B., & Bernard, W.T. (2012). "With God in our lives he gives us the strength to carry on": African Nova Scotian women, spirituality, and racism-related stress. *Mental Health, Religion & Culture, 15*(2), 103–120.

Bernard, W.T. (2000). *Beyond inclusion: Diversity in women's health research.* Maritime Centre of Excellence for Women's Health Policy Forum, Halifax, Nova Scotia. Maritime Centre of Excellence for Women's Health.

Bernard, W.T. (2001). *Including Black women in health and social policy development: Winning over addictions, empowering Black mothers with addictions to overcome triple jeopardy.* Maritime Centre of Excellence for Women's Health.

Bernard, W.T. (2002). Beyond inclusion. In C. Amaratunga (Ed.), *Race, ethnicity, and women's health* (pp. 1–14). Halcraft.

Bernard, W.T., & Smith, H. (2018). Injustice, justice, and Africentric practice in Canada. *Canadian Social Work Review*, 35(1), 149–157.

Bryson, J.E., Wilson, J., Plimmer, G., Blumenfeld, S., Donnelly, N., Ku, B., & Ryan, B. (2014). Women workers: Caring, sharing, enjoying their work – or just another gender stereotype? *Labour & Industry: A Journal of the Social and Economic Relations of Work*, 24(40), 258–271.

Codjoe, H. (2001). Fighting a "public enemy" of Black academic achievement – the persistence of racism and the schooling experiences of Black students in Canada. *Race Ethnicity and Education*, 4(4), 343–375.

Collins, P.H. (1990). *Black feminist thought.* Routledge.

Collins, P.H. (2000a). *Black feminist thought: Knowledge, consciousness and the politics of empowerment* (2nd ed.). Routledge.

Collins, P.H. (2000b.) Gender, Black feminism, and Black political economy. *The Annals of the American Academy of Political and Social Science*, (568)4, 41–53.

Crawford, C. (2007). Black women, racing and gendering the Canadian nation. In N. Massaquoi & N.N. Wane (Eds.), *Theorizing empowerment: Canadian perspective on Black feminist thought* (pp. 119–128). INANNA Publications and Education.

Crenshaw, K. (1991). Mapping the margins: Intersectionality, identity politics, and violence against women of color. *Stanford Law Review*, 43(6), 1241–1299

Davis-Murdoch, S. (2005). *A cultural competence guide for primary health care professionals in Nova Scotia.* Unpublished report. https://multiculturalmentalhealth.ca/wp-content/uploads/2019/07/Cultural_Competence_guide_for_Primary_Health_Care_Professionals-Nova-Scotia-.pdf.

DeGruy, J. (2005). *Post traumatic slave syndrome: America's legacy of enduring injury and healing.* Uptone Press.

Dickens, D., & Chavez, E. (2018). Navigating the workplace: The costs and benefits of shifting identities at work among early career US Black women. *Sex Roles*, 78, 760–774.

Dobbins, J., & Skillings, J. (2000). Racism as a clinical syndrome. *American Journal of Orthopsychiatry*, 70(1), 14–27.

Dotson, K. (2011). Tracking epistemic violence, tracking practices of silencing. *Hypatia*, 26(2): 236–257.

Edmonds, S. (2001). *Racism as a determinant of women's health.* Retrieved from http:/// www.yorku.ca/nnewh/english/nnewhind.html.

Enang, J. (1999). The childbirth experiences of African Nova Scotian women. (Unpublished master's thesis). Dalhousie University, Canada.

Essed, P. (1991). *Understanding everyday racism. An interdisciplinary theory.* Sage.

Este, D., & Bernard, W.T. (2006). Spirituality among African Nova Scotians: A key to survival in Canadian society. *Critical Social Work*, 7(1), 1–22

Etowa, J.B. (2005). *Surviving on the Margin of a Profession: Experiences of Black Nurses.* (Unpublished doctoral dissertation). University of Calgary, Canada

Etowa, J. (2007). Negotiating the boundaries of difference in the professional lives of Black nurses. *The International Journal of Diversity in Organizations, Communities and Nations*, 7(3), 214–226.

Etowa, J.B., Beagan, B.L., Eghan, F., & Bernard, W.T. (2017). "You feel you have to be made of steel": The strong Black woman, health, and well-being in Nova Scotia. *Health Care for Women International*, 38(4), 379–393, doi:10.1080/07399332.2017.1290099 http://dx.doi.org/10.1080/07399332.2017.1290099.

Etowa, J., Keddy, B., Beagan, B., Eghan, F., Loppie, C., Bernard, W.T., Davis-Murdoch, S., Gahagan, J., Houston, A., & Edmonds, S. (2005). *Menopause and midlife health of the strong Black women: African Canadian women's perspective.* Health Association of African Canadians, Nova Scotia.

Etowa, J., Keddy, B., Egbeyemi, J., & Eghan, F. (2007). Depression: The "invisible grey fog" influencing the midlife health of African Canadian women. *International Journal of Mental Health Nursing, 16*, 203-213.

Etowa, J., Thomas W.B., Oyinsan, B., & Clow, B. (2007). Participatory action research: An approach for improving Black women's health in rural and remote communities. *Journal of Transcultural Nursing*, 18(4), 349–357.

Etowa, J., Wiens, J., Bernard, T.W., & Clow, B. (2007). Determinants of Black women's health in rural and remote communities. *Canadian Journal of Nursing Research*, 39(3), 56–76.

Fraser, R., & Reddick, T. (1997). *Black women's health program: Building Black women's capacity on health.* Final report. North End Community Health Center, Halifax, Nova Scotia.

Fricker, M. (2010). *Epistemic injustice. Power and the ethics of knowing.* Oxford University Press.

Gaunt, R. (2013). Ambivalent sexism and perceptions of men and women who violate gendered family roles. *Community, Work & Family*, 16(4), 401–416.

Gee, G.C., Walsemann, M.K., & Brondolo, E. (2012). A life course perspective on how racism may be related to health inequities. *American Journal of Public Health*, 102(5), 967–974.

Hamilton-Hinch, B. (2016). Surviving the impact of the experience of racism on health and well-being: An exploration of women of African ancestry living in Nova Scotia. (Unpublished doctoral dissertation.) Dalhousie University.

Henry, A. (1993). Missing: Black self-representations in Canadian educational research. *Canadian Journal of Education*, 18(3), 206–222.

Henry, A. (2015). "We especially welcome application from members of visible minority groups": Reflections on race, gender, and life at three universities. *Race Ethnicity and Education*, 1–13.

hooks, b. (2000). *Feminist theory: From margin to center.* Pluto Press.

hooks, b. (2003). *Rock my soul: Black people and self-esteem.* Atria Books.

Jackson, F., & Naidoo, K. (2012). "Lemeh check see if meh mask on straight": Examining how Black women of Caribbean descent in Canada manage depression and construct womanhood through being strong. *Southern Journal of Canadian Studies*, 5(1–20), 223–240

James, C. (2012). *Life at the intersection: Community, class and schooling.* Fernwood Publishing.

James, C., Este, D., Bernard, W.T, Benjamin, A. Lloyd, B., & Turner, T. (2010). *Race & well-being: The lives, hopes and activism of African Canadians.* Fernwood Publishing.

Jones, C., & Shorter-Gooden, K. (2003). *Shifting: The double lives of Black women in America.* Harper Collins.

Jones, L. (2008). Preventing depression: Culturally relevant work with Black women. *Research on Social Work Practice,* 18(6), 626–634.

Juster, R.P., & Lupien, S. (2012). A sex-and gender-based analysis of allostatic load and physical complaints. *Gender Medicine,* 9(6), 511–523.

Krieger, N. (2003). Does racism harm health? Did child abuse exist before 1962? On explicit questions, critical science, and current controversies: An ecosocial perspective. *American Journal of Public Health,* 93, 194–199.

Lorde, A. (1984). Age, race, class, and sex: Women redefining difference. In *Essays and speeches* (pp. 114–123). The Crossing Press.

Lynam, J.M., & Cowley, S. (2007). Understanding marginalization as a social determinant of health. *Critical Public Health,* 17(2), 137–149.

McGibbon, E., & Etowa, J. (2009). *Anti-racist health care practice.* Canadian Scholars Press.

Maxwell, J. (2012). Leveraging the courts to protect women's fundamental rights at the intersection of family-wage work structures and women's role as wage earner and primary caregiver. *Duke Journal of Gender Law & Policy,* 20(1), 127–172.

Mogadime, D. (2008). Racial differential experiences of employment equity for women teachers: One teacher's narrative of resistance and struggle. *Journal of Black Studies,* 39(1), 85–108.

Office of African Nova Scotian Affairs. (2014). *African Nova Scotia Affairs Statistics and Research.* Retrieved from https://ansa.novascotia.ca/sites/default/files/inline/documents/ansa-stats-research-2014-11.pdf.

Raphael, D. (Ed.). (2004, 2009). *Social determinants of health: Canadian* perspective (2nd ed.). Canadian Scholars Press.

Rice, C. (2010). *Extraordinary, ordinary people: A memoir of family.* Crown Publishers.

Schatzki, R.T., & Natter, W. (Eds.). (1996). *The social and political body.* Guilford Press.

Seeleman, C., Suurmond, J., & Stronks, K. (2009). Cultural competence: A conceptual framework for teaching and learning. *Medical Education,* 43, 229–237

Sharif, J.R., Dar, A.A., & Amaratunga, C. (2000). *Ethnicity, income and access to health care in the Atlantic region: A synthesis of literature.* Maritime Centre of Excellence for Women's Health: IWK Grace Health Centre.

Spivak, G. (1998). Can the subaltern speak? In C. Nelson & L. Grossberg (Eds.), *Marxism and the interpretation of culture* (pp. 271–313). University of Illinois Press

Thomas, A., Hacker, J., & Hoxha, J. (2011). Gendered racial identity of Black young women. *Sex Roles,* 64(7), 530–542.

Utsey, S.O., Bolden, M.A., Williams III, O., Lee, A., Lanier, Y., & Newsome, C. (2007). Spiritual well-being as a mediator of the relation between culture-specific coping and quality of life in a community sample of African Americans. *Journal of Cross-Cultural Psychology,* 38(2), 123–136.

Veenstra, G. (2009). Racialized identity and health in Canada: Results from a nationally representative survey. *Social Science & Medicine,* 68, 538–542.

Waldron, I. (2012). Out from the margins: Centring African-centred knowledge in psychological discourse. *The Australian Community Psychologist,* 24(1), 38–51.

Waldron, I.R.G. (2019). Archetypes of Black womanhood: Implications for mental health, coping and help-seeking. In M. Zangeneh and A. Al-Krenawi (Eds.), *Culture, diversity and mental health: Enhancing clinical practice* (pp. 21–38), Springer.

Waldron, I.R.G. (2020). Black women's experiences with mental illness, help-seeking and coping in the Halifax regional municipality: a study conducted to inform NSHA's Nova Scotia Sisterhood Initiative. Dalhousie University.

Waldron, I.R.G. (2021). The wounds that do not heal: Black expendability and the traumatizing aftereffects of anti-Black police violence. *Equality, Diversity and Inclusion: An International Journal*, 40(1), 29–40. doi: 10.1108/EDI-06-2020-0175.

Wallace, D., & Bell, A. (1999). Being Black at a predominantly White university. *College English*, 61(3), 307–327.

Wells-Wilbon, R. (2021). Reclaiming our right to wholeness and wellness. In R. Wells-Wilbon & A. Estreet (Eds.), *Trauma and mental health social work with urban populations: African-centered clinical interventions*. Routledge.

West, L., Donovan, R., & Daniel, A. (2016). The price of strength: Black college women's perspectives on the strong Black women stereotype. *Women & Therapy*, 39, 390–412.

Wharton, A.S., & Erickson, R. (1995). The consequences of caring: Exploring the links between women's job and family emotion work. *The Sociological Quarterly*, 36(2), 273–296.

Williams, D.R., & Sternthal, M. (2010). Understanding racial-ethnic disparities in health: Sociological contributions. *Journal of Health and Social Behavior*, 51, 15–S27.

Williams, D.R., & Williams-Morris, R. (2010). Racism and mental health: The African American experience. *Ethnicity & Health*, 5(3–4), 243–268.

World Health Organization (WHO). (1948). Preamble to the Constitution of WHO as adopted by the International Health Conference, New York, June19 –July 22,1946; signed on July 22, 1946, by the representatives of 61 States (Official Records of WHO, no. 2, p. 100) and entered into force on April 7, 1948.

World Health Organization. (2001). *WHO's contribution to the world conference against racism, racial discrimination, xenophobia and related intolerance: Health and freedom from discrimination*. Health & Human Rights Publication Series (2). Retrieved from http://www.who.int/hhr/activities/q_and_a/en/Health_and_Freedom_from_ Discrimination_English_699KB.pdf.

World Health Organization. (2014). *Social determinants of mental health*. World Health Organization.

Wortley, S., & Owusu-Bempah, A. (2011). The usual suspects: Police stop and search practices in Canada. *Policing and Society*, 21(4), 395–407.

Wright Myers, L. (2002). *A broken silence: Voices of African American women in the academy*. Praeger.

Yosso, T.J., & Solórzano, D.G. (2005). In M. Romero & E. Margolis (Eds.), *The Blackwell companion to social inequalities* (pp. 117–146). Blackwell Publishing.

# 12

# ALWAYS POLITICAL – INDIGENEITY, COLONIZATION AND TRAUMA WORK

## Reclaiming Worldviews

*Mareese Terare*

## Introduction

The common assumption that all people should be free and equal in dignity and rights is embedded in the United Nations (UN) Human Rights, "Article 1: All human beings are born free and equal in dignity and rights" (United Nations General Assembly, 1948). This reality is far from this truth for many Australians, and, more specifically, First Nations women, who experience institutional and interpersonal/intimate partner violence.[1] The extent of institutional and interpersonal violence like domestic violence trauma experiences is extremely high in Australia generally and more specifically in Australian First Nations communities and families (Australian Institute of Health and Welfare, 2018, 2023).[2] Institutional violence and trauma must be considered within the Australian sociopolitical and historical context. This context relates to post-1788, and, more recently, the post-1901 Federation of Australia – the historical experiences of colonization and genocide enacted on First Nations Australians. The legislation "Immigration Restriction Act 1901 or Immigration Restriction Bill 1901" (Australian House of Representatives, 1901), ensured the ongoing oppression, colonization and genocide against First Nations Australians as well as ensuring Australia is nationally and internationally defined as a White nation.

This chapter will discuss the implications and outcomes of colonization, or more specifically genocidal, policies, which sanctioned severing of connection and relatedness to First Nations worldviews to ensure a White Australia. The wisdoms of Aunty Lilla Watson resonate the aim of this chapter: "If you have come to help me you are wasting your time. But if you have come because your liberation is bound with mine, then let us work together" (Watson, circa 1985).

DOI: 10.4324/9781003379591-13

Trauma is defined as an event or process that overwhelms an individual, a family or a community and the ability to cope in mind, body, soul and spirit. Trauma is often the effect of violent crime and a violation of human rights. It is critical to understand the impact of trauma on First Nations women and families.

The characteristics within human services to address human rights violations against First Nations people (including institutional/systemic violence; racism, discrimination and implicit bias and interpersonal violence; family/domestic violence, sexual assault and child maltreatment – neglect and physical, sexual, emotional and psychological harm of children and young people) will be discussed within the context of the right to culturally safe responses.

This chapter will discuss and define the nature of complex and compounded trauma and First Nations Australians' experiences, the implications and uncertainty of this on the capacity of human and community services to provide equitable access to First Nations women. First Nations people are highly represented regarding trauma/violence experiences, family/domestic violence, sexual assault and child maltreatment (including neglect and physical and emotional abuse). The extent of interpersonal traumas such as domestic violence within First Nations communities is extreme.

Within the National Aboriginal and Torres Strait Islander Survey (NATSISS), the section on Aboriginal and Torres Strait Islander Women's Experiences of Family and Domestic Violence quotes Tracey Dillon (Chief Executive Officer, South East Tasmanian Aboriginal Corporation), who states, "Abused and battered mother, abused and battered kids, abused and battered grandparents, abused and battered generation. It sticks with you for generations and doesn't leave. It becomes an acceptable practice. In my work I've seen violence in different generations of our people."

Reporting on family and domestic violence it was found that, in the past year, 1 in 10 (10 percent) of Indigenous women had experienced family and domestic violence. Women in the age groups 25–34 years and 35–44 years were most likely to have experienced family and domestic violence (at 14 percent). It is further reported that more than two-thirds (72 percent) of the women who experienced violence identified an intimate partner or family member as at least one of the perpetrators in their most recent experience. In comparison, the rate reported by Aboriginal and Torres Strait Islander men was 35 percent. Research consistently shows that those who experienced physical violence reported that the perpetrator of the most recent incident was a family member, including a current or previous partner (Australian Bureau of Statistics, 2013, 2016, 2022a, 2022b; Australian Human Rights Commission, 2017; Australian Health Ministers' Advisory Council, 2017).

In the survey on Aboriginal and Torres Strait Islander Women's Experiences of Family and Domestic Violence (2014–2015) almost 6 in 10 (57 percent) women who had experienced family and domestic violence endured physical injuries. In the study, women who had experienced family and domestic violence were more likely than women who had not experienced any physical violence to experience at least one long-term health condition (79 percent compared with 68 percent) or to experience mental health concerns (53 percent compared with 31 percent); they were also less likely to rate their own health as excellent or very good (27 percent compared with 38 percent) or to experience homelessness at some time in their lives (55 percent compared with 26 percent); and alter their overall life satisfaction rating. The life satisfaction rating among women who had experienced family and domestic violence was 6.2, which was lower than the rating of 7.4 out of 10 for women who had not experienced domestic violence. There is no question that experiences of violence and trauma have a significant impact on Indigenous women's lives. The report quotes Cheryl Axleby, Co-Chair, National Aboriginal and Torres Strait Islander Legal Services who emphasizes that it is important to "ensure survivors of family violence have access to Aboriginal and Torres Strait Islander community-controlled, culturally safe services that can negotiate with police, courts and child protection services on their behalf".

The ongoing annihilation of First Nations knowledge within colonial constructs provides us with two options: (1) to maintain the status quo of oppression and living out the indoctrinated worldview, or (2) to continue ongoing decolonizing by reinforcing commitment to human rights and reclaiming worldviews. Fast-forward and we are seeing the rates of experiences of violence and trauma increase, yet only slight improvements in human services addressing the extent of violence and applying First Nations worldviews to policy and practice frameworks.

## Worldviews

It is important to understand First Nations worldviews when providing a service to First Nations people, more specifically to people who are surviving within colonial and Western structures, where colonization is continuing, and genocidal practices were enacted. Genocidal practice under the guise of colonial rule came about in the invasion of Australia in 1788 and the enactment of laws to stop First Nations people practicing their worldviews, their knowledge, beliefs and ceremonies. First Nations people were legislatively forbidden and systemically discouraged to speak their tribal language.

We often hear the term "worldviews", but rarely do we understand the nature and significance of it in the human services. In the Australian human service sector, worldview is being referenced to define the way First Nations or Aboriginal people live in the world and that this lens is different to a Western or colonial way of looking at the world. Worldviews in this context refer to an inherent human right. Wilson (2001) describes worldviews or epistemology as what we know, ontology what we believe and axiology what we do.

Sherwood explains worldviews as "frameworks for interpreting and exploring the world, supporting the way we act and relate to our world" (Sherwood, 2010, p. 57). I concur. In essence, worldviews inform how one sees, interacts and engages in the world. Different Australian nations/tribes had their individual worldviews, which explain their definition and the significance of relatedness, often articulated differently. However, commonalities also surround their epistemology – ways of knowing. This ensured that elders were revered, and children were collectively loved, cared for, nurtured and protected (Terare, 2020). Children were respected and trusted to learn from their actions. Mother Earth and all her connections provided the opportunity for reciprocal responsibilities to love care and protect her entities (Martin, 2009).

"Worldview" defines what is important and provides core understandings of what is right and what is wrong for individuals and communities. Taken-for-granted, everyday accepted ways of how to communicate and behave within certain social groups, societies and cultures are all part of the way of knowing. Among First Nations worldviews, this allowed for ontological principles: caring, connections, belonging and relatedness are established and practiced, ensuring survival of the individual, family and tribe/nation.

Human services generally practice from a White/Western lens without scope of change of altering service delivery to meet First Nations needs – they are leaving their policy and practice frameworks open for interpretation as not being accessible or potentially racist to First Nations women. This could explain the lack of access to human services around domestic violence.

### Nature and Extent of Violence

The worldwide movement against gendered violence started with the women's movement in the early 1970s. Fast-forward to the 1980s and 1990s when the emergence of grassroots Aboriginal women's movements across Australia provided agency for governments to act against the scourge of interpersonal violence. Most governments provided funding to explore the extent of violence in First Nations communities. This led commonwealth, state and territory governments to explore the cause, extent and prevalence of sexual assault, domestic violence and child maltreatment within First Nations families and communities.

Australian states and territories commissioned numerous reports exploring the prevalence and extent of interpersonal violence impacting First Nations people (domestic violence, sexual assault and child maltreatment) (Anderson and Wild, 2007; Australian Law Reform Commission, 2010, 2011; Centre for Aboriginal Health, 2011; Commonwealth of Australia, 1997; D'Eatough, 2002; New South Wales Attorney General's Department – Aboriginal, 2006) New South Wales Department of Health, 2010; New South Wales Department for Women, 1996; Robertson, 2000; Victorian Indigenous Family Violence Task Force, 2003).

Australian New South Wales legislation surrounding domestic violence states that is a crime to physically assault, sexually assault, stalk, intimidate, coerce, harass, kidnap, deprive of liberty or breach a protection order (Australian Law Reform Commission, 2011). Each state and/or territory have their respective laws and legislation, like New South Wales, prohibiting domestic violence. The offences include, for example, murder, manslaughter, wounding or causing grievous bodily harm with intent, assault, sexual assault, kidnapping, child abduction and destroying or damaging property. This also includes narrower offences such as discharging a firearm with intent, causing bodily injury by gunpowder, or setting traps (Australian Law Reform Commission, 2011). Generally, offences include a set of behaviors that are used to maintain control of another person. Put simply, they are actions that completely violate women and children's (where there are children) human rights.

Violence against women and children is a significant problem and has reached epidemic proportions (Marcus & Braaf, 2007). We are losing up to one woman every ten days to homicide (Serpell, Sullivan, & Doherty, 2022). They are usually murdered by a man they know, whereby the majority are from intimate relationships or have become recently separated. In 2021, girls between the ages of 10 and 17 made up 42 percent of female sexual assault cases (Australian Bureau Statistics, 2022a). One in three women have experienced physical abuse since the age of 15, and one in five have experienced sexual abuse (Australian Bureau Statistics, 2022a). Women are more likely to experience violence at different stages through their life – and they are often at risk of violence when they are pregnant or separating from a relationship (Australian Institute of Health & Welfare, 2018).

The statistics are staggering. They clearly demonstrate the need to do better at keeping all women and children safe from domestic violence. However, what we know is that First Nations women experience intimate partner violence at even higher rates than any other Australian group. This has been consistent across three decades. Lawrie and Matthews, in their report to the New South Wales Attorney General, found the extent of violence against women to be highest in Aboriginal communities (Lawrie & Matthews, 2002). Marcus and Braaf (2007) found a combination of oppressive and violent experiences were prevalent in Indigenous communities and families. Rethinking human services delivery to First Nations communities is critical, especially with regard to experiences of interpersonal violence (sexual assault, family violence and child abuse). Indigenous women reported three times as many life-changing incidents of sexual violence than non-Indigenous women. New South Wales Health found "Aboriginal females are twelve times more likely to be hospitalized due to violence compared to the non-Aboriginal population" (New South Wales Department of Health, 2010, p. 7).

The "Heroines of fortitude" evaluation report by the New South Wales Women's Department (1996) found extremely disturbing information about the treatment of women who were witnesses in sexual assault cases generally. Further, cross-examination experiences were overtly excessive for Aboriginal women. Aboriginal women were cross-examined for longer periods and ultimately required more breaks due to the level of their distress. Cross-examination questions reflected extensive reference to the women's alcohol use. Narratives of "Aboriginal women as promiscuous, drunken liars" were evident (Puren, 1997,

p. 138). The cross-examination practices reflect the omnipresence of racism in Australia, where the defense counsel "rely explicitly on racist and sexist stereotypes of Aboriginal women, which the right of the accused to 'a fair trial' apparently legitimates" (ibid., p. 137). This information is challenging, to say the least, and glaringly indicates our need to do better.

In my own research, First Nations human service workers identified key issues about the status of Aboriginal women around racism and sexism in the trauma context. They identify five themes that guide their practice: belonging, connections, always being political, sharing knowledge and challenging theories. Aboriginal women are significantly overrepresented in their frequent experiences of domestic violence and sexual assault (Terare, 2020). First Nations human service workers also expressed significant concern about the shockingly high rates of imprisonment for First Nations women. While we want to believe that all women are equal, and/or women are equal to men, it is clear when we look at Aboriginal women's experiences of violence and trauma that they are not treated equally.

## Sociopolitical and Historical Contexts

Deeper and broader understandings of the historical and political contexts affecting diverse communities is essential for effective human service practice frameworks. Policy and practice approaches should reflect the needs revealed by research findings. This is even more critical when working with Australian First Nations people, whose countries have been colonized and where genocidal policies have been part of their clans' and families' history. This is critical knowledge to understand when providing services.

Key knowledge includes understanding trauma generally and, more specifically, understanding the nature and definition of compound, complex and cumulative trauma where institutional and systemic violence is significant due to historical contexts. The extent of institutional violence on First Nations people is evident in the high rates of social issues, including high rates of incarceration of both adult and children (Enns, 2016).

## Institutional and Systemic Violence/Trauma

The effects of trauma associated with violence on Aboriginal people are profound and can be linked to the current health status of adults. Racism denies us access to and equity within human service provision (Herring, Spangaro, Lauw, & McNamara, 2013; Parter et al., 2021; Gatwiri, Rotumah, & Rix, 2021). Australia's colonial history and the co-existing ideologies have provided the foundation for oppression, abuse and ongoing human rights violations against Aboriginal people. This history of violence and oppression includes being removed from the country and herded into missions; Aboriginal babies and children being abducted; the massacre of clans; and the forbidding and outlawing of traditional practices of culture and ways of knowing (Terare, 2020). The pathologization of Aboriginal people defines them as the "problem". Aboriginal struggles are individualized and decontextualized. This dominant approach reflects a White/Western lens and adopts ongoing paternalistic colonial constructs and services policy and practice frameworks that are not effective in working with First Nations people.

Racist practices within mainstream human services are rarely considered within trauma discourses. When racism is ignored and not discussed, Aboriginal and Torres Strait Islander people experience disproportionate adverse impacts across human services, including the whole spectrum of the justice system. This includes discriminatory and racist policing practices, intergenerational trauma and systemic failures leading to the gross overrepresentation of First Nations people, especially males, in the prison system (Australian Bureau of Statistics, 2014–2015a, 2014–2015b).

Given the extent of violence against Aboriginal women and the omnipresence of racism in service users' communities, the human service providers who participated in my research (Terare, 2020) have insisted that historical knowledge is essential and must underpin the development and application of practice frameworks for trauma. This includes an extensive understanding and knowledge of the destructive and adverse events that took place post-1788 by colonialists, including the declaration of Terra Nullius (land belonging to no one), to ensure the colonization of Australian First Nations people, their families and communities.

The assimilation era – now known as the Stolen Generations – were devastating to First Nations people and culture. During these times child abduction was established as a way of "breeding out the race" under the guise of offering the children protection through the "Aboriginal Protection Board". The 1915 amendments to the Aborigines Protection Act 1909 extended the power of the government and their helpers to remove any child at any time and for any reason. Helpers in this context are those who followed the instructions of the government in power, including human services workers and members religious and other groups. The rationale for the forced removal of Aboriginal children from their parents was part of a broader policy framework known as assimilation. White Australians had convinced themselves that Aboriginal people were a "dying race", and that those remaining, especially those of mixed parentage, would be better off assimilated into "White" society (Commonwealth of Australia, 1997).

Indeed, First Nations families, clans and communities experienced systemic criminal actions of having their babies and children abducted. The abduction of babies and children left parents, families and clans devasted. The effects are still experienced today. Babies and children were sent to training homes, run mostly by religious groups, to prepare the girls for domestic servitude and the boys for hard labor.

## Cumulative, Compounded and Complex Trauma

We need to recognize and address the impact of cumulative, compounded historical and political institutional abuse alongside ongoing violence and the lack of access to adequate culturally safe human services. When First Nations people's human rights continue to be violated, women experiencing violence and abuse have no safe place to go. A lack of access to adequate health care and protection within the criminal justice system leads women to try escape with their children to a safe place within their extended family or friends. This is not always appropriate or secure, as family does not always understand or know how to respond to women and children who have been violated in a safe and secure way – a way that supports their well-being. Although unintended, this can create more stress for the women and their children. The combination of traumas created by historical abuse, lack of access to safe, appropriate health and justice services and support, domestic violence, set alongside a sense of isolation and fear of being judged, creates profound insidious cumulative and compound trauma. Cumulative, compounded trauma, or exposure to multiple traumas, can lead to more complex symptoms or effects (Cloitre et al., 2009).

Complex or post-traumatic stress disorder (PTSD) trauma reactions are often expressed through intrusive, avoidant or constrictive and hyperarousal reactions. According to Herman (1992b) intrusive reactions include dreams/nightmares, flashbacks, obsessive thoughts, physiological reactions, and other ways of re-experiencing traumatic events. Often in reaction to the difficulty and persistence of intrusive reaction, people develop avoidant reactions that help to numb them from the persistence and intensity of intrusive thoughts, feelings and memories related to trauma. And hyperarousal reactions or hypervigilance is a form of self-protection, where a traumatized person is watchful and on the alert for any future danger. They may find themselves having difficulty concentrating in all these responses. The backward-and-forward relationship between intrusion and constriction is referred to as the dialectic of trauma (Herman, 1992b), which can impact on one's sense of self and consciousness.

There can be a tremendous sense of overall loss and pain, which may include a loss of confidence in oneself, and significant loss or distrust in the family, community and human services or government (Wagner, Wolfe, Rotnitsky, Proctor, & Erickson, 2000). This can lead to chronic social and emotional struggles. These struggles are often pathologized as individual problems through a *Diagnostic and Statistical Manual of Mental Disorders* (DSM-5) diagnosis (American Psychiatric Association, 2013), which does not account for the social context of domestic violence or the ongoing impact of historical trauma and colonial violence. This approach is unlikely to be helpful.

## What has Worked?

Effective practice with people who have experienced institutional and interpersonal trauma such as domestic violence generally requires a unique set of skills that directly respond to contextualized individual and community needs. Knowledge and understanding of a communities' sociohistorical and political context is more likely to support and develop effective policy and practice frameworks. When working with First Nations people we need to be open to learning about and listening to their individual needs through cultural humility and genuine listening. In Bundjalung language we call this *ningenah* ("shush and listen") (Terare, 2020). My research with Australian First Nations human services workers, both male and female, found that when working with First Nations people and their communities around sensitive issues like domestic violence, sexual assault and child maltreatment, they need to work from human rights policy and practice frameworks.

Research participants who work with interpersonal trauma described clear links and deep understanding of human rights and extended that to the nature of humanity, as it was linked to participants' ancestral way and identity. This approach emphasized the need for human service values to be based on a commitment to equality. This led to an understanding that the effects of social political/historical legacies are often pathologized and fail to be understood as inter- and transgenerational trauma (Atkinson, 2002; Menzies, 2019; Terare, 2020). Effective interactive communication approaches reflected an emphasis on equality and collaboration with attention to positive, supportive body language and on challenging barriers to access and equity. Research participants were unwavering about the challenges they saw within their agencies regarding access and equity for First Nations clients and support for First Nations colleagues. They strongly argued that managers and colleagues were unclear and uncertain about how to appropriately recognize the needs of diverse communities and how to provide services among First Nations people, specifically about the worldviews of First Nations people (Terare, 2020, p. 110). They also had very little understanding of complex trauma and how this plays out with First Nations people experiencing domestic violence.

The research draws compelling links from historical contexts to current social emotional well-being issues of grief and loss. "You've got to go back – for us to be able to come through everything – you have to pinpoint where the trauma started" (ibid., p. 103). Historical and intergenerational trauma extends across oppressed social groups and deeply impacts contemporary First Nations families. Menzies (2019) states:

It was first conceptualized in relation to Holocaust survivors and their families and has since been recognized in a range of other racial or ethnic groups who have experienced extreme violence, segregation, economic deprivation and cultural dispossession, such as Cambodians, Palestinians, and colonized Indigenous peoples.

*(p. 2)*

Historical knowledge is essential and must underpin the development and application of policy and practice frameworks. This knowledge impacts greatly on women and their families and is important to working in the area of domestic violence and complex trauma. The nature and prevalence of racism in the shape of institutional trauma in Australia is rarely publicly discussed outside of those that experience it. The intergenerational traumatic experience is rarely discussed and understood as a trauma experience and, further, needs to be understood in relation to ongoing oppression and violence against women and children. Too often intergenerational and complex trauma is interpreted as an individual acute reaction rather than a reaction firmly situated in a sociopolitical and historical context. Frequently, the historical and contemporary context of First Nations people can produce chronic health problems that impact their overall social, emotional and physical well-being.

Research participants identified their client's common experiences of institutional racism, and these experiences were not limited to individuals, as these adverse experiences also impacted on their families (Terare, 2020). If a human service practitioner has been racist, it is this unsafe and oppressive practice that is remembered and subsequently these services are avoided (ibid.).

The aim of human service practice according to First Nations service practitioners is to ensure that humane policy and practice frameworks include the principle of connection and working collaboratively. Social connection from a First Nations worldview is reflected in meaningful and purposeful relationships. It extends beyond initial engagement to the development of respectful, transparent and honest processes of establishing and maintaining connections.

The research participants' First Nations identity supports their practice, and their worldview supports their understanding of the importance of their knowledge and understanding of identity and the nature of sharing, caring and respect. Their practice is based on the ethos of human rights, equity and justice for all First Nations people. More specifically supporting those living or escaping personal war zones, to justly access service. "Always political" is one of the themes that arose from the research. Research participants defined their work as "always political" by working to disrupt and change oppressive systems. The very nature of "understanding Aboriginal people in context of human rights and equity by understanding the histories", establishes the principle of "always political" work (Terare, 2020, p. 110).

Research participants are determined to develop policy and practice frameworks that empower and/or re-empower. Through their optimism they develop a clear path for the future by clearly defining their roles and responsibilities. They identify attitudes and values of working innovatively, proactively and collaboratively to meet the needs of their target group. The key to establishing successful work across their scope of service delivery extends to counseling, the facilitation of women and men's "yarning circles" and participating in proactive and collaborative community development projects. Yarning circles in this context relate to the development of cultural safety, which is critical to their practice. The reality of not relying on governments and bureaucracy to meet their clients' needs is a classic example of research participants' empowerment and re-empowerment. They work toward self-determination, which provides them with purpose. According to Terare and Rawsthorne (2020), "Yarning is Australian First Nations people storytelling and is based on reciprocal relations where respect is assumed. The contribution within yarning is guided by individuals and can consists of loud and silent energy" (p. 953).

Research participants aim to support and encourage clients to consider where they come from pre-invasion and colonization. This allows clients to deeply reflect on their sovereign power and that respective countries have never been ceded. The "always political" principle is demonstrated by research participants' practice, which consists of strategies based on empowerment, reinforcing rights and healing, to move forward from their current issues – the importance of applying a practice framework for First Nations people where empowerment is key. They discuss the nature of power and what this looks like. This is where they can define with intent to mitigate power dynamics. Their vision is to provide opportunities for clients to re-create their futures. Continuing themes in our yarning circles were reclaiming personal autonomy and self-determination. The belief that everyone has the right to be treated equally is foundational in their approach to developing policy and establishing practice frameworks.

This process recognizes equity and social justice as key practices that must be incorporated in policy development. This is especially crucial when working with Australian First Nations people, and especially those women, men and children who are experiencing interpersonal violence. The importance of human rights and First Nations worldviews – epistemologies – ways of knowing, ontologies (ways of being) and axiology (ways of doing) are foundational and fundamental to providing service to First Nations women' experience domestic violence.

## Cultural Safety and Cultural Humility

### Cultural Safety

Extending the wisdoms and work of Ramsden (2002) and Williams (1999), the First Nations service practitioners who participated in this research argued that First Nations groups are marginalized and, as a result, have had every aspect of their human rights violated. The framework of cultural safety and cultural humility emerged as a way forward. Their provision of services relied on developing safe and secure relationships with clients and their families. Cultural safety is in essence about ensuring human service workers make sure their structures and systems are culturally responsive and that they feel safe and secure in their personal, social and professional spheres (Papps & Ramsden, 1996). Feeling safe is possible when there is no attack on your being. I am emphasizing several principles in this process: (1)

Cultural safety is important. It is a basic human right to be treated equally within the context of your culture. This is especially important for groups that do not fit into the popular/dominant culture. (2) Cultural safety provides "opportunities" for people to critique, engage, debate and discuss relevant issues like ideologies and social structure that reify racism, sexism, homophobia, "classism" and ableism without fear of retribution. And (3) Overall cultural safety enhances human rights. Cultural safety is measured by the enhancement of human rights (Terare, 2019).

### Cultural Humility

Cultural humility requires personal commitment to ensure skills and knowledge are constantly updated and reflective of a target group's needs. The research participants follow the three dimensions outlined by Tervalon and Garcia (1998), which include lifelong learning and self-reflection and mitigate power imbalance and institutional accountability.

Critical self-reflection is key to responsive practice, where we deeply reflect on aspects of our practice that may need revising. This is essential terms of reference to ensure we are aware of our professional development needs and that they respond to relevant emerging research findings. Service accountability is key to good practice. We need policy frameworks that are responsive to the needs of the clients, which are informed by current reliable and authentic research.

Lifelong learning includes an awareness that we are not experts – only partial knowers. This encourages comfort in seeking new knowledge and skills and ongoing growth, especially if people feel out of their depth. This process initiates client-focused approaches. When service providers are stuck or uncertain about what to do, they may, problematically, focus on the client as deficient. Seeking ongoing support either via different learning environments, like classroom or yarning circles or via cultural or clinical supervision, may be helpful.

Mitigating power is key to social justice and human rights. Human service workers in essence are duty bearers for human rights. While important to all human service work, this is especially critical for child protection in First Nations communities given historical trauma in child protection. Similarly, being a duty bearer for human rights applies to working with mothers and women who have experienced violence and abuse.

The nature and characteristics of cultural humility includes being open to learning; developing an ability to express feeling; adopting a human equity and rights philosophical approach; understanding the connection between knowledge, power and privilege and the importance or disrupting and challenging unhelpful, oppressive discourse and practice; a commitment to social justice; establishment of self-agency in order to advocate for social change; ongoing commitment to work toward inclusive equity and equality; and willingness to learn from diversity and difference.

## Conclusion

This chapter has argued that responses to institutional abuse and domestic violence trauma affecting Australian First Nations women requires the incorporation of Indigenous worldviews. First Nation worldviews are not currently articulated as a critical component within the trauma field. Trauma-informed practice ideas emphasize connection, developing therapeutic alliances and relationships, and working collaboratively, especially where there has been relational injury (Herman, 1992a, 1992b, 1998, 2015). A focus on connections is a significant principle embedded in a First Nations worldview. It is important to consider how violence and abuse has created a trauma response, also in the context of other historical forms of abuse. Services need to reflect on their strengths and deficits in the context of access and equity for First Nations women and their families. Women are not the deficit. Service providers also need to identify and reflect on positions of privilege that may impact on clients.

First Nations women survivors of domestic violence need to be able to access human services that have a deep understanding of First Nation worldviews and the sociohistorical and political context that has impacted greatly on First Nations people (aspects of these strategies may also support all women). In line with self-determination and re-empowerment, service providers need to be guided by their clients' worldviews – their ways of knowing about what services they need. Supporting clients to reclaim their First Nations worldview is a strategy to re-empower – this may provide a client with a sense of meaning and purpose.

Cultural safety and cultural humility are important ways forward. Human service workers need to encompass practice and knowledge and understanding of human rights and what it means to have these rights continuously violated. Services need to demonstrate their ability to decolonize aspects of their service delivery. Whilst flying the flag and having Aboriginal arts and crafts visible is helpful, services can extend this to developing cultural safety and maintaining cultural humility and congruency. Demonstrating publicly the importance of resistance to colonial ways supports the ongoing resilience of First Nations people. First Nations human service workers acknowledge this within equity and social justice frameworks by reclaiming their tribal strengths from over 65,000 years of living in the moment.

## Notes

1  I will be using the term domestic violence and this relates to intimate partner abuse where gender roles play a big part; males are primarily the offenders and females are primarily the victims. This does not mean that all males are offenders, nor does it mean that all females are victims. I will be using the terms First Nations and Aboriginal interchangeably to refer to Australian First Nations people.
2  Although most of my work has focused on women and children, I am aware of the challenge for services to provide accessible and relevant support to First Nations men

as well. The experiences of male children, male community members and male human service workers need their voices heard.

## References

American Psychiatric Association. (2013). *Diagnostic and statistical manual of mental disorders* (5th ed.). https://doi.org/10.1176/appi.books.9780890425596.

Anderson, P., & Wild, R. (2007). *Ampe Akelyernemane Meke Mekarle ("Little children are sacred")*: Report of the Northern Territory Board of Inquiry into the protection of Aboriginal children from sexual abuse. https://apo.org.au/sites/default/files/resource-files/2007-06/apo-nid8402.pdf.

Atkinson, J. (2002). *Trauma trails, recreating song lines: The transgenerational effects of trauma in Indigenous Australia*. Spinifex Press.

Australian Bureau of Statistics (ABS). (2013). Defining the data challenge for family, domestic and sexual violence. https://www.abs.gov.au/statistics/people/crime-and-justice/defining-data-challenge-family-domestic-and-sexual-violence/latest-release.

Australian Bureau of Statistics. (2014–2015a). National Aboriginal and Torres Strait Islander social survey (NATSISS). Aboriginal and Torres Strait Islander women's experiences of family and domestic violence. http://www.abs.gov.au/AUSSTATS/abs@.nsf/mf/4714.0.

Australian Bureau of Statistics. (2014–2015b). National Aboriginal and Torres Strait Islander Social Survey (NATSISS). http://www.abs.gov.au/AUSSTATS/abs@.nsf/mf/4714.0.

Australian Bureau of Statistics. (2016). Personal safety survey (PSS): Statistics for family, domestic, sexual violence, physical assault, partner emotional abuse, child abuse, sexual harassment, stalking and safety. https://www.abs.gov.au/statistics/people/crime-and-justice/personal-safety-australia/2016.

Australian Bureau Statistics. (2022a). Personal safety, Australia (2021–2022). Recorded crime. https://www.abs.gov.au/statistics/people/crime-and-justice/personal-safety-australia/2021-22.

Australian Bureau of Statistics. (2022b). Personal safety, Australia (2021–2022). https://www.abs.gov.au/statistics/people/crime-and-justice/personal-safety-australia/latest-release.

Australian Health Ministers' Advisory Council. (2017). Aboriginal and Torres Strait Islander Health Performance Framework 2017 Report, AHMAC, Canberra. http://www.dpmc.gov.au/hpf.

Australian House of Representatives. (1901). Immigration Restriction Act. https://www.legislation.gov.au/C1901A00017/asmade/text.

Australian Human Rights Commission, (2017). Annual report 2016–2017.

Australian Institute of Health and Welfare. (2018). Family, domestic and sexual violence data in Australia. Report. https://www.aihw.gov.au/reports/family-domestic-and-sexual-violence/family-domestic-sexual-violence-data.

Australian Institute of Health and Welfare. (2023). Report.

Australian Law Reform Commission. (2010). Family violence: A national legal response. ALRC Report 114. Current definitions in family violence legislation. https://www.alrc.gov.au/publication/family-violence-a-national-legal-response-alrc-report-114/5-a-common-interpretative-framework-definitions-in-family-violence-legislation-3/current-definitions-in-family-violence-legislation/.

Australian Law Reform Commission. (2011). Family violence and Commonwealth laws: Social security law. IP 39. Definition of family violence. https://www.alrc.gov .au/publication/family-violence-and-commonwealth-laws-social-security-law-ip-39/ definition-of-family-violence/.

Centre for Aboriginal Health. (2011). Booklet. Aboriginal family health strategy, 2011–2016: Responding to family violence in Aboriginal communities. New South Wales Health Department.

Cloitre, M., Stolbach, B.C., Herman, J.L., Kolk, B.V.D., Pynoos, R., Wang, J., & Petkova, E. (2009). A developmental approach to complex PTSD: Childhood and adult cumulative trauma as predictors of symptom complexity. *Journal of Traumatic Stress*, 22(5), 399–408.

Commonwealth of Australia. (1997). *Bringing them Home Report*. Report of the National Inquiry into the separation of Aboriginal and Torres Strait Islander children from their families. https://humanrights.gov.au/our-work/bringing-them-home-report-1997.

D'Eatough, T.R. (2002). Inquiry into response by government agencies to complaints of family violence and child abuse in Aboriginal communities (The Gordon Inquiry), Western Australia – 2002, Western Australia. *Developing Practice: The Child, Youth and Family Work Journal*, (5), 50–52.

Enns, P.K. (2016). *Incarceration nation*. Cambridge University Press.

Gatwiri, K., Rotumah, D., & Rix, E. (2021). Black Lives Matter in healthcare: Racism and implications for health inequity among Aboriginal and Torres Strait Islander peoples in Australia. *International Journal of Environmental Research and Public Health*, 18(9), 4399.

Herman, J.L. (1992a). Complex PTSD: A syndrome in survivors of prolonged and repeated trauma. *Journal of Traumatic Stress*, 5(3), 377–391.

Herman, J. (1992b). *Trauma and recovery: The aftermath of violence – From domestic abuse to political terror* (1st ed.). Basic Books.

Herman, J.L. (1998). Recovery from psychological trauma. *Psychiatry and Clinical Neurosciences*, 52: S98–S103. https://doi.org/10.1046/j.1440-1819.1998.0520s5S145.x.

Herman, J. (2015). *Trauma and recovery: The aftermath of violence – From domestic abuse to political terror*. (3rd ed.). Basic Books.

Herring, S., Spangaro, J., Lauw, M., & McNamara, L. (2013). The intersection of trauma, racism, and cultural competence in effective work with Aboriginal people: Waiting for trust. *Australian Social Work*, 66(1), 104–117.

Lawrie, R., & Matthews, W. (2002). Holistic community justice: Proposed response to family violence in Aboriginal communities. *University of New South Wales Law Journal*, 25(1), 228.

Marcus, G., & Braaf, R. (2007). *Domestic and family violence studies, surveys and statistics: Pointers to policy and practice*. Australian Domestic and Family Violence Clearinghouse.

Martin, K. (2009). Ways of knowing, being and doing: A theoretical framework and methods for Indigenous and Indigenist research. *Australian Studies*. https://doi.org/0 .1080/14443050309387838.

Menzies, K. (2019). Understanding the Australian Aboriginal experience of collective, historical and intergenerational trauma. *International Social Work*, 62(6), 1522–1534.

New South Wales Attorney General's Department – Aboriginal. (2006). Child Sexual Assault Taskforce. *Breaking the silence: Creating the future: Addressing child sexual assault in Aboriginal communities in New South Wales*. https://www.indigenousjustice .gov.au/wp content/uploads/mp/files/resources/files/54.pdf.

New South Wales Department for Women. (1996). *Heroines of fortitude: The experiences of women in court as victims of sexual assault*. http://www.women.nsw.gov.au/publications/publica2.html.

New South Wales Department of Health. (2010). Mortality and hospitalisation due to injury in the Aboriginal population of New South Wales. Centre for Aboriginal Health, Sydney.

Papps, E., & Ramsden, I. (1996). Cultural safety in nursing: The New Zealand experience. *International Journal for Quality in Health Care*, 8(5), 491–497.

Parter, C., Murray, D., Mohamed, J., Rambaldini, B., Calma, T., Wilson, S., ... & Skinner, J. (2021). Talking about the "r" word: A right to a health system that is free of racism. *Public Health Research and Practice*, 31(1): e31121022021. https://doi.org/10.17061/phrp3112102.

Puren, N. (1997). Bodies/ethics/violence: Review of heroines of fortitude: The experiences of women as victims of sexual assault and the crimes (Rape) Act 1991 (NSW): An evaluation report. *Australian Feminist Law Journal*, 9, 134–142.

Ramsden, I. (2002). Cultural safety and nursing education in Aotearoa and Te Waipounamu (Doctoral dissertation, Victoria University of Wellington).

Robertson, B. (2000). Aboriginal and Torres Strait Islander women's task force on violence report. Queensland Government (Department of Aboriginal and Torres Strait Islander Policy and Development).

Serpell, B., Sullivan, T., & Doherty, L. (2022). Homicide in Australia 2019–20. Statistical Report no. 39. Australian Institute of Criminology (AIC), 2022. doi:10.52922/sr78511.

Sherwood, J.M. (2010). Do no harm: Decolonising Aboriginal health research. Doctoral dissertation, University of New South Wales, Sydney.

Terare, M.R. (2019). Transforming classrooms: Developing culturally safe learning environments. In D. Baines, B. Bennett, S. Goodwin, & M. Rawsthorne, M. (Eds.), *Working across difference: Social work, social policy and social justice* (pp. 26–37). Bloomsbury.

Terare, M.R. (2020). "It hasn't worked so we have to change what we are doing": First Nations worldview in human service practice. Doctoral dissertation, University of Sydney.

Terare, M., & Rawsthorne, M. (2020). Country is yarning to me: Worldview, health and well-being amongst Australian First Nations people. *The British Journal of Social Work*, 50(3), 944–960.

Tervalon, M., & Murray-Garcia, J. (1998). Cultural humility versus cultural competence: A critical distinction in defining physician training outcomes in multicultural education. *Journal of Health Care for the Poor and Underserved*, 9(2), 117–125.

United Nations General Assembly (1948). Universal Declaration of Human Rights. https://www.un.org/en/about-us/universal-declaration-of-human-rights.

Victorian Indigenous Family Violence Task Force. (2003). Final Report, December 2003. Aboriginal Affairs, Victoria (Department for Victorian Communities).

Wagner, A.W., Wolfe, J., Rotnitsky, A., Proctor, S.P., & Erickson, D.J. (2000). An investigation of the impact of posttraumatic stress disorder on physical health. *Journal of Traumatic Stress*, 13, 41–55.

Watson, L. Aunty (circa 1985). "Let us work together". Aboriginal Movement, Queensland, Australia. https://uniting.church/lilla-watson-let-us-work-together/.

Williams, R. (1999). Cultural safety – What does it mean for our work practice? *Australian and New Zealand Journal of Public Health*, 23(2), 213–214.

Wilson, S. (2001). What is Indigenous research methodology? *Canadian Journal of Native Education*, 25(2).

# 13

# COLLECTIVE CARE FOR COLLECTIVE TRAUMA

*Tanya Turton*

## Introduction

Conversations about trauma are often rooted in discussions and reflections about individual trauma. These conversations do not leave enough space for acknowledging the impact of intergenerational trauma, community traumas and the community care needed for continued recovery. This chapter is a first voice look at the experiences of Black communities and intersectional identities, and the use of collective care within our communities as an active tool for engaging with trauma. This chapter is an invitation to interrogate mainstream conversations about trauma and explore the ways communities have been caring for each other. These community-based approaches provide a helpful template for community-based care and engagement.

Conversations on trauma over the past decade have centered individualistic solutions, leaving out the valuable role of collective care. Over two decades ago, bell hooks (1952–2021) wrote about the importance of a love ethic, one rooted in integrity; this ethic translates to care rooted in community, actively working to decrease isolation (hooks, 2001). When working with intersectional communities, primarily those who have not only experienced personal trauma, but collective trauma over the course of multiple generations, there is a need for validating the wisdom rooted in the collective understanding. Technologies of joy, gathering, mutual aid, care circles, storytelling and witnessing are intrinsic to Black queer healing justice spaces and have been handed down as sacred to survival. Practitioners who hope to be impactful would benefit from considering collective care as a valid approach for engaging in trauma talk. Care that promotes agency, dignity and interdependence, void of savior complexes and filled with mutual trust, can only be built with an understanding of the role of

DOI: 10.4324/9781003379591-14

collective care as a survival tool. For many marginalized communities, collective care was the only option when medical spaces either abandoned them or provided inadequate care (Piepzna-Samarasinha, 2018). Talking about trauma within these communities and providing adequate care requires engaging with care as a collective initiative, incorporating not only the individual seeking care, but also their communities.

Communities have used collective methods to survive trauma, but these methods have been delegitimized in professional clinical spaces, leaving communities such as Black queer women further marginalized, and the individualist care provided ultimately becomes inaccessible. Addressing this mistrust and engaging with collective care is a vital step in working with communities who have navigated race-, gender-, or sexuality-based traumas.

## Collective Care as an Ancestral Practice

Collective care or community care refers to the ways Black and queer communities have survived as a result of various forms of mutual aid for generations, through looking out for and supporting each other. This form of care is built into our communities as a necessary practice for surviving systemic neglect and being underresourced (Piepzna-Samarasinha, 2018). This form of care was not only birthed from our resilience, but is also rooted in the ancestral principles of Afrocentric teachings, which prioritizes an interconnected approach to life. As a Jamaican woman, I grew up learning about the importance of mutual aid. We did not call it that though. We called it "pawdna" which is a microfinancing system birthed out of West African Indigenous methods of community economics. Once I was old enough to work, I began "throwing" my first hand, as it is referred to in the Jamaican culture. As early as I can remember I understood my mother to be a central matriarch in our community, because she was responsible for ensuring we had systems for saving the money necessary for paying school fees and medical fees and for caring for loved ones back home. My work is rooted in an Afrocentric paradigm. Using this approach provides the necessary framework for understanding social work and providing trauma support rooted in both helping individuals and working toward healthy communities.

Within the African diaspora, the word love is a central tenet to how we relate to each other and the language used to represent our commitment to engaging with each other. Yet, in professional circles, love is a taboo word or construct. My intention in this chapter is to interrogate the current model of trauma support and provide alternative examples, particularly for how to work with diverse communities, those filled with Black people and intersectional identities. Communities of Black women, queer people and gender-diverse people require an approach rooted in love – a community-centered vision and an ethic of connection and support. This approach moves away from individualized approaches to care and the limitations of romantic concepts of love, embracing principles of interconnection.

The chapter draws on the Black feminist teachings of bell hooks, who states, "living by a love ethic we learn to value loyalty and a commitment to sustained bonds over material advancement" – which means "while careers and making money remain important agendas, they never take precedent over valuing and nurturing human life and well-being" (hooks, 2001, p. 88). A love ethic is inherently rooted in interconnectedness: "we see our lives and our fate as intimately connected to those of everyone else on the planet" (hooks, 2001, p. 88). Building on the foundations of hooks' teachings, I offer this chapter as an opportunity to reflect on our approach to working with trauma and building tools for care.

## My Path to the Work

When I was 10 years old, I watched my sister struggle with displacement, grief and trauma. She was a brilliant, caring and beautiful young woman, but my family was unable to find the necessary support for her. Desperate for help my mother brought my sister to the hospital, but they sent her home. According to those who engaged with her, they saw nothing wrong. My family did everything we knew to do, and yet still on a cold winter night while 11- year-old me sat in my parents' bedroom, my 22-year-old sister died by suicide in the same apartment. I was devastated. Many years later, I found myself in a similar space to my own sister. I was struggling with emotional regulation and described these struggles to a mental health provider, who told me I was fine. She brushed off my concerns, calling them "growing pains". My experience of engaging with mental health providers has been a revolving door of "you are fine", "you are so strong", or "you are resilient". Perhaps thinking they are adopting a strengths-based approach to care, they have tended to lean on the side of telling me about how amazing I am, rather than listening and offering tools.

For Black women, mental health and trauma support is often made more challenging because of the pervasive nature of the "strong Black woman" trope. It is assumed that, because we have coped thus far, we will and should find the means to sort through the experiences on our own. Baker-Bell (2017) explains this phenomenon well: "Black women have a different interpretation of our social reality, and we are continuously negotiating our sense of self against images projected onto us by others" (p. 532). Black women negotiating and navigating trauma are contending with their own perceptions and expectations of what it means to cope, while also attempting to make sense of the messages provided to us by the rest of the world. Baker-Bell (2017) goes on to explain: "Black women, by virtue of our race and gender, are socially conditioned to believe that we have to be strong, be self-sacrificing and act with super strength" (p. 533). For Black women navigating trauma, we are often told to turn inward and make peace with our pain and struggles. The systems we turn to for support, turn back at us and utter the words that are dangerous for us to hear "you have been so strong, just keep doing what you are doing". In my experience, strong is code for, "stuff it down and pretend to be fine".

In my work, I notice that the rhetoric about strength is rooted in individualism. This encourages people to believe that all the things that hurt are their own to deal with. For me personally, each time I found myself facing unbelievable pain, it was through the collective support of others that I found the needed care that enabled me to breathe deeper again. When my sister passed, my family banded tighter together. In coming closer, we were able to help each other make sense of a loss that we could barely even speak about. In addition to the rhetoric of strong Black womanhood, I have also heard conversations that suggest Black people are not interested in talking about mental health. This is often paired with further assumptions that Black communities do not need mental health support due to their investment in spirituality and religion. For many marginalized communities, collective care was the only option when medical spaces either abandoned them or provided inadequate care (Piepzna-Samarasinha, 2018). Religion and spirituality for many was and is a means of building collective spaces where they can be seen and witnessed.

When I think about people like my sister and myself, I am reminded of the times we sought out the support of mental health professionals and were told our ability to seemingly cope meant we were fine. Rooted in this knowledge, I created a grassroots non-profit in 2018 called Adornment Stories Collective. My intention is to provide spaces where intersectional communities like us can engage in activities such as movement, photography, film, yoga and many more as an entrance to conversations on mental health. More than skill development, we provide safer spaces for communities to process life events, build community connections and be supported on their own transformative journeys. Adornment Stories Collective engages Black women, gender-diverse identities, queer and trans communities. We provide a plurality of creative means for engaging with mental health discourse, decrease stigma and create a platform for the stories of intersectional Black communities.

Our work continues to be impactful not only because of its deep roots in collective care, but the presence of critical hope in all our curriculum and engagement tools. *Critical hope* can be understood as "hopeful action that is based on the critical analysis of a situation and the recognition that wishing alone is not sufficient enough to make change" (James et al., 2010, p. 27). In my work, collective care and *critical hope* are intertwined. It is because of critical hope that I am reminded that acts of solidarity and working together have the power to transform, liberate and provide the needed support sometimes lacking in other mental health forms of engagement. Collective care is both an ancestral practice rooted in culture and a responsive practice needed because of historical neglect. Critical hope reminds us this is a valid way to care for our communities.

## Collective Trauma

Unfortunately, trauma is an experience that connects some communities. While trauma is often understood as an individual experience, many of us know that it happens collectively as well. While collective disasters such as hurricanes and other natural disasters can cause collective trauma, I am speaking of the ones caused by social conditions. Collective trauma rooted in colonization and its impact has ramifications for various communities. The term *anti-Black racism* was coined by Dr. Akua Benjamin in 2003 to speak to this specific experience, explaining "the specific and distinct experiences of Black people and their unique subjection to discriminatory practices and exclusion in Canada" (Mullings, Clarke, Bernard, Este & Giwa, 2021, p. 8). The trauma of anti-Black racism ripples through various institutions, such as social policies and economic and political spaces, and results in a lack of opportunities for the Black community. The impact of racial trauma can be felt for members in the Black community, not only socially but physically (ibid., 2021).

In 2020, the entire world watched George Perry Floyd Jr. being murdered across their social media timeline. This racial violence registered in the lives of Black people as a reminder of our collective trauma and affirmation that any one of us could be next. As I write this in 2023, we mourn the loss of O'Shae Sibley, and we form collective spaces to process the realities of living as an openly Black queer person. Black communities have watched name after name be added in the hashtag call for justice, and with each name the story of how they lost their lives is filled with anti-Black racism and a complete disregard for the Black community as a whole. These instances of racial trauma are not individual experiences, they are symptoms of multi-generational trauma and reminders of what our ancestors had to endure for our survival. The implications of this ongoing trauma are profound.

Trauma can be understood as an "overarching term which refers to an event, series of events or experiences that occurs over time involving threats to life or encounters with death and causing intense, lasting adverse effects on individuals' physical, social, emotional or spiritual well-being and overall ability to function" (Blakey & Glaude, 2021, p. 216). The nature of the collective trauma that people experience because they may be Black, a woman, queer or various other identities, means that they are not only experiencing personal trauma in their own lives, but they are also living in relationship to others within their families and communities who are having similar experiences. In addition to personalized moments of unimaginable pain, they are living with collective ones. *Complex trauma* can be understood as "another type of trauma that results from exposure to multiple, recurrent and prolonged traumatic events that tend to be invasive, interpersonal and have wide-ranging long-term effects" (ibid., p. 216). Complex trauma enhances the likeliness of "internalizing problems, post-traumatic stress, and other clinical diagnoses" and can impact every aspect of a person's life, even long after they are no longer experiencing the traumatic event itself (ibid., p. 216).

An impact of anti-Black racism within the medical system is that many Black community members have lost trust in the systems that should be caring for them. According to Mullings, Clarke, Bernard, Este and Giwa (2021), "research has shown that Black people are much less likely to report trust in physicians' and hospitals' health care practitioners; thus, they are less likely to seek treatment or adhere to recommended treatment plans" (p. 246). The historical trauma and contemporary neglect within the medical system for Black communities has resulted in, "eighty-one percent of the Black women surveyed across Toronto felt that their physician would involve them in research without their knowledge" (ibid., p. 247). The distrust that exists reflects that "the biomedical model is inherently racist, discriminatory, short-sighted, hostile and limited in providing health care" (ibid., p. 247). Those whose identities are diverse and intersecting such as women, queer, trans, non-binary, (dis)Abled, neurodivergent, living in poverty or racialized may avoid a mental health care system with providers and researchers who "have a preconceived notion of what a 'normal' body is and fail to recognize that bodies and people's health needs are not universal"(ibid., p. 247). Social workers in Canada providing mental health care report that many diverse and marginalized clients face significant barriers in receiving adequate care, particularly trauma care, and that the social contexts and inequities experienced are not being addressed (Brown, C., Johnstone, & Ross, 2021; Doll, Brown, C., Johnstone, & Ross, 2023; Brown, C., Johnstone, Ross, & Doll, 2022; Ross, Brown, C., & Johnstone, 2023). The current system of care reflects neoliberal, poorly funded, inaccessible care, with an emphasis on individual pathology, diagnosis, short-term, one-size-fits-all care.

   The legacy of systemic racism within communities can be "historical trauma", "cultural legacy burdens" or collective trauma (Gutiérrez, 2022, p. 24). This type of trauma is rooted in the legacy of colonialism, racism, patriarchy and capitalist class structure. These structures are reflected in multiple forms of prejudice and discrimination including misogynoir, transphobia, homophobia and fatphobia. Systemic and institutional harm cause dehumanization and have real implications on people's lives. This is the kind of trauma "Black, Indigenous and brown femme people, who have kept our communities alive after being both abandoned and policed by the state, and in the face of medical experimentation and denial of health insurance" face and continue to live through (Piepzna-Samarasinha, 2018, p. 37). *Collective care* became intrinsic to communities not only because of the ineffectiveness of individualism, which focuses on individual deficit, blame, pathology and responsibility, but also due to the violence experienced within the health care systems, which has taught entire communities of Black people that we could not rely on health care support. Fear and distrust of the health care system is rooted in reality and we often experience it as trauma.

## Liberation Rooted in Collective Care

In response to systemic abandonment and trauma, many of the communities previously mentioned learned how to centre "interdependence" as a means of care (Gutiérrez, 2022, p. 26). *Collective care* is birthed from the technologies of Black communities, disability justice movements and queer communities, aimed at "collective care that lifts us instead of abandons us" (Piepzna-Samarasinha, 2018, p. 33). While various communities engage with community care as a cultural experience, in this context we are specifically speaking to the innovative organizing done "in a way where we are in control, joyful, building community, loved, giving, and receiving, that doesn't burn anyone out, abuse or underpay anyone in the process" (ibid., 2018, p. 33). This form of care moves away from traditional non-profit and medical engagement because it believes in "solidarity not charity"- this form of care moves away from the dichotomy of the helper and helped (ibid., p. 41).

Collective care depends on the belief that we are all in need of care and will occupy both roles at various points in our life through various relationships, therefore the hierarchies and sympathy often imposed on those in need of care are counter to the actual process of caring. hooks (2001) affirms we must all "see our lives and our fate as intimately connected to those of everyone else on the planet" (p. 88). Collective care requires relinquishing moral superiority. I adopt a collective care approach because I want to engage with others in a way that allows them to show-up whole. As a practitioner, social worker and community member, it is all of our responsibilities to ask each other how we must show-up to ensure mutual care. hooks (2001) uses the language of *love ethic* rather than *collective care*, but the sentiments remain and are parallel to my intentions. For hooks (2001) "a love ethic presupposes that everyone has the right to be free, to live fully and well" (p. 87).

Collective care as a tool of engaging with trauma is not easy. It is hard. It is important we acknowledge this together so as to avoid a false narrative of superiority or of being a savior. Many of us have been indoctrinated into the belief that those who provide care are experts and morally superior. Collective care requires relinquishing this colonial framework while acknowledging the importance of ethically engaging with the power we do have when in a care provider position.

We are socialized to process the world through the Western worldview of individualism, especially today within the neoliberal biomedical fields of providing health and mental health care. This means our critical thought needs to be reflected in critical practice. Critical theories of collective care must be integrated into intentional critical practices of collective care. A holistic framework for collective care centers humanity and is one that makes space for the emotional, spiritual, physical and cognitive interconnections of knowledge, practice and action. While the language continues to evolve, writers and scholars of the past have engaged with these concepts and provided blueprints stating, "embracing a love ethic means that we utilize all the dimensions of love – care, commitment, trust, responsibility, respect and knowledge" (hooks, 2001, p. 95). Embracing a practice of collective care and moving away from individualism that reinforces social structures of power and dominance requires a willingness to learn how others would like us to support them and "cultivating courage [and] the strength to stand up for what we believe in, to be accountable both in word and deed" (ibid., p. 92).

## Collective Care within Trauma Intervention Work

Collective care in communities is important, and particularly meaningful for trauma work. This will shift current models of intervention both in professional spaces and self-help spaces rooted in individualism toward thinking collectively. This takes additional innovation, world-building and strategizing for those of us who aim to engage with a collective, centered model of support work.

My team and I planned a retreat for Black queer and trans communities. This retreat offered access to a group of peers, with nature, meaningful conversation about mental health, instructors for relationship-building, sound baths, meditation, yoga, and catered dinners during which we ate together. While the various modalities and nature certainly offered healing, the primary impactful factor was the time together with others.

Surveys of people's experiences were filled with touching stories of what the retreat meant to them, but the one most relevant to this discussion is a participant who reported a decrease in post-traumatic stress disorder (PTSD) symptoms. They shared with us that for the weekend they were able to experience safety, which brought feelings of validation and happiness. While no doubt influenced by the social world, happiness is a subjective feeling. I would like to focus on how they discussed it for a moment. They went on to confirm that they usually feel happiness when using drugs or alcohol or when self-harming, but the retreat led to feelings of happiness brought on by feeling safe. This translated into better sleep and a decrease of symptoms over the weekend we spent together. While I recognize not every intervention or support strategy will be rooted in something as immersive as a Black queer and trans retreat, what I urge us as practitioners to consider is how can we actively work to ensure the people we are working with feel safe and how we can foster feelings of connection. – particularly for those who have felt neglected within our sector.

I have outlined how the historical trauma many Black people, Indigenous people and people of color have experienced navigating the health care system. I have advocated for the importance and value of collective care and the need for building trust. As practitioners we should engage with communities in ways that encourage and fulfill the expectation of a safe space for connection and care.

## Theoretical Frameworks for Practice

Collective care as a tool for liberation, resistance and holistic living is not an academic tool and should be understood as a practice rooted in Black and people of color communities, and birthed from healing justice movements. I provide this foundational understanding in hopes of honoring the roots of this knowledge and ensuring it is not forgotten. I would like to guide those interested to various theoretical underpinnings that they can engage with to help support their practice and understanding of collective care. My practice is primarily informed by Afrocentric teachings and guided by this paradigm of understanding the world.

Collective care in my practice is rooted in critical hope, narrative theory, and Afrocentric and Black feminist thought.

## Critical Hope

Within the context of supporting communities that have been historically and contemporarily traumatized, *critical hope* is foundational to building strategic practice rooted in "hopeful action that is based on the critical analysis of a situation" (James et al., 2010, p. 27). Within Black communities, critical hope has historically been used as a means of liberation and empowerment, because it teaches "a commitment to engagement in a process of liberation from oppression" (ibid., p. 28). Trauma work rooted in collective care must engage with critical hope as a means of making sense of how people cope rather than framing coping mechanism as "maladaptive". Critical hope reminds us that everyone is deserving of care that believes in their capacity and supports their dignity.

## Narrative Therapy

Narrative therapy encourages collaborative conversations about unhelpful stories, counterviews where these come from and helps to produce alternative counterstories (Brown, C. & Augusta-Scott, 2007). Viewing therapy as political, it encourages us to clarify our positionality and avoid the myth of neutrality (White, 1994). While it acknowledges that traditional therapy power dynamics usually meaning the therapist has more institutional power and authority than the client, it seeks to emphasize the client's story and what it means to them. It focuses on a collaborative process of re-storying. Collective care provides a framework for ethically engaging in power dynamics and encourages us to name these dynamics when providing care. Using the tool of naming, engaging in meaningful discussion and building a shared understanding of power we are able to dismantle the learned dichotomy of superior versus inferior, while validating the human need for care. Narrative therapy maintains that "it is never a matter of whether or not we bring politics into the therapy room, but it is a matter of whether or not we are prepared to acknowledge the existence of these politics, and it is a matter of the degree to which we are prepared to be complicit in the reproduction of these politics" (White, 1994, p. 1). It is crucial to consider the power in your role, the social constructs of your identities and the impact of this power on the person in front of you. Power is bestowed upon us, often without our own consent, and acquired via titles and social identity. Regardless of how we acquire power, we are responsible for its impact. Collective care provides a framework for how to act accountably. When working with a person in need of care, a practical means of engaging in this conversation is asking questions, explaining what your role is and the intention of your time together. It is important to emphasize to those seeking care that the work is collaborative and that their voice, experiences, values and thoughts are central. This affirmation is vital for those who may believe that their need for care makes them powerless. A White practitioner for instance, may not be trusted because of the harms and silencing done by others who look like them, therefore effort needs to be made to encourage people of color and Black communities to ask questions, or seek ways to better understand how they are relating to the information shared and bridge the gaps. The practitioner may also need to work at finding ways to help clients feel more comfortable in the space. This might include offering time for clarification, reflecting back what you have heard, checking on how the process is going, making plans together on next steps, and being clear that you want to hear what their thoughts and feelings are. It is vital to take steps to remember how to pronounce the names of clients, be informed of their pronouns and avoid generalizations. Care and mindfulness require not only procedural attempts at client care, but intentional actions to recognize personhood. Many Black, Indigenous and people of color, particularly Black women and Black gender-diverse people, have not experienced care rooted in dignity and autonomy. Many clients have felt dehumanized and ultimately not received the care they needed. Engaging with a collective care framework requires being mindful of power and ultimately providing opportunities to uplift the humanity of clients who have not experienced trauma support in this fashion.

Narrative therapy emphasizes *double listening*, which is foundational to collective care. For instance, in terms of trauma, narrative therapy is aware that trauma stories often feel very dangerous. They are often difficult to tell, and it is often dangerous to speak (Brown, C., 2018). This makes it important for narrative therapy to listen beyond the words, to listen to what is not spoken, partially spoken, or yet to be spoken (Brown, C., 2014, 2020, 2022; Brown, C. & MacDonald, 2022). Further, there are no neutral stories, and there is no neutral telling or hearing of stories. Coping with trauma can be very hard and the ways people cope are often pathologized. In narrative approaches, when we double listen to trauma stories, we are listening for how they make sense (Brown, C., 2018). This approach is similar to the respectfulness and positive regard of a critical hope stance. White (2004) explains "the ways in which people respond to trauma, the steps that they take in response to trauma, are based on what they give value to, on what they hold precious in life" (p. 47). Narrative therapy reminds us that both the telling of and the hearing of stories are part of the therapeutic conversation. Together, critical hope, narrative theory and communities of care are consistent in understanding how important it is to acknowledge the important impact of how we receive communities' stories. When clients offer meaning rooted in their own cultural understanding or life experiences, double listening offers a commitment to deeply tune in and engage with what is being shared, without judgment of what it means to them.

Collective care emphasizes that a collaborative and connected relationship alongside double listening allows for prioritizing human connection, non-judgmental and co-created solutions via the listening process. Collective care values the experience of the person being listened to and not just the information shared.

## Afrocentric Framework and Black Feminist Thought

An Afrocentric framework is rooted in "African ancestral knowledge systems, practices and ways of being" (Mullings, Clarke, Bernard, Este & Giwa., 2021, p. 10). Narrative and storytelling are ancestral tools within the African diaspora and have been essential to the process of making-meaning for generations. Afrocentric principles remind us of the value of connection, which enhances and deepens understanding. Afrocentric storytelling is not linear and leans on circular discussion techniques for building understanding. This means "letting stories flow" and encouraging "anecdotal" or "illustrative" language, which can be essential to building an environment of care (ibid., p. 80). A primary premise of an Afrocentric worldview is the value for collectivity and community. Conversations about trauma are only effective in this worldview if they consider both the impact on the individual and on the entire community. In the context of working with trauma as researchers, community workers, educators or practitioners, Afrocentric ways of knowing rely on notions of truth and meaning that are grounded in "the experiences of community" (Reviere, 2001, p. 713).

An Afrocentric worldview is positioned. As such, objectivity is impossible and as people working with and on behalf of others we must situate ourselves in the conversation. Embodied in the collective care practice means sharing appropriate information as a practitioner about who you are and what brings you to the work. The vulnerable act of showing who one is, should not only be relegated to those in need of care, but is a reciprocal action of grounding the conversation in transparency. Within Black communities this action can be seen when we share what neighborhood we grew up in, or the last name of our families.

Influenced by Black feminist thought, practitioners should situate themselves in relation to those we are caring for. While doing so, practitioners will need to assess what information may be unhelpful or potentially harmful for a client to hear – we must be mindful when sharing transparently. While my work is rooted in community, and I do not often work one-on-one with clients, I still intentionally share what informs how I see the world. I am transparent about my Jamaican background, that I lost a family member to suicide, and that I identify as queer. This is helpful in building a caring and transparent environment about what I bring to the room with me. This helps build a collaborative relationship and disrupts the traditional hierarchy between service providers and service users. I often share ideas I have about working together, sometimes simply by saying, for example, "I hope to create a space where you feel more able to explore your struggles", additionally contextualizing why I am in the space and what my role will be. The inclusion of a personal identity is important for avoiding a false sense of objective presence in the space. Situating oneself in this way allows for "self-reflection", "introspection" and "retrospection", aiding in accountability to self and those sharing space with us in that moment (Reviere, 2001, p. 715). Collective care rooted in an Afrocentric framework and influenced by Black feminist thought carves out time for meaningful connection that goes both ways and values the community.

## Barriers in Practice

The primary barrier I have seen in practice is the lack of trust. This lack of trust moves in two directions. Marginalized service users do not trust service providers, and service providers do not trust service users. When working with various organizations who are aiming to connect with Black women and queer communities in transformative ways, one of the challenges is the practitioners do not trust the communities they work with. When it comes to working with intersectional communities and those navigating the stigma of mental health problems, service providers engage with service users with a heightened caution and discomfort that communicates distrust. I share this insight both as someone who is a service user and someone who has collaborated with organizations over a decade, witnessing the distrust of service providers. In order to develop connection and deep-rooted care, there needs to be trust. We need to assume the best of people and be centered in *critical hope* and patience. We need to find opportunities for building mutual trust. Essentially, if we treat people as though we do not trust them, they have no reason to trust us.

It is also important not only to offer collective care principles via the approach I have discussed, but also for providers to show respect to the communities of care and those who operate from this worldview. I have witnessed and experienced practitioners dismissing the role of family, both chosen and biological, in building a strong care plan. Allowing care circles to be present, when consented to and appropriate, can shift the experience of those seeking care. Simple acts like asking if there is anyone they would like to be present with them as a support person, and then speaking to both people, can communicate a much-needed respect for their care circle. Moving away from a focus only on the individual will require not only seeing the whole person, but also valuing their entire circle of care in any plans considered and developed with them.

## Conclusion

Building frameworks for collective care is rooted in supporting people holistically and making space for differences and nuances of experience. It calls on us to take the extra time to imagine what their unique experience may be and offer deeper curiosity as to how folks are making meaning in their lives. Collective care is about agency, autonomy and believing it is possible to provide more meaningful care. Collective care calls for a more circular approach to care because individualistic and linear approaches are leaving too many people behind.

# References

Baker-Bell, A. (2017). For Loretta: A Black woman literacy scholar's journey to prioritizing self-preservation and Black feminist–womanist storytelling. *Journal of Literacy Research*, 49(4), 526–543. https://doi.org/10.1177/1086296X17733092.

Blakey, J.M., & Glaude, M.W. (2021). Complex trauma among African American mothers in child protective services. *Traumatology*, 27(2), 215–226. https://doi.org/10.1037/trm0000288.

Brown, C. (2014). Untangling emotional threads, self-management discourse and women's body talk. In M. LaFrance & S. McKenzie-Mohr (Eds.). *Women voicing resistance. Discursive and narrative explorations* (pp. 174–190). Routledge.

Brown, C. (2018). The dangers of trauma talk: Counterstorying co-occurring strategies for coping with trauma. *Journal of Systemic Therapies*, 37(3), 42–60.

Brown, C. (2020). Feminist narrative therapy and complex trauma: Critical clinical work with women diagnosed as "borderline". In C. Brown & J. MacDonald (Eds.), *Critical clinical social work: Counterstorying for social justice* (pp. 82–109). Canadian Scholars Press.

Brown, C. (2022). Postmodern theory: The case of narrative theory in social work. In R. Hugman, D. Holscher, & D. McAuliffe (Eds.), *Social work theory and ethics* (pp.79–100). Springer.

Brown, C. & Augusta-Scott, T. (2007). Introduction: Postmodernism, reflexivity, and narrative therapy. In C. Brown & T. Augusta-Scott (Eds.), Narrative therapy: Making meaning, making lives (pp. ix–xliii). Sage.

Brown, C., Johnstone, M., & Ross, N. (2021). Repositioning social work practice in mental health in Nova Scotia. *Report*. Nova Scotia College of Social Workers. https://nscsw.org/wp-content/uploads/2021/01/NSCSW-Repositioning-Social-Work-Practice-in-Mental-Health-in-Nova-Scotia-Report-2021.pdf.

Brown, C., Johnstone, M., Ross, N., & Doll, K. (2022). Challenging the constraints of neoliberalism and biomedicalism: Repositioning social work in mental health. *Qualitative Health Research*, 32(5), 771–787. https://doi.org/10.1177/10497323211069681

Brown, C., & MacDonald, J. (2022). Critical clinical social work in the context of trauma and (dis)Ability. In D. Baines (Ed.). *Doing anti-oppressive practice: Building transformative, politicized social work* (4th ed.) (pp. 118–140). Fernwood Press.

Doll, K., Brown, C., Johnstone, M., & Ross, N. (2023). Neoliberalism, control of trans and gender diverse bodies and social work. *Journal of Evidence-Focused Social Work*, 20(4), 568–594.

Gutierrez, N. (2022). *The pain we carry*. New Harbinger Publications.

hooks, b. (2001). *All about love: New visions*. William Morrow.

James, C., Este, D., Bernard, W.T., Benjamin, A., Lloyd, B. & Turner, T. (2010). *Race and well-being: The lives, hopes, and activism of African Canadians*. Fernwood Books.

Mullings, D.V., Clarke, J., Bernard, W.T., Este, D., & Giwa, S. (Eds.) (2021) *Africentric Social Work*. Fernwood Publishing.

Piepzna-Samarasinha, L. (2018). *Care work: Dreaming disability justice*. Arsenal Pulp Press.

Reviere, R. (2001). Toward an Afrocentric research methodology. *Journal of Black Studies*, 31(6). Sage. https://www.jstor.org/stable/2668042.

Ross, N., Brown, C., & Johnstone, M. (2023). Beyond medicalised approaches to violence and trauma: Empowering social work practice. *Journal of Social Work*. 1–19.

White, M. (1994). The politics of therapy: Putting to rest the illusion of neutrality. *Dulwich Centre Newsletter*, 1, 1–4. Dulwich Centre.

White, M. (2004). Working with people who are suffering the consequences of multiple trauma: A narrative perspective. *International Journal of Narrative Therapy and Community Work*, 2004(1), 45–76.

# 14

# UNDERSTANDING THE POLITICS OF EMOTION IN GENDERED VIOLENCE

## A Feminist Critique of Trauma and Cognitivist Discourses in Research and Practice

*Nicole Moulding*

## Introduction

This chapter critically examines the use of two of the most dominant theoretical approaches used in intimate partner violence research and practice – trauma-informed and cognitivist perspectives. Trauma-informed and cognitivist approaches have become increasingly influential over time in gendered violence research and practice and have been taken up within some strands of feminist research. In this chapter, I argue that the dominance of trauma-informed and cognitive-behavioral approaches has contributed to a lack of attention to the role of gendered, socially embodied emotions and affects as drivers of violent and controlling gender practices in everyday relationships. In turn, this has worked to limit the scope of prevention and the nature and effectiveness of men's perpetration programs and restricted the development of therapeutic support for perpetrators and victim-survivors that engages with the gendered nature of trauma.

To elaborate the rationale for focusing on socially embodied emotion and affect in gendered violence research and practice, I draw on Ahall's (2018) concept of the "politics of emotion", which is defined as the effort to capture "the political effects of emotional practices", where "emotion" refers to representations of bodily feelings or sensations and "affect" points to "energies transmitted through bodily encounters" (ibid, p. 38). While both emotion and affect are understood to be social and gendered, emotion is largely conscious and affect generally non-conscious (or less-conscious) (ibid., p. 40). I do not want to get overly caught up with the potential differences between "emotion" and "affect" because the two are commonly used interchangeably. But I do adopt Wetherell's (2012) concept of *affective practice*, which "focuses on the emotional as it appears in social life and tries to follow what participants do" (Wetherell, 2012, p. 5). Here, then, affect

DOI: 10.4324/9781003379591-15

involves *doing* while emotion is more about the *felt*. Later in the chapter, selected findings from my own and others' research are presented to illustrate how interactive emotions and affects help to drive intimate partner violence, drawing on the specific example of emotions and affects related to gendered forms of honor and abjection. This is followed by a consideration of future pathways for research.

The discussion in this chapter is relevant to diverse gender identities and sexualities because I am interested in how masculinities and femininities frame and shape abuse, and this is pertinent not only to cis-gendered individuals in ostensibly heterosexual relationships but also LGBT individuals. Hence, when reference is made in this chapter to "women" or "men", I am usually pointing to historical trends in gendered violence research and practice, or to the findings from past research that predominantly focused on cis-gendered individuals in heterosexual relationships. When the terms "women" and "men" are used more generally than this, all individuals who identify as "women" or "men" are being referred to; otherwise, the language of "perpetrators" and "victim-survivors" is used because this does not presume any particular gender identity and captures individuals who identify as non-binary, gender-fluid and intersex, in addition to other groups.

## Intimate Partner Violence: What We Think We Know

The body of knowledge about gendered violence is large and includes research across gender studies, social work, psychology, sociology, nursing, public health and criminology, as well as a number of other smaller disciplines. I am not about to attempt a detailed review of this work discipline-by-discipline but, rather, I seek to provide a general picture of the dominant threads, their theoretical orientations, and the contemporary policy and practice approaches they speak to. Feminists in Western countries were the first to draw attention to violence against women as a significant and widespread social problem during the second wave of the women's movement in the 1970s and 1980s. However, other disciplines became increasingly involved in the gendered violence space from the late 1980s onward, including feminist therapy (Breckenridge, 1999), sociology (Straus & Gelles, 1986), and epidemiology/public health (Bowman et al., 2015).

Since the 1970s, we have particularly seen a burgeoning of psychological research into gendered violence. Psychological research predominantly focuses on the individual drivers and impact of abuse, such as: the influence of cognitive schemas on perpetration and victimization; trauma and the relationship between growing up in intimate partner violence or child maltreatment and later perpetration or victimization; the impact of violence on neural pathways; and the role of mental health problems and drug and alcohol use in intimate partner violence (for example, Bonomi et al., 2009; Calvete, Estévez, & Corral, 2007; Goldenson, Geffner, Foster, & Clipson, 2007; Machisa, Christofides, & Jewkes, 2016; Rees et al., 2011; Romito, Molzan Turan, & De Marchi, 2005; Semiatin, Torres, LaMotte, Portnoy, & Murphy, 2017; Senkans, McEwan, & Ogloff, 2020).

With few exceptions, psychological approaches are presented as if they are gender-neutral, but they are actually at once gender-blind *and* profoundly gendered in their underlying masculinist assumptions about gender and mental illness, often falling into pathologizing both victim-survivors and perpetrators (Moulding, Franzway, Wendt, Zufferey, & Chung, 2021). As such, few connections are made in the bulk of psychological research between violence and its gendered social context, meaning or impact, leaving unexplained why it is cis-gendered heterosexual men who are the main abusers when so many more women, and individuals with diverse gender and sexual identities, report histories of trauma and mental illness (ibid.). Without eliding that some men who use violence and control have experienced trauma, casting their later violence entirely as a consequence of this often overlooks the role of gender inequalities and cultures in intimate partner violence (ibid.).

In contrast to the individualistic focus of much psychological research, feminists have historically understood patriarchy as the structural and ideological basis for gendered violence (for example, Brownmiller, 1975; Dobash & Dobash, 1978; Kelly, 1988; MacKinnon, 1993; Millet, 1970), enabling and driving all forms, from domestic violence and child sexual abuse to rape, sexual harassment and the proliferation of violent pornography (Berggren, Gottzen, & Bornas, 2021; Breckenridge, 1999; McPhail, 2002; Reavey & Warner, 2003). While there is some theoretical variability in the contemporary feminist research into intimate partner violence (IPV), most researchers primarily situate the problem in unequal gender power relations and, depending on the theory, related gendered norms, ideologies, beliefs or discourses (for example; Franzway, Moulding, Wendt, Zufferey, & Chung ,2020; Kelly & Rehman, 2013; Taylor & Jasinski, 2011; Walby, 2009; Wendt & Zannettino, 2015; Westmarland & Kelly, 2013). Over the past decade, intersectional feminist analytic frameworks have also been widely applied, bringing important insights into how gender intersects with other social inequalities in the experience and impact of intimate partner violence, such as those related to class, race, (dis)Ability, and sexual and gender diversity (see, for example, Thiara & Gill, 2010; Thiara, Hague & Mullender, 2011).

Feminist research has made, and continues to make, a critically important contribution to how we understand gendered violence and respond to it. Beginning in the early 1970s, feminists were responsible for the development of women's shelters (Pizzey, 1974) and have advocated over decades now for increased services and resourcing to support women who leave violent relationships, including the establishment of domestic violence leave and coercive control legislation in some jurisdictions (Franzway, Moulding, Wendt, Zufferey, & Chung, 2020). However, unlike the earlier radical feminists, contemporary feminist research has increasingly focused on the *impact* of intimate partner violence on women, often without addressing the *drivers* of violence (Berggren, Gottzen, & Bornas, 2021).

Masculinities scholarship, which is often feminist-informed, has also grown over the past few decades, yet there has been surprisingly little attention directed specifically toward gendered violence despite its high prevalence and heavily gendered nature (Berggren, Gottzen, & Bornas, 2021). Well-known masculinities scholars, such as Connell, Hearn, Kimmel and others touch on violence against women, but there are few who focus specifically on it (Berggren, Gottzen, & Bornas, 2021). Berggren, Gottzen and Bornas (2021) provide a very useful summary of the main strands of masculinities scholarship in the gendered violence area, which is drawn on here. Key early masculinities scholars drew, and continue to draw, on socialist feminism's engagement with Marxism and the concept of hegemony, as in Connell's idea of hegemonic masculinity and masculinity as a practice (Connell, 1995). Hegemonic masculinity is understood as representing the most highly valued way of "doing masculinity" and sits in a hierarchical relation to other masculinities and, of course, to all femininities and other non-binary gender identities (ibid.). Within this perspective, violence against women is understood as one of a myriad of gender practices reflective of hegemonic masculinity (Connell, 1995; Hearn, 1996, 2012; Messerschmidt, 1986, 1997, 2004, 2012). Other research into gendered violence and masculinities focuses more specifically on men's own accounts of abuse to explore how they discursively justify their problematic behavior (Kelly & Westmarland, 2016; Ptacek, 1988; Stokoe, 2010). A further group of masculinities scholars draw on social network theory to understand how men's relations with other men enable violence against women (Hearn & Whitehead, 2006; DeKeseredy, Schwartz, & Donnermeyer, 2009; Kimmel, 2010). Intersectional masculinities research focuses on how interpersonal violence is shaped by the different ways that gender intersects with class, race, sexuality and age (Boonzaier & van Niekerk, 2019; Langenderfer-Magruder, Whitfield, Walls, Kattari, & Ramos, 2016).

Lastly, some masculinities researchers have explored how early family relations might be critical to masculine subject formation and the later perpetration of violence against intimate partners, sometimes referred to as the "cycle of violence" or as the "intergenerational transmission of violence" (Gadd, 2000, 2003; Gadd & Jefferson, 2007). Some studies have focused more specifically on how early trauma among men might be implicated in violence against female intimate partners (for example, Brown, J., 2004; Kaplenko, Loveland, & Raghavan, 2018; Seymour, Wendt & Natalier, 2023). Whilst most of this research attempts to retain a feminist understanding of the social construction of gender, it also assumes that trauma related to either growing up in domestic violence or experiencing childhood abuse is the substantive driver of later partner abuse, rather than structural and symbolic gender inequality, including gender relations in the family of origin. More significantly, though, less than a third of men who perpetrate violence against their partners grow up in domestic violence (Roberts, Gilman, Fitzmaurice, Decker & Koenen, 2010) whilst evidence for clear-cut links between trauma related to childhood abuse and later interpersonal violence perpetration is highly contested. For example, a matched prospective study using a population sample (rather than a retrospective design using a clinical sample) found that individuals with and without backgrounds of child abuse actually report equal rates of intimate partner violence perpetration as adults (Widom, Czaja & Dutton, 2014). Moreover, it is important to be aware that perpetrators could report past abuse to justify their violent behavior (Romans, Martin, & Anderson, 1995) and that many perpetrators never come to the attention of authorities because they do not live in circumstances of social disadvantage with high rates of childhood adversity. Some of the research into trauma in perpetrators also relies on psycho-analytic, psychodynamic and attachment theories, which assume universal (and unproven) intrapsychic structures and dynamics (for example, Brown, J., 2004). As such, there is a tendency, despite good intentions, to slide into an intrapsychic focus, losing touch with the sociocultural and structural dimensions of violence (Berggren, Gottzen, & Bornas, 2021).

Much of the masculinities research into gendered violence also tends to pre-sume and over-emphasize *conscious* individual psychological processes in the attempt to understand the drivers of men's violence (Berggren, Gottzen, & Bornas, 2021), such as the role of gendered thoughts, attitudes and beliefs or the individual discursive narratives offered by perpetrators to justify their violence. In this way, perpetrators are understood to be "overly instrumental, and men are positioned as essentially strong and powerful", which is "neither intellectually coherent nor recognisable to the men themselves" (ibid., p. 42).

## How Do Current Understandings Speak to Violence Rehabilitation and Prevention?

Psychological, feminist and masculinities perspectives on intimate partner vio-lence have commonly been brought together in the main approaches to policy and practice. As a case in point, men's behavior change programs are almost univer-sally premised on a pro-feminist social learning model that is usually cognitivist in orientation, with behavior change understood to flow from changed beliefs, attitudes, thoughts and feelings (Gadd, 2004; Morran, 2011). Even programs that use a post-structural feminist lens and a narrative-discursive approach to thera-peutic change (for example, Wendt, Natalier, Seymour, King, & Macaitis, 2020) are nonetheless essentially cognitivist in nature through their focus on individual men's explanations, justifications and conscious understandings of their violence, perhaps in an effort to try and hold men accountable for their violence. Other programs take a more trauma-informed approach, focusing on the role of trauma-related shame in the perpetration of abuse and drawing on an intergenerational understanding of trauma (Haines et al., 2022). However, such programs have been shown to have at best modest (Arias, Arce, & Vilariño, 2013) to poor outcomes (Augusta-Scott & Dankwort, 2002; Bowen & Gilchrist, 2006; Bowen, Gilchrist, & Beech, 2005).

In a similar vein to perpetrator programs, primary prevention – usually in the form of anti-domestic violence education campaigns – employ a public health behavior change approach that is almost always informed by pro-feminist social psychology and the assumption that changes in gendered attitudes and beliefs will lead to reductions in gendered violence (Salter, 2016). In spite of many such campaigns, no such reductions have occurred (World Health Organization (WHO), 2010) and they are unlikely to in the future through such an approach (DeGue et al., 2012). It has been well-established for decades now that health promotion campaigns do not change behavior on their own in the absence of structural change (Baum & Miller, 2014).

However, reductions in some measures of structural gender inequality and shifts in gender roles and expectations in some countries over the past five decades have not brought about any concomitant decrease in the rates of violence either (Australian Bureau of Statistics (ABS), 2017; Gracia & Merlo, 2016). Even more concerningly, there are indications that sexual violence (including within intimate relationships) has actually increased in some places, including Australia, over the past few years (ABS, 2017). It is almost certainly the case that more could have been done, given the sheer extent of the problem and the unwillingness of many neoliberal governments to properly step up.

Since the 1990s, and outside of intersectional studies and research into family violence within Aboriginal and other First Nations communities, there has been remarkably little advancement in our understanding of the core drivers of gendered violence and coercive control in everyday relationships. While there has arguably been a lack of attention to structural gender inequalities in intimate partner violence research and practice (Salter, 2016), I argue that the cultural "gender norm" side of the gendered violence equation is also somewhat bereft due to underexploration of the less-conscious, more subliminal emotional and affectual aspects of intimate partner violence, limiting insight into the everyday drivers and responses and thereby hindering the scope for ending it (Berggren, Gottzen, & Bornas, 2021).

## What We Do Not Know: Emotion and Affect as Underexplored Areas of Inquiry

Gendered violence involves interactions *between bodies* that are profoundly visceral, intersubjective, embodied, socially situated and political. Yet the body – its sensations, desires, affects and emotions and its interactions with other bodies that are also in the grip of culture – have received surprisingly little attention from researchers. As such, when the focus is on "trauma", the emotional dimensions of gendered violence are reduced to intrapsychic psychological distress that is not relevant to many perpetrators, overlooks the sociopolitical aspects of *specific* emotions and affects, constructs violent men as "victims", and has little to offer in terms of prevention. In contrast, the cognitive bias in the bulk of the gendered violence research – that is, the emphasis on gendered thoughts, attitudes, beliefs or individual discursive narratives – positions emotion as simply a bodily aftereffect of cognition that is not particularly meaningful or influential in its own right, resulting in a focus on attitudinal (or discursive) change at the expense of other preventive and rehabilitative strategies (Salter, 2016).

While suffering from the above limitations, the existing research into gendered violence nevertheless provides important clues as to what some of the more specific and nuanced affective drivers of everyday violence might be beyond individualistic, generalized notions of "trauma". As case in point, it is not uncommon for perpetrators to say that they feel disrespected by their partners when they attempt to explain their violent and controlling behavior (for example, Hill, 2019; Oddone, 2020). In a study by Oddone (2020), some men say that their violence is a way of "saving face" with partners in interactions where they believe there is "degradation of their status [as] 'men'", with their reputations with other men understood to be part of this (p. 255). Such comments are often analysed by researchers as symptomatic of attitudes or discourses consistent with hegemonic masculinity and a related belief in male superiority and entitlement to deference from others, especially women (ibid.). However, the relationship between subscribing to traditional gender inequities and violence-condoning discursive narratives (or attitudes, norms or beliefs, if you like), and the violent and controlling practices themselves, is not necessarily a straightforward one. In fact, there can be marked ruptures between "thinking", "believing", "saying" and "doing". Hence, while men who use violence more commonly admit to hegemonic masculinities and violence-condoning attitudes than other men (Flood & Pease, 2009), their violence is not always reflected in explicit gender-inequitable or violence-condoning views (Fulu, Jewkes, Roselli, & Garcia-Moreno, 2013; Gibbs et al., 2020). It is of course possible that some violent men are not straightforward about their beliefs or too ashamed to admit to them (Zapata-Calvente, Moya, Bohner, & Megías, 2019). However, recent evidence suggests that gender inequities and violence-condoning attitudes are usually so well-established by the time violence is enacted as to be automatic, implicit, habituated and not necessarily fully "conscious" (see Pornari, Dixon, & Humphreys, 2021; Zapata-Calvente, Moya, Bohner, & Megías, 2019). It is therefore necessary to go much further than looking to cognition or individual trauma to properly unpack the socially embodied nature of masculine sense of entitlement and its relationship to abusive practices.

While masculinized forms of honor and pride are almost never named in explorations of gendered violence in Western contexts, violent men's oft-cited comments about "feeling disrespected" by their partners seem to point to a sense of feeling dishonored in some way in their intimate relationships and, perhaps, in their wider lives too. I am not suggesting that emotions and affects related to a masculinized sense of entitlement to honor and pride are the *only* emotions driving violence perpetration, but they serve as an illustration of how dominant trauma or cognitivist theoretical frameworks have become. Nor am I suggesting that the perpetrator's responsibility for their violence is lessened because the emotional drivers may not be fully conscious. The next section begins to tease apart how the affective and emotional dimensions of male sense of entitlement to honor might play a role in driving gendered violence in everyday relationships.

## Violence Perpetration and Socially Embodied Emotion

As has been pointed out by Connell and Messerschmidt (2005), hegemonic masculinity can be understood as "the most honored way of being a man" (p. 832). While the authors themselves use the language of honor here, the concept has not been much studied in Western masculinities research more generally (ibid.), and not at all in relation to gendered violence outside of research into so-called "honor killings" and "honor-based violence" in some migrant communities and countries of origin (Cooney, 2014, 2019; Gill & Brah, 2014; Idriss, 2017; Rosen, 2008; Vandello & Cohen, 2008).

Honor is a multidimensional construct and is somewhat slippery to pin down. The *Oxford Dictionary* defines honor as "the quality of knowing and doing what is morally right". Here, honor is quite simply a positive individual quality or virtue. I acknowledge that some violent men *believe* that their abuse is motivated by the need to morally correct their errant partners (Stark, 2007). For example, Oddone (2020) documents one violent man justifying his violence through the idea that he needs to "give her a lesson" in appropriate female behavior (p. 252) – but such observations do not mean that violent men's behavior is actually honorable in any way. However, the *Oxford Dictionary* also defines honor as "a quality that combines respect, being proud and honesty" and "something that you are very pleased or proud to do because people are showing you great respect". Here, honor involves feelings of high personal regard and pride in oneself that are dependent on a show of esteem – or honoring – on the part of others. It is this more social, relational, emotional and hierarchical version of honor and honoring that I am concerned with here, not the virtue *per se*. Indeed, some in the gendered-violence field refuse to use the language of "honor killings" or "honor-based violence" because, as they rightly point out, there is nothing conceivably virtuous about abusing and killing partners, ex-partners or children. So let me be crystal clear here that I am *not* talking about honor as a virtue. Rather, I am talking about hegemonic forms of *masculinist-defined honor* and associated emotions and affects, and how these might help to drive and shape gendered violence and its impact.

Masculinist forms of honor that presume that men are entitled to respect, deference and esteem from others simply because they are men most certainly emerge from a historical hierarchical gender order, sustained by long-standing and intertwined gender discourses and continuing unequal structural gender power relations. But masculinized honor and honoring do not reside in thought, belief, ideology, discourse or structure alone. A sense of entitlement to honoring and pride as a man is also socially embodied in a state of being that is *felt* and *sensed* as well as (sometimes) thought and believed, with related actions or practices of honoring embedded in oftentimes concealed systems of "prestige, esteem, standing [and] distinction" (Bourdieu, 1979 cited in Hatch, 1989, p. 341); here, then, *dis*honoring (or disrespecting) is experienced as an "attack on self-esteem" (Bourdieu, 1979, p. 107) within the hierarchical gender order, just as many violent men's testimonies seem to attest to.

While masculinities scholars and psychological researchers have looked to individual histories of trauma-related shame and anger when they do examine perpetrator emotion, a cocktail of other socially situated affects and emotions are also likely to be involved in feeling *"dis*honored" (or disrespected) by a partner, and a perpetrator will not need to have suffered individual "trauma" in order to feel them. Hence, in addition to anger and shame, this mix is likely to include humiliation, indignation, rage, *out*rage, fear, a desire for revenge, disgust toward oneself and/or the intimate partner and, when there is a fear of infidelity, extreme jealousy – this last emotion is extremely common in violent, controlling men and has been underresearched. Feelings of jealousy also have little to do with actual transgressions on the part of the partner (Franzway, Moulding, Wendt, Zufferey, & Chung, 2020; Stark, 2007). Moreover, these emotions, sensations and affects are likely to be experienced as immediate, in the moment, habituated and not always fully conscious or consciously thought through (Pornari, Dixon, & Humphreys, 2021).

Certainly, in previous studies, some violent men describe their rage building in response to perceived criticisms from partners, read as slights to their status as men, until the rage suddenly explodes in violence and abuse (Oddone, 2020). Similarly, some violent men also say that their abusive and controlling behavior seems to occur in the absence of specific thought (Whiting, Merchant, Bradford, & Smith, 2020), and that it feels *bodily* and *instinctual* (Oddone, 2020). Lastly, some violent men indicate that, for these reasons, their abusive behavior is often perplexing to them and feels out of control (ibid.; Whiting, Merchant, Bradford, & Smith, 2020). This seems to suggest that less-conscious, socially embodied, highly gendered and deeply ingrained emotions, desires, sensations and affects related to masculinized honoring and face-saving may be important drivers of gendered violence for some male perpetrators. Following Connell and Messerschmidt (2005), I argue that to understand the social embodiment that is part-and-parcel of these masculinities, it is necessary to attend to its physical, emotional and sensual elements, and its intersectional and interactive aspects. These require further exploration more broadly, but particularly so in relation to gendered violence.

As briefly noted earlier, honor and related injuries to male self-esteem, pride and reputation are considered to be the central drivers of "honor killings" or "honor-based violence" in more explicitly patriarchal migrant communities and countries (Cooney, 2014, 2019; Gill & Brah, 2014; Idriss, 2017; Rosen, 2008), as if the protection of male honor through gendered violence is relevant *only* to these groups (Grewal, 2013; Hamad, 2019). Yet the existence of male-defined family honor systems in some migrant groups does not mean that male-defined honor is not in play in other contexts (Hamad, 2019). Moreover, if more masculinized honor systems and practices in non-migrant communities are somewhat hidden and unacknowledged, long-standing and deeply ingrained, they might be particularly resistant to change in the face of shifting gender mores and gender power relations. Observations of "backlash violence" in the face of women's equality gains (Stark, 2007; Gracia & Merlo, 2016) and the escalation and increasing severity of domestic violence in migrant communities' post-migration to Westernized countries (Erez, Adelman, & Gregory, 2009) may point to this. More individualistic and concealed forms of male-coded honour in Westernized contexts, therefore, arguably warrant dedicated investigation (Baker, Gregware, & Cassidy, 1999).

## Victim-survivors and the Social Construction and Embodiment of Emotion

To effect change, it is undoubtedly crucial to consider what is felt by and drives perpetrators in the moments when they enact violence and control. However, gendered violence is inherently intersubjective and interactive (Anderson, 2009), so it is equally important that the emotions and affects experienced by victim-survivors are considered at the same time. In saying this, I am not suggesting that the behavior of victim-survivors "causes" or "triggers" intimate partner violence. Rather, I am arguing that it is important to properly understand victim-survivors' responses, because there has been a long history of casting women as passive victims without agency, victim-blaming them as causing the violence, or falling into misguided notions about victim-survivors seeking out violent and controlling partners as a result of pre-existing trauma (Moulding, 2016; Moulding, Buchanan, & Wendt, 2015).

While fear is certainly a central emotion experienced by victim-survivors in response to intimate partner violence, my previous research with colleagues has found that many women often emphasize a range of other emotions as perhaps equally or even more troubling (Franzway, Moulding, Wendt, Zufferey, & Chung, 2020; Moulding, Franzway, Wendt, Zufferey, & Chung, 2021). In particular, many women place greater emphasis on how they come to feel like different *persons* because of the dehumanizing and objectifying nature of coercive control, fragmented within themselves, no longer confident, with no clear sense of who they are or their agency (Franzway, Moulding, Wendt, Zufferey, & Chung, 2020; Moulding, Franzway, Wendt, Zufferey, & Chung, 2021). This is in many ways the point of gendered violence and particularly of coercive control (see also Stark, 2007). Previous research with colleagues has also demonstrated how very particular femininity discourses are mobilized and enacted through these controlling abusive practices to strip women of their sense of self by variously constructing them as irrational and mad, stupid, weak and dependent, dirty, ugly and fat, disgusting (particularly during pregnancy, a time when violence often commences or worsens) or as sexually out of control and dangerous (see Franzway, Moulding, Wendt, Zufferey, & Chung, 2020; Moulding, Franzway, Wendt, Zufferey, & Chung, 2021).

The positioning of women and the feminine as mad, bad, irrational and out of control in violent and controlling practices occurs through the historical hierarchical gender binary that simultaneously positions men and masculinity as superior, rational, moral and in control. As has been pointed out by Stark (2007), violent and controlling men often define their own attitudes, views and behavior as reasonable, rational and morally correct, while their female partners are cast as emotional, irrational and immoral. However, men who use violence experience many of the very same emotions and vulnerabilities they deny and project onto women, so their violence can be understood as a way of reproducing gender difference and the hierarchical gender binary or gender order (Anderson, 2009). Taking this argument further, I argue that practices of violence and control effectively locate women and the feminine as *abject* (Kristeva, 1982), the shame-ridden counter-opposite to honored forms of hegemonic masculinity. The idea of the "abject" was developed by Julia Kristeva and literally means "to cast off, exclude or prohibit" (Warin, 2010, p. 112). Kristeva's notion of the abject seeks to:

> describe and account for temporal and spatial disruptions within the life of the subject and in particular those moments when the subject experiences a frightening loss of distinction between themselves and objects/others. The abject describes those forces, practices and things which are opposed to and unsettle the conscious ego, the "I". It is the zone between being and non-being, "the border of my condition as a living being".
>
> *(Kristeva, 1982, p. 3)*

Drawing on the idea of abjection to theorize violence and control, Tyler (2009) argues that "battered women's idea of themselves as individuals is gradually obliterated until they are literally pushed 'toward the place where meaning collapses' [(Kristeva, 1982: p. 2, cited in Tyler, 2009] ..., a state which she describes as *'being* on the edge of non-existence' or 'abjection lived'" (Tyler, 2009, p. 90). However, women do not necessarily take up these positions of abjection lightly. In my previous research with colleagues, we have detailed the often-unacknowledged anger and betrayal that many women feel toward the men who have pushed them toward the edge (Franzway, Moulding, Wendt, Zufferey, & Chung, 2020; Moulding, Franzway, Wendt, Zufferey, & Chung, 2021; Moulding, Chung, Zufferey, Franzway, & Wendt, 2023). Our research has also shown how many women experience enormous shame and guilt in response to partner abuse, often staying in violent relationships because they are trying to live up to the gendered social expectations about keeping the family together and ensuring that their children have a father, in line with hegemonic mothering and femininity discourses (Franzway, Moulding, Wendt, Zufferey, & Chung, 2020; Moulding, Buchanan & Wendt, 2015).

Feminist scholars have theorized women's efforts along these lines as "doing femininity" (Wendt & Zannetino, 2015), that is, as attempting to meet hegemonic femininity ideals, just as violent men are understood to be attempting to meet, however misguidedly, hegemonic masculinity ideals by "doing masculinity" through violence and coercive control (Oddone, 2020). However, the idea of "doing femininity" (or "doing masculinity", for that matter) does not go far enough in identifying the gendered emotions and affects involved in these practices. When women talk about trying to keep the family together and attempting to meet other gendered femininity and motherhood ideals, their narratives point to feminized forms of honor and the desire to circumvent abjection, shame, guilt and dishonor. Hence, while honor is mainly presumed to be a masculine preserve, women's narratives of living with violence and abuse point to the role of feminine-coded forms of honor and recognition (see Churcher & Gatens, 2019), represented in their efforts to meet gendered expectations as partners and mothers (Moulding, Buchanan & Wendt, 2015).

In light of the above discussion of how gendered forms of honor and abjection, and their associated affects, might help to drive gendered violence in everyday relationships, I would argue that trauma-based and cognitivist theories are simply unequal to the task of capturing or theorizing such dynamic, nuanced social phenomena. As a result, the social embodiment and intersubjective dynamics of these gendered affects and emotions in gendered violence remains relatively unexplored in research and overlooked in practice.

## A Way Forward: Feminist Affective-Discursive Approaches to Gendered Violence

While many important insights have been gained from previous research into gendered violence, an individual-society dualism continues to beset research in ways that limit theorization and the development of effective, integrated policy and practice. Within this dualism, trauma models and cognitivist theories about individual attitudes, beliefs and discursive narratives sit to one side, while wider social structures, gender discourses and ideologies sit to the other. As a result of this, most research to date has directed effort toward the (also worthy and necessary) project of making gendered violence *understandable* and *knowable* through examination of the individual discursive narratives and beliefs used by perpetrators and victim-survivors to rationalize and explain it, the "trauma" thought to both trigger and result from it, and the structural gender inequalities and related discourses that enable and support it. To better understand gendered violence, it is also necessary to journey into the so-called "irrational" meaning-making realm where the social meets the body. After all, gendered violence is often ultimately self-defeating for those who use it, even if there are immediate gains to be had, driving many intimate partners away and, in the worst-case scenarios, escalating to the murders of partners, ex-partners and their children (Johnson, 2006). Hence, to better understand how to intervene more effectively in the epidemic of gendered violence in Australia and other countries around the world, the role of less-conscious, socially embodied affects and emotions, and their political effects, requires further elaboration and theorization.

Drawing on Ahall (2018), there is scope for a feminist affective-discursive approach to researching practices of gendered violence that includes attention to discourse but also to "what goes without saying" and is "beyond words" because "the logic of gender works affectively, emotionally and performatively" – that is, it works *between bodies* – with much occurring at a level below full consciousness (Ahall, 2018, p. 43). Moreover, any exploration of the politics of emotion in gendered violence requires sensitivity to the different ways these politics play out in different groups in line with an intersectional framework (Crenshaw, 1991), taking into account diverse emotions and affects related to gender, sexualities, class, culture and other social differences and identities.

## Conclusion

In closing, while this critique of current theoretical and practice approaches to gendered violence has particularly placed trauma and cognitivist discourses in the spotlight, I am not suggesting that these approaches have no relevance to understanding gendered violence perpetration or victimization. Rather, I want to caution, first, that an uncritical engagement with trauma theory incorrectly assumes that individual trauma is virtually universal among both perpetrators and victim-survivors and, from there, often slides into an individualistic intrapsychic orientation that loses sight of the gendered social processes driving abuse. I also argue that trauma theory is simply unequal to the task of capturing the highly gendered, nuanced, intersubjective emotions and affects embodied in gendered violence. I have used the example of emotions and affects related to gendered forms of honor and abjection to illustrate this. On the other hand, cognitivist approaches often naively assume that gendered social norms or discourses are reflected unproblematically in explicit, conscious attitudes, beliefs or individual discursive narratives, which then translate rather seamlessly into violent practices. This relationship is not necessarily so straightforward, and to assume that it is ignores less-conscious embodied emotions, affects and sensations and, along with them, all that is *not* said or explicit. To address this gap, there is scope for feminist inquiry into how socially embodied emotions and affects also drive gendered violence to inform the development of more effective multidimensional interventions that simultaneously address the intertwined discursive, affective and structural drivers of intimate partner violence in everyday relationships.

## References

Ahall, L. (2018). Affect as methodology: Feminism and the politics of emotion. *International Political Sociology*, 12(1), 36–52. https://doi.org/10.1093/ips/olx024.

Anderson, K.L. (2009). Gendering coercive control. *Violence Against Women*, 15(12), 1444–1457. doi: 10.1177/1077801209346837.

Arias, E., Arce, R., & Vilariño, M. (2013). Batterer intervention programmes: A meta-analytic review of effectiveness. *Psychosocial Intervention*, 22(2), 153–160. https://doi.org/https://doi.org/10.5093/in2013a18.

Augusta-Scott, T., & Dankwort, J. (2002). Partner abuse group intervention: Lessons from education and narrative therapy approaches. *Journal of Interpersonal Violence*, 17(7), 783–805. https://doi.org/10.1177/0886260502017007006.

Australian Bureau of Statistics (ABS) (2017). *Personal Safety Survey*, Australia, 2016, ABS Cat. no. 4906.0. ABS, Canberra.

Baker, N.V., Gregware, P.R., & Cassidy, M.A. (1999). Family killing fields. *Violence Against Women*, 5(2), 164–184. https://doi.org/10.1177/107780129952005.

Baum, F., & Miller, M. (2014). Why behavioural health promotion endures despite its failure to reduce health inequities. In S. Cohen (Ed.), *From health behaviours to health practices: Critical perspectives* (pp. 213–225). Wiley-Blackwell. https://doi.org/10.1002/9781118898345.

Berggren, K., Gottzen, L., & Bornas, H. (2021) Theorising masculinity and intimate partner violence. In L. Gottzen, M. Bjornholt and F. Boonzair (Eds.). *Men, masculinities and intimate partner violence*. Routledge. https://doi.org/10.4324/9780429280054.

Bonomi, A.E., Anderson, M.L., Reid, R.J., Rivara, F.P., Carrell, D., & Thompson, R.S. (2009). Medical and psychosocial diagnoses in women with a history of intimate partner violence. *Archives of Internal Medicine (1960)*, 169(18), 1692–1697. https://doi.org/10.1001/archinternmed.2009.292.

Boonzaier, F., & van Niekerk, T. (2019). Discursive trends in research on masculinities and interpersonal violence. *Routledge International Handbook of Masculinity Studies*, 457–466.

Bourdieu, P. (1979). Symbolic power. *Critique of Anthropology*, 4(13–14), 77–85. https://doi.org/10.1177/0308275X7900401307.

Bowen, E., & Gilchrist, E. (2006). Predicting dropout of court-mandated treatment in a British sample of domestic violence offenders. *Psychology, Crime & Law*, 12(5), 573–587. https://doi.org/10.1080/10683160500337659.

Bowen, E., Gilchrist, E.A., & Beech, A.R. (2005). An examination of the impact of community-based rehabilitation on the offending behaviour of male domestic violence offenders and the characteristics associated with recidivism. *Legal and Criminological Psychology*, 10(2), 189–209. https://doi.org/10.1348/135532505X36778.

Bowman, B., Stevens, G., Eagle, G., Langa, M., Kramer, S., Kiguwa, P., & Nduna, M. (2015). The second wave of violence scholarship: South African synergies with a global research agenda. *Social Science & Medicine (1982)*, 146, 243–248. https://doi.org/10.1016/j.socscimed.2015.10.014.

Breckenridge, J. (1999). Subjugation and silences: The role of the professions in silencing victims of sexual and domestic violence. In J. Breckenridge and L. Laing (Eds.), *Challenging silence: Innovative responses to sexual and domestic violence* (pp. 6–30). Allen & Unwin.

Brown, J. (2004). Shame and domestic violence: Treatment perspectives for perpetrators from self-psychology and affect theory. *Sexual and Relationship Therapy*, 19(1), 39–56. https://doi.org/10.1080/14681990410001640826.

Brownmiller, S. (1975). *Against our will*. Bantam Books.

Calvete, E., Estévez, A., & Corral, S. (2007). Intimate partner violence and depressive symptoms in women: Cognitive schemas as moderators and mediators. *Behaviour Research and Therapy*, 45(4), 791–804. https://doi.org/10.1016/j.brat.2006.07.006.

Churcher, M., & Gatens, M. (2019). Reframing honour in heterosexual imaginaries. *Angelaki: Journal of Theoretical Humanities*, 24(4), 151–164. https://doi.org/10.1080 /0969725X.2019.1635834.

Connell, R.W. (1995). *Masculinities*. Polity Press.

Connell, R.W., & Messerschmidt, J.W. (2005). Hegemonic masculinity. *Gender & Society*, 19(6), 829–859. doi: 10.1177/0891243205278639.

Cooney, M. (2014). Death by family: Honor violence as punishment. *Punishment & Society*, 16(4), 406–427. https://doi.org/10.1177/1462474514539537.

Cooney, M. (2019). *Execution by family: A theory of honor violence*. Routledge. https://doi .org/10.4324/9781351240659.

Crenshaw, K. (1991). Mapping the margins: Intersectionality, identity politics, and violence against women of color. *Stanford Law Review*, 1241–1299. https://doi.org/10 .2307/1229039.

DeGue, S., Holt, M.K., Massetti, G.M., Matjasko, J.L., Tharp, A.T., & Valle, L.A. (2012). Looking ahead toward community-level strategies to prevent sexual violence. *Journal of Women's Health*, 21(1), 1–3. https://doi.org/10.1089/jwh.2011.3263.

DeKeseredy, W., Schwartz, M., & Donnermeyer, J. (2009). *Dangerous exits: Escaping abusive relationships in rural America*. Rutgers University Press. https://doi.org/10 .36019/9780813548609.

Dobash, R.E., & Dobash, R.P. (1978). Wives: The "appropriate" victims of marital violence. *Victimology: An International Journal*, 2(3–4), 426–442.

Erez, E., Adelman, M., & Gregory, C. (2009). Intersections of immigration and domestic violence. *Feminist Criminology*, 4(1), 32–56. https://doi.org/10.1177/1557085108325413.

Flood, M., & Pease, B. (2009). Factors influencing attitudes to violence against women. *Trauma, Violence & Abuse*, 10(2), 125–142. https://doi.org/10.1177/1524838009334131.

Franzway, S., Moulding, N., Wendt, S., Zufferey, C., & Chung, D. (2020). *The sexual politics of gendered violence and women's citizenship*. Policy Press.

Fulu, E., Jewkes, R., Roselli, T., & Garcia-Moreno, C. (2013). Prevalence of and factors associated with male perpetration of intimate partner violence: Findings from the UN multi-country cross-sectional study on men and violence in Asia and the Pacific. *The Lancet Global Health*, 1(4), e187–e207. https://doi.org/10.1016/S2214-109X(13)70074-3.

Gadd, D. (2000). Masculinities, violence and defended psychosocial subjects. *Theoretical Criminology*, 4(4), 429–449. https://doi.org/10.1177/1362480600004004002.

Gadd, D. (2003). Reading between the lines: Subjectivity and men's violence. *Men and Masculinities*, 5(4), 333–354. https://doi.org/10.1177/1097184X02250838.

Gadd, D. (2004). Evidence-led policy or policy-led evidence? Cognitive behavioural programmes for men who are violent towards women. *Criminal Justice*, 4(2), 173–198. https://doi.org/10.1177/1466802504044913.

Gadd, D., & Jefferson, T. (2007). *Psychosocial criminology: An introduction*. Sage. https:// doi.org/10.4135/9781446211496.

Gibbs, A., Dunkle, K., Ramsoomar, L., Willan, S., Jama Shai, N., Chatterji, S., et al. (2020). New learnings on drivers of men's physical and/or sexual violence against their female partners, and women's experiences of this, and the implications for prevention interventions. *Global Health Action*, 13(1), 1739845. https://doi.org/10.1080/16549716 .2020.1739845.

Gill, A.K., & Brah, A. (2014). Interrogating cultural narratives about "honour"-based violence. *The European Journal of Women's Studies*, 21(1), 72–86. doi: 10.1177/1350506813510424.

Goldenson, J., Geffner, R., Foster, S.L., & Clipson, C.R. (2007). Female domestic violence offenders: Their attachment security, trauma symptoms, and personality organization. *Violence and Victims*, 22(5), 532–545. https://doi.org/10.1891/088667007782312186.

Gracia, E., & Merlo, J. (2016). Intimate partner violence against women and the Nordic paradox. *Social Science and Medicine*, 157, 27–30. doi:10.16/j.socscimed.2016.03.040.

Grewal, I. (2013). Outsourcing patriarchy. *International Feminist Journal of Politics*, 15(1), 1–19. https://doi.org/10.1080/14616742.2012.755352.

Haines, A., Andary, S., Amos, J., Louth, R., Mannik, P., et al. (2022). Men working with men in intensive family services: Reflections on violence, trauma lifeworlds, and organic interventions. *Australian and New Zealand Journal of Family Therapy*, 43, 442–461. https://doi.org/10.1002/anzf.1517.

Hamad, R. (2019). *White tears/brown scars: How white feminism betrays women of colour.* Melbourne University Publishing

Hatch, E. (1989). Theories of social honor. *American Anthropologist*, 91(2), 341–353. https://doi.org/10.1525/aa.1989.91.2.02a00040.

Hearn, J. (1996). Deconstructing the dominant: Making the one(s) the other(s). *Organization*, 3, 611–626.

Hearn, J. (2012). A multi-faceted power analysis of men's violence to known women: From hegemonic masculinity to the hegemony of men. *The Sociological Review (Keele)*, 60(4), 589–610. https://doi.org/10.1111/j.1467-954X.2012.02125.x.

Hearn, J., & Whitehead, A. (2006). Collateral damage: Men's "domestic" violence to women seen through men's relations with men. *Probation Journal*, 53(1), 38–56. https://doi.org/10.1177/0264550506060864.

Hill, J. (2019). *See what you made me do.* Black.

Idriss, M.M. (2017). Not domestic violence or cultural tradition: Is honour-based violence distinct from domestic violence? *The Journal of Social Welfare & Family Law*, 39(1), 3–21. doi:10.1080/09649069.2016.1272755.

Johnson, C.H. (2006). Familicide and family law: A study of filicide: Suicide following separation. *Family Court Review*, 44(3), 448–463. https://doi.org/10.1111/j.1744-1617.2006.00099.x.

Kaplenko, H., Loveland, J.E., & Raghavan, C. (2018). Relationships between shame, restrictiveness, authoritativeness, and coercive control in men mandated to a domestic violence offenders program. *Violence and Victims*, 33(2): 296–309. doi: 10.1891/0886-6708.VV-D-16-00123.

Kelly, L. (1988). What's in a name? Defining child sexual abuse. *Feminist Review*, 28, 65–73. https://doi.org/10.2307/1394895.

Kelly, L., & Rehman, Y. (2013). *Moving in the shadows: Violence in the lives of minority women and children.* Routledge. https://doi.org/10.4324/9781315596198.

Kelly, L., & Westmarland, N. (2016). Naming and defining "domestic violence": Lessons from research with violent men. *Feminist Review*, 112(1), 113–127. https://doi.org/10.1057/fr.2015.52.

Kimmel, M. (2010). *Misframing Men: The Politics of Contemporary Masculinities.* Rutgers University Press. https://doi.org/10.36019/9780813549750

Kristeva, J. (1982). *Powers of horror: An essay on abjection.* Columbia University Press.

Langenderfer-Magruder, L., Whitfield, D.L., Walls, N.E., Kattari, S.K., & Ramos, D. (2016). Experiences of intimate partner violence and subsequent police reporting among lesbian, gay, bisexual, transgender, and queer adults in Colorado. *Journal of Interpersonal Violence*, 31(5), 855–871. https://doi.org/10.1177/0886260514556767.

MacKinnon, C.A. (1993). *Only words*. Harvard University Press.

McPhail, B.A. (2002). Gender-bias hate crimes: A review. *Trauma, Violence & Abuse*, 3(2), 125–143. https://doi.org/10.1177/15248380020032003.

Machisa, M.T., Christofides, N., & Jewkes, R. (2016). Structural pathways between child abuse, poor mental health outcomes and male-perpetrated intimate partner violence (IPV). *PloS One*, 11(3), e0150986–e0150986. https://doi.org/10.1371/journal.pone.0150986.

Messerschmidt, J.W. (1986). *Capitalism, patriarchy, and crime: Toward a socialist feminist criminology*. Rowman & Littlefield.

Messerschmidt, J. (1997). *Crime as structured action: Gender, race, class, and crime in the making*. Sage. https://doi.org/10.4135/9781452232294.

Messerschmidt, J.W. (2004). *Flesh and blood: Adolescent gender diversity and violence*. Rowman & Littlefield.

Messerschmidt, J.W. (2012). Engendering gendered knowledge: Assessing the academic appropriation of hegemonic masculinity. *Men and Masculinities*, 15(1), 56–76. https://doi.org/10.1177/1097184X11428384.

Millet, K. (1970). *Sexual politics*.: Doubleday.

Morran, D. (2011) Re-education or recovery? Re-thinking some aspects of domestic violence perpetrator programmes. *Probation Journal*, 58(1): 23–36. https://doi.org/10.1177/0264550510388968.

Moulding, N.T. (2016). *Gendered violence, mental health and recovery in everyday lives: Beyond trauma*. Routledge. https://doi.org/10.4324/9781315816630.

Moulding, N.T., Buchanan, F., & Wendt, S. (2015). Untangling self-blame and mother-blame in women's and children's perspectives on maternal protectiveness in domestic violence: Implications for practice. *Child Abuse Review*, 24(4), 49–260.

Moulding, N.T., Chung, D., Zufferey, C., Franzway, S., & Wendt, S. (2023). Social participation after intimate partner violence: Investigating the impact on women's citizenship. *Violence Against Women*, 27(8), 1064–1090. https://doi.org/10.1177/1077801220921937.

Moulding, N., Franzway, S., Wendt, S., Zufferey, C., & Chung, D. (2021). Rethinking women's mental health after intimate partner violence. *Violence Against Women*, 27(8), 1064–1090. https://doi.org/10.1177/1077801220921937.

Oddone, C. (2020). Perpetrating violence in intimate relationships as a gendering practice: An ethnographic study on domestic violence perpetrators in France and Italy. *Violence: An International Journal*, 1(2), 242–264. https://doi.org/10.1177/2633002420962274.

Pizzey, E. (1974). *Scream quietly or the neighbours will hear*. Penguin Books.

Pornari, C.D., Dixon, L., & Humphreys, G.W. (2021). A preliminary investigation into a range of implicit and explicit offense supportive cognitions in perpetrators of physical intimate partner violence. *Journal of Interpersonal Violence*, 36(3–4), NP2079–2111NP. https://doi.org/10.1177/0886260518755487.

Ptacek, J. (1988). Why do men batter their wives? In K. Yllö & M. Bograd (Eds.), *Feminist perspectives on wife abuse* (pp. 133–157). Sage.

Reavey, P., & Warner, S. (2003). Introduction. In P. Reavey & S. Warner (Eds.), *New feminist stories of child sexual abuse: Sexual scripts and dangerous dialogue* (pp. 1–12). Routledge. https://doi.org/10.4324/9780203361573.

Rees, S., Silove, D., Chey, T., Ivancic, L., Steel, Z., Creamer, M., Teesson, M., Bryant, R., McFarlane, A.C., Mills, K.L., Slade, T., Carragher, N., O'Donnell, M., & Forbes, D.

(2011). Lifetime prevalence of gender-based violence in women and the relationship with mental disorders and psychosocial function. *JAMA : The Journal of the American Medical Association*, 306(5), 513–521. https://doi.org/10.1001/jama.2011.1098.

Roberts, A.L., Gilman, S.E., Fitzmaurice, G., Deckerf, M.R., & Koenen, K.C. (2010). Witness of intimate partner violence in childhood and perpetration of intimate partner violence in adulthood epidemiology. *Epidemiology*, 21(6): 809–818. doi:10.1097/EDE.0b013e3181f39f03.

Romans, S.E., Martin, J.L., & Anderson, J.C. (1995). Sexual abuse in childhood and deliberate self-harm. *The American Journal of Psychiatry*, 152(9),1336-1342. doi: 10.1176/ajp.152.9.1336.

Romito, P., Molzan Turan, J., & De Marchi, M. (2005). The impact of current and past interpersonal violence on women's mental health. *Social Science & Medicine*, 60(8), 1717–1727. https://doi.org/10.1016/j.socscimed.2004.08.026.

Rosen, D. (2008). Honour killings an expression of immigrant alienation. *Eureka Street*, 18(6), 12–13. https://doi//10.3316/informit.048774839776998.

Salter, M. (2016). "Real men don't hit women": Constructing masculinity in the prevention of violence against women. *Australian & New Zealand Journal of Criminology*, 49(4), 463–479. https://doi.org/10.1177/0004865815587031.

Semiatin, J.N., Torres, S., LaMotte, A.D., Portnoy, G.A., & Murphy, C.M. (2017). Trauma exposure, PTSD symptoms, and presenting clinical problems among male perpetrators of intimate partner violence. *Psychology of Violence*, 7(1), 91–100. https://doi.org/10.1037/vio0000041.

Senkans, S., McEwan, T.E., & Ogloff, J.R.P. (2020). Conceptualising intimate partner violence perpetrators' cognition as aggressive relational schemas. *Aggression and Violent Behavior*, 55, 101456. https://doi.org/10.1016/j.avb.2020.101456.

Seymour, K., Wendt, S., & Natalier, K. (2023). *Responding to domestic violence: Difficult conversations*. Routledge. https://doi.org/10.4324/9781003171355.

Stark, E. (2007). *Coercive control: The entrapment of women in personal life*. Oxford University Press.

Stokoe, E. (2010). "I'm not gonna hit a lady": Conversation analysis, membership categorization and men's denials of violence towards women. *Discourse & Society*, 21(1), 59–82. Doi: 10.1177/0957926509345072.

Straus, M.A., & Gelles, R.J. (1986). Societal change and change in family violence from 1975 to 1985 as revealed by two national surveys. *Journal of Marriage and Family*, 48(3), 465–479. https://doi.org/10.2307/352033.

Taylor, R., & Jasinski, J.L. (2011). Femicide and the feminist perspective. *Homicide Studies*, 15(4), 341–362. https://doi.org/10.1177/1088767911424541.

Thiara, R.K., & Gill, A.K. (2010), Understanding violence against South Asian women: What it means for practice. In R.K. Thiara & A.K. Gill (Eds.), *Violence Against Women in South Asian Communities; Issues for Policy and Practice* (pp. 28–54). Jessica Kingsley Publishers.

Thiara, R.K., Hague, G., & Mullender, A. (2011). Losing out on both counts: Disabled women and domestic violence, *Disability & Society*, 26: 6, 757–771, doi: 10.1080/09687599.2011.602867.

Tyler, I. (2009). Against abjection. *Feminist theory*, 10(1), pp.77–98.

Vandello, J.A., & Cohen, D. (2008). Culture, gender, and men's intimate partner violence. *Social and Personality Psychology Compass*, 2, 652–667. https://doi.org/10.1111/j.1751-9004.2008.00080.x.

Walby, S. (2009). *Globalization and inequalities complexities and contested modernities.* Sage.

Warin, M. (2010). *Abject relations: Everyday worlds of anorexia.* Rutgers University Press. https://doi.org/10.36019/9780813548210.

Wendt, S., Natalier, K., Seymour, K., King, D., & Macaitis, K. (2020). Strengthening the domestic and family violence workforce: Key questions. *Australian Social Work*, 73(2), 236–244. https://doi.org/10.1080/0312407X.2019.1638429.

Wendt, S., & Zannettino, L. (2015). *Domestic violence in diverse contexts: A re-examination of gender.* Routledge. https://doi.org/10.4324/9781315751894.

Westmarland, N., & Kelly, L. (2013). Why extending measurements of "success" in domestic violence perpetrator programmes matters for social work. *The British Journal of Social Work*, 43(6), 1092–1110. https://doi.org/10.1093/bjsw/bcs049.

Wetherell, M. (2012). *Affect and emotion: A new social science understanding.* Sage. https://doi.org/10.4135/9781446250945.

Whiting, J.B., Merchant, L.V., Bradford, A.B., & Smith, D.B. (2020). The ecology of family violence: Treating cultural contexts and relationship processes. *The Handbook of Systemic Family Therapy*, 4, 153–190. https://doi.org/10.1002/9781119438519.ch89.

Widom, C.S., Czaja, S., & Dutton, M.A. (2014). Child abuse and neglect and intimate partner violence victimization and perpetration: A prospective investigation. *Child Abuse and Neglect*, 38, 650–663. doi:10.1016/j.chiabu.2013.11.004.

World Health Organization (WHO). (2010). *Preventing intimate partner and sexual violence against women: Taking action and generating evidence.* World Health Organization, Geneva. Retrieved from: https://apps.who.int/iris/handle/10665/44350.

Zapata-Calvente, A.L., Moya, M., Bohner, G., & Megías, J.L. (2019). Automatic associations and conscious attitudes predict different aspects of men's intimate partner violence and sexual harassment proclivities. *Sex Roles*, 81, 439–455. https://doi.org/10.1007/s11199-019-1006-0.

# 15

# TRAUMA- AND VIOLENCE-INFORMED CARE

## A Restorative and Just Response to Family Violence

*Nancy Ross and Ann Schumacher*

## Introduction

Overwhelming evidence suggests that 60 to 70 percent of the people who experience violence in their intimate partnership wish to stay in the relationship (Cravens, Whiting, & Aamar, 2015; Kulkarni, 2019; Ross & Ryan, 2021), but they do not have adequate access to resources, including an adequate basic income, nor do they have tools for developing their social and emotional literacy skills that would support that aspiration. Once they become part of the judicial system, which places them in adversarial roles, opportunities are limited for reconciliation or restoration of the relationship. Responses to intimate partner violence in Canada rely heavily on law enforcement officers, and the state and child welfare systems, which have already been subject to significant critique. Police officers, lawyers, survivors, allied professionals and even those who perpetrated the harm have all expressed concern about the emotional damage experienced by individuals and families while engaged with these systems (Ross & Ryan, 2021). This is no doubt an unanticipated and unintended effect of the earlier advocacy of the women's movement's efforts to develop greater awareness of violence against women, services for these women, and more effective responses by the criminal justice system to ensure their safety. We argue for an alternative, family-centered restorative approach that is founded on trauma- and violence-informed care.

In this chapter, we will outline the ways in which the pro-arrest, pro-charge and pro-prosecution policies have been experienced as unhelpful and frequently harmful by introducing a case example of "Charlotte" and "Joe" (pseudonyms). Charlotte reflects the experiences described by 23 women cumulatively and Joe, the voice of 14 men charged for domestic violence. Their experiences, described in a report entitled *A Review of Pro-Arrest, Pro-Charge and Pro-Prosecution*

DOI: 10.4324/9781003379591-16

*Policies: Redefining Responses to Domestic Violence* (Ross & Ryan, 2021), highlight what happens when a frightened individual calls the police during family violence. We then suggest how restorative approaches could better support families suffering from domestic violence if they are built upon a caring trauma- and violence-informed infrastructure that is well-resourced and substantive.

## Description of Pro-arrest Policies

In Canada, when a victim or concerned bystander calls the police to report an incident of domestic violence, the response is guided by pro-arrest, pro-charge and pro-prosecution policies. These policies were implemented by the government of Canada in the 1980s and 1990s with the hope they would serve as a deterrent and, thereby, reduce the rates of domestic violence. In cooperation with the solicitor general and local police departments across the country, these policies criminalized domestic violence by giving legal authority to the police and prosecution to lay criminal charges if reasonable evidence of family violence was found (Barata & Schneider, 2004; Davidson, 2004; Department of Justice, 2010). These policies immediately removed the responsibility and choice of survivors to either pursue or not pursue criminal action against the person causing the harm (Davidson, 2004). Furthermore, the dictate to arrest and lay a charge resulted in reducing the discretion of the police, setting in motion a one-size-fits-all approach to interpersonal violence. The initiation of these policies was largely the result of advocacy efforts by mainstream White feminists who hoped carceral responses to domestic violence would ultimately lower the rates and increase public awareness of domestic violence as a serious and criminal offence (ibid.).

While it is helpful to appreciate the motivating factors around the creation of law enforcement policies, there have been significant critiques of their impact over the last 40 years. As noted by the substantive review of the literature on the efficacy of judicial processes for interpersonal violence by Ryan and colleagues (Ryan, Silvio, Borden, & Ross, 2022), almost 60 percent of the articles either failed to support these policies or recommended significant revisions. Notably, using police as first responders has become a substantial barrier in calling for help during interpersonal violence. In a report that summarized findings from over 900 service providers' responses about police interventions in the United States, 76 percent of the respondents said the police acted in a demeaning and biased manner (Coker, Park, Goldscheid, Neal, & Halstead, 2015). In a Canadian review of the literature related to the implementation of pro-arrest, pro-charge and pro-prosecution policies, 25.4 percent of the articles noted that the negative implications of these policies intensified for individuals and communities who are socially, racially and economically oppressed (p. 224).

As mentioned above, the fear of becoming involved in the carceral system is sometimes a deterrent to phoning the police, and this, in certain cases, can have adverse effects. The primary wish of those who call the police is for the violence to stop. However, they are often not prepared for the invasive system responses this call can set in motion. Again, this is especially true for those who are racially, socially and economically marginalized and who already feel an increased vulnerability to experiencing further harm once they become part of the criminal justice system (Ryan, Silvio, Borden, & Ross, 2022). The "Charlotte and Joe" case study presented below highlights what can happen once a survivor calls the police. These experiences are portrayed in greater detail in the above-mentioned report, which chronicles Charlotte and Joe's journey through multiple segments of the judicial system (Ross & Ryan, 2021). While the project portrayed in this report did not include interviews with children, both Charlotte and Joe noted the negative impact of family violence on children, highlighting the frequency of intergenerational trauma, and the absence of supportive system responses for their children.

## Charlotte and Joe: A Case Study

In our discussion of Charlotte and Joe's case, we will describe their experience with the multiple layers of the judicial process after Charlotte called the police for help. Overall, the process was largely negative and overwhelmingly stressful. Just calling the police was a difficult choice, followed by challenges with the family court, Child Protection Services, a women's shelter, defense counsel, victim services, the criminal justice system, mandatory pediatric assessment on family dynamics, offender/family programs, and the Crown.

### Charlotte Calls the Police for Help

After experiencing intimate partner violence, Charlotte described how the decision to call the police was very scary, and how she was worried that it would only make things worse by setting in motion a criminal justice system response that would be at odds with what she wanted and needed. Frequently, survivors are reluctant to call the police and, according to the Public Health Agency of Canada (2018a), at least 80 percent do not. The police have not always received specialized training in defusing highly charged domestic situations or in conflict management skills when responding to interpersonal violence calls. The police, on the other hand, have also stated that the pro-arrest policies limit their ability to be discretionary in their responses (Ross & Ryan, 2021). Joe shared that, when a police officer arrests someone, whether it is the best response at the time or not, the policies dictate the same response for everyone.

### Charlotte Goes to Family Court

Once Charlotte made the call for help, she was told by the police to contact the family court. This meant filling out a significant amount of tedious and time-consuming paperwork that was often confusing and not coordinated with the criminal

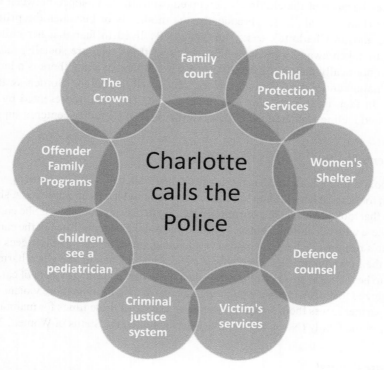

**FIGURE 15.1** Calling the police.

court system. This placed additional stress and responsibility on Charlotte, who was already traumatized by the domestic violence event (Ross & Ryan, 2021).

When Joe was advised to not have any contact with his partner or their children and to leave the home, he felt the focus was on him receiving a sentence and not on providing him with support. Following his arrest, Joe became suicidal.

### Child Protection Services

After Charlotte phoned the police, Child Protection Services came to her house and told her that if her partner was allowed to return home, they would have reason to remove her children from her care. Everything moved quickly for Charlotte, including the interviews the Child Protection Services held with her boys. Just the appearance of Child Protection Services in the home can create fear and further emotional distress, especially for families who wish to remain together. The fear is based on the reality that possibly witnessing violence could be a rationale for removing children from their home. In Ontario, for example, 48 percent of the children in the care of the state were removed from their home by Child Protection

Services because of the children's perceived exposure to violence between their parents (Fallon et al., 2015). Frequently, the mother is or becomes the primary parent; and, in Charlotte's case, she continually lived in fear that her children might be taken away by the state. Furthermore, those who are socially, racially and economically marginalized are especially vulnerable when there is a lack of coordination and infrastructure between systems (Ryan, Silvio, Borden, & Ross, 2022). In fact, many survivors feel revictimized. The men, represented by Joe, expressed feeling alienated from their families with little father-centered support.

## Women's Shelter

The police told Charlotte that the local women's shelter was a temporary viable option for her and her children to be safe, but she found it was an unpleasant, shared space that looked much like a dormitory, lacking in privacy or comfort. She chose to stay there with her children but was not allowed to take her pets. She felt the carceral system's response in her case made her and other survivors feel like refugees away from their own home. She asked why she should be the one to flee when harm was done to her? During this period, Joe would have benefited from a system of care that recognized that many people who perpetuate harm may become more violent when their partner leaves them, and support can be critical at these times for maintaining safety of the family (Nova Scotia Advisory Council on the Status of Women, 2022).

## Defense Counsel

The criminal lawyer representing Charlotte's partner, Joe, in the judicial system was the one who informed her that Joe expected her to leave the house. Charlotte also feared that Joe's goal was to discredit her on the stand. In this type of adversarial system, Joe was discouraged from accepting any responsibility for the interpersonal violence and Charlotte experienced both fear and trauma as her credibility was systematically dismantled (Ross & Ryan, 2021).

## Victim Services

Charlotte received counseling services from Victim Services (sometimes called Survivor Services in the United States), but her partner, Joe, did not. She wanted him to go to counseling, but the criminal justice system and the court trial process supported an adversarial process in which Joe took steps to prove his innocence and/or minimize the scope of harm perpetrated. This, in turn, reduced opportunities and possibilities for Joe, the person who caused the harm, to be held accountable and to accept responsibility for his actions. It was only after he was found guilty that he could enter the counseling services if they were available and recommended. Charlotte, in contrast, believed that Joe should have counseling services immediately and that such services should not be dependent on a guilty plea.

## Criminal Justice System

Joe had a history of adverse childhood experiences, as he had witnessed intimate partner violence between his parents as well as consistent substance abuse within his childhood home. All he knew when growing up, he said, was violence; and he had also experienced incarceration, another form of violence. During the intake consultation, he openly expressed feeling like a victim in the judicial system, which had no understanding of his emotions and, at one point, he mentioned wanting to end his life. Counseling was not offered to him, even though he said he would appreciate any support available and expressed the desire to learn new skills.

## Impact of Mandatory Pediatric Assessment on Family Dynamics

Charlotte was required to take her children for an evaluation with a pediatrician, who indicated they would experience emotional ups and downs, in part because of being separated from their father. It is important to keep in mind that the emotional and mental well-being of children can be compromised with the criminalization of a parent or when the family system is suffering from intergenerational trauma, including historical childhood abuse of one or both parents. Such was the case with Joe.

## Offender/Family Programs

Neither Joe nor Charlotte were offered any programs for developing their social and emotional literacy or conflict management skills within the carceral system, nor were they offered any restorative alternatives to the adversarial system. Services that were family-centered were largely absent throughout each of the stages of the application of these policies. As a result of the one-size-fits-all approach, the different needs of families were not addressed within the standardized judicial process.

## The Crown

Charlotte's lawyer believed that the adversarial court system pitted partners against one another, which was certainly not helpful for those who wanted to stay together. In fact, most of the lawyers who were research participants acknowledged the need for more relational, family-centered, trauma- and violence-informed approaches (Ross & Ryan, 2021).

## Trauma- and Violence-informed Family-centered Care

We propose a trauma- and violence-informed approach to intimate partner violence because it takes into consideration the partners' intention for relational restitution and has the potential to support the healing process both for those who have been harmed and for those who have caused harm. At the same time, this restorative approach can introduce families to non-violent forms of communication and help them develop conflict resolution and peacemaking skills (Packer, 2021).

Trauma can significantly alter the way a person sees the world, serving as a filter through which many daily events are experienced and interpreted. Too often individuals feel shame, self-blame and stigma for the challenges they face in attempting to cope with trauma. In neoliberal contexts, community supports are often diminished while, at the same time, emphasis on individual responsibility is increased (Brown, C., 2021). This means that, for many individuals as well as the public in general, the understanding of trauma can be narrow – limited to individuals and families – without a critical analysis of the structural and cultural factors that have created the stressed environments and heighten vulnerability to the levels of trauma and violence.

When trauma's tendrils reach back into an individual's childhood, or even further, deep within the ancestral lineage, it is identified as intergenerational trauma. Research shows there is often an intergenerational component to adverse childhood experiences and intimate partner violence (Bethell et. al. 2017; Bombay, Matheson, & Anisman, 2014; Hubl, 2020). Not only is the occurrence of violence in a partner relationship traumatic, but many of the individuals who experience intimate partner violence have grown up with their own childhood traumas, including parental substance-use problems with drugs and alcohol, poverty and neglect. In some families who experience intimate partner violence, trauma has been discretely transmitted from prior generations through attachment relationships and, unbeknownst to the offspring – either because it is unconscious or because it is triggered by earlier experiences of childhood adversity, for example – he or she reacts to a stressor in a way that may be disproportional to the incident that has occurred. According to Hubl (2020, p. 4), trauma brings about separation and fragmentation, which is the energy of the unmet or unintegrated past, distorting the present moment. An unintegrated past or trauma becomes "a preprogrammed path along which every individual or culture sets out until the contents of that past have been brought into the light of consciousness, reconciled and healed" (ibid., p. 5). Remembering the words of philosopher George Santayana, "Those who cannot remember the past are condemned to repeat it." Since unconscious trauma is bound to repeat, maladaptive survival strategies are often created to endure the unbearable suffering. Substance-use problems, self-harm, and interpersonal violence – all seen in Joe – are some of the primary coping strategies (Bethell et al., 2017; Hughes et al., 2017; Maté, 2008).

The fundamental principles of trauma-based care include relational procedures that support a participant's sense of safety, trust, choice-making, empowerment and partnership, as well as helping them understand the impact that trauma often has across their lifespan, and even intergenerationally (Herman, 1992; 2015; Levenson, 2017; Substance Abuse and Mental Health Services Administration, 2014). Whilst these principles constitute what is commonly referred to as "trauma-informed" approaches, there are scholars who have challenged the recent exponential rise of this term because it has led to standardized practices that are often depoliticized, degendered, medicalized and individualized within systems subject to neoliberal constraints (Johnstone, Brown, C., & Ross, 2022; Tseris, 2013). These practices do not include analysis and responses to cultural and structural violence that had been an important component of the feminist movement's trauma-based responses (Brown, C., 2021). Insertion of the word "violence" in the term "trauma- and violence-informed" serves as an attempt to address this lack of regard and to emphasize the connections between trauma and cultural, structural and direct forms of violence (Galtung, 1990; Government of Canada, 2021). Trauma is both the experience of, and response to, an overwhelming series of events, including violence. Violence can take many forms and may be an ongoing cause of trauma responses. The inclusion of the term "violence" may help reduce the tendency to blame or judge people for their psychological or behavioral reactions to experiences of violence and recognize that these responses may be a result of trauma (Public Health Agency of Canada, 2018b).

Expanding this term to include "violence-informed" provides a critical lens that is aligned with peace-building frameworks that identify and link structural, cultural and systemic inequity, including experiences of racism and colonization, to trauma and violence (Boulding, 2002; Clark, 2016; Curle, 1996, 1999; Galtung, 1990; Galtung & Webel, 2007; Woodhouse & Santiago, 2012). These frameworks recognize that the establishment of peace is dependent on the establishment of "just relations" and, therefore, must address social inequity and asymmetrical power relationships that are essential to a critical feminist intersectional and anti-oppressive lens.

Attention to structural and cultural violence contributes to a move from biomedical and pathologizing responses to trauma by indicating that it is the violence experienced within social contexts that must be acknowledged and contested, as was demonstrated within the feminist movement (Burstow, 2003; Ellis & Dietz, 2017; Herman, 2015; Larkin, Felliti, & Anda, 2014; Tseris, 2013). This emphasis on social context is essential for moving beyond the narrow understanding of trauma as located only within individuals, to allow for the complex interplay of structural and cultural factors that cumulatively influence the stressed environments in which violence and abuse occur.

The structural and cultural violence wheel in Figure 15.2 highlights many of the factors that can contribute to stressed environments causing violence and trauma (Ross, 2017). The chart notes that forms of structural violence seen in the upper half of the circle can include systemic injustice fueled by colonialism, neoliberalism, globalized capitalism and patriarchy. These factors can contribute to long-standing histories of racism, poverty and oppression, which have been highlighted by the experiences of Indigenous peoples in Canada (*In Plain Sight*, 2021). The four quadrants of the lower half of the circle depict factors of cultural violence, which are aspects of a culture that validates and obscures violence

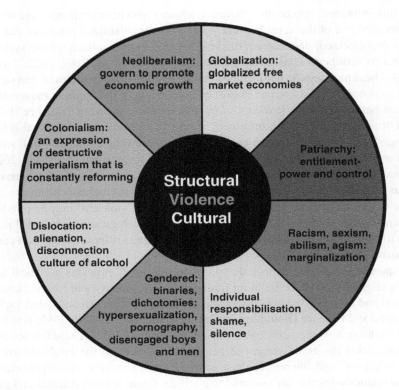

**FIGURE 15.2** Structural and cultural violences.

(Galtung, 1990). These factors are used to justify or legitimize structural violence. For example, in Halifax, Nova Scotia, the removal of the bronze statue of Edward Cornwallis – who was known for his cruel violence toward Indigenous peoples – signified an act of reconciliation by acknowledging that the presence of his statue rendered his violence not only invisible but also served as a form of validation.

Recent work that acknowledges new frameworks for addressing the prevalence of adverse childhood experiences and trauma also emphasizes the importance of building community resilience as a response to cultural and structural violence (Bethell et al., 2017; Creative Interventions, 2021; Ellis & Dietz, 2017; Thompson & O'Dea, 2011). These models aim to address gaps and strengthen community support structures for families, including clinical, public health, social welfare, education and other relevant resources that promote health and social well-being. They require the government's commitment to work proactively and upstream. Such models signal the need for a paradigm shift from punitive, adversarial and surveillance of risk models that place greater emphasis on individual responsibility as opposed to those that prioritize community organizing and social change.

An initial step for individuals to move forward is to understand what happens to their body, mind and emotions when faced with stressful situations and how they can learn to control their triggered responses. According to Hubl (2020), when someone shuts down or emotionally isolates, their ability to receive information and communicate in certain aspects of their lives can be affected and negatively impact their health and well-being. "Healing is the work of opening or returning connection" to themselves and to others (Hubl, 2020, p. 4), which can only occur when participants feel supported and respected in a non-adversarial, safe and trusting environment as mentioned above. Throughout this chapter, we have taken steps to broaden the lens of what is considered trauma- and violence-informed care by including community well-being. Trauma-resilient communities respond to structural violence by providing safe environments where individuals feel a sense of belonging and connection, which are primary supports for healing from the trauma (Vides et al., 2022). The Trauma Resilient Communities (TRC) model aims to disrupt structural violence and is currently being tested in Louisville, Kentucky, to respond to increased rates of community violence and racial trauma (ibid.). This model, which is grounded in constructivist, structural violence and organizational social context theories, utilizes a resilient framework to promote healing within individuals, organizations and communities (ibid.).

Trauma and Violence-Informed Restorative Processes

Restorative justice is a relational approach to justice that is focused on mediating interpersonal relationships and on the establishment of just relations. Justice viewed restoratively is fundamentally about just and caring relations. In simple terms, as an approach to justice, it says relationship matters in the way we understand justice and the issues at stake, as well as how we respond. This relational view extends beyond interpersonal relationships to relations at the level of groups, of institutions, of systems and of society.

Restorative justice can offer a set of principles to guide practices and processes and is not one fixed model or practice. Through a principle-based approach, restorative justice can respond to the nature of the situation and needs of the parties. This factor could be the one that could make the greatest difference for criminal justice reform. These principles would reshape responses within the criminal justice system to become more relationship-centered. They provide directives to implement comprehensive and inclusive measures that are participatory and focused on individual and collective responsibility. A focus on non-adversarial collaboration that envisions a more positive and just future is essential to reform (Llewellyn, 2018). Becoming more relationship-centered would focus on understanding and promoting just interconnections between individuals, groups and communities. A comprehensive and holistic approach would consider the social and historical contexts and causes of harm and its impacts.

To become more inclusive and participatory would enable culturally appropriate and trauma- and violence-informed practices that would be attentive to the safety and well-being of participants. To be responsive would enable systems to become human centered, contextual and flexible in practice. A focus on individual and collective responsibility would rest on the ability to offer safe spaces that are trauma- and violence-informed. As noted above, an adversarial system can limit acceptance of accountability. Collective responsibility would imply a critical analysis of social, political, economic and patriarchal colonial structural factors that contribute to violence and a willingness to work upstream to advocate for social equity and social justice.

Collaborative and non-adversarial work implies a need to reduce silos and to work together to address the root causes of the issues that are troubling within the current criminal justice system and to imagine transformative responses outside of it. A forward-focused response implies a paradigm shift, as we have argued for throughout this paper. It calls for the provision of supports in a non-punitive approach that could be empowering and could include education, problem-solving and preventative and proactive advocacy efforts.

## Paradigm Shifts

Currently, in Nova Scotia, there is a moratorium on restorative justice programs for intimate partner violence being processed in the criminal justice system. However, August-Scott, Harrison & Singer (2017) argue that the current uniform assumptions that women who are victims of interpersonal violence are terrorized, are powerless to stop the violence and should leave their partners are disempowering to the survivors (primarily women). These assumptions include the recognition that many victims of interpersonal violence remain in the relationship because they may have no place to go, they may be concerned about their children not having their father live with them, or they may be concerned about financial security. However, these assumptions can obscure the understanding that many survivors hope their relationship can improve with access to supportive networks and services and that change is possible (ibid.). This is particularly true for those who wish to stay in a relationship with their partner because they know there is more to their partner than their choice to abuse. Leadership in the Intimate Partner Violence Movement has prioritized women's safety when advocating for using restorative alternatives. As noted by Augusta-Scott and colleagues (2017), a restorative approach can engage men who have perpetrated harm in certain restorative processes (such as counseling and social and emotional learning (SEL) training) to create greater safety for women. For example, follow-up research on RESTORE, a four-year demonstration project that implemented restorative justice in response to adult sexual assault cases in Arizona, found more than 90 percent of participants agreed or strongly agreed that they felt safe because of their participation (Koss, 2014). Additionally, Pennell, Burford, Sasson, Packer and Smith (2021) address issues of safety in their overview of restorative programs in the United States that incorporated family and community approaches to intimate partner violence. Their research shows that when men participated actively and voluntarily in restorative programs, women did feel safer.

A restorative process – whose principles are grounded in connection and caring – as opposed to the current adversarial judicial process, has the potential to give voice to those most directly affected by interpersonal violence and the breakdown of their partner relationship. However, the appropriateness of restorative justice; particularly for sexual violence has been contested due to the concern for continued power imbalances between the victim and offender and that these would be reinforced in their participation in restorative programs. According to Jülich and Thorburn (2017, p. 42), "the recognition of entrenched societal structures and concurrent efforts to ameliorate these during participation is therefore integral to the notion of equality withing restorative responses". Therefore, a restorative process must prioritize substantive equality when offering the person harmed and the one causing harm a new channel of structured communication where they can safely express their emotions, problem-solve and learn how to manage conflict points in their relationship. The first step, however, is acknowledging that trauma has occurred within the couple relationship and then both partners must voluntarily agree that they want to create and will respect a safe environment where they can each address their pain. "Whenever we provide a safe space for things to come out, it is the beginning of trauma being transformed. Trauma that is not transformed is transmitted" (RYSE Center, n.d. – a youth-empowered social justice community in Oakland, California). A safe, trusting environment encourages accountability, compassion and hope for those couples and families wanting to stay together.

From our perspective, the current judicial approach to addressing interpersonal violence harms relationships and perpetuates further emotional violence, especially when children are separated from their parents. There are couples who regret their actions but have no way of addressing their regret, and the multiple bureaucratic hoops with extensive paperwork simply compound the situation. As mentioned above, the judicial process can be especially challenging for minority or impoverished families who do not have reliable transportation to attend appointments, available resources for replacing lost work time, or even alternative housing if deemed necessary by the court system.

This suggests that we need a paradigm shift when responding to interpersonal violence. A paradigm shift is a phrase meant to imply a shift in the way we view the world, our overall concept or understanding of reality. In this case, we need to see a profound shift from punishment to support and a fundamental belief that people can change if provided with appropriate and timely professional resources as well as support from a network of family and community. For instance, consistently connecting people who do harm with resources and counseling, while still remaining survivor-centered, would be a fundamental shift in addressing intimate partner violence. This approach informed the development of the *Safety and Repair Manual* (Augusta-Scott, 2023), which responded to the voices of many women who had experienced intimate partner violence but who wanted their partner or ex-partner to be part of the repair process. The manual is based on feminist and trauma-informed principles. Another supportive shift for those who have chosen to go through the legal process, would be offering comprehensive services that assist them in understanding each stage of the judicial system and how it will impact them.

Most importantly, for those families who have experienced interpersonal violence but wish to stay together, we should expand our constellation of care and move away from the goal of separating them. In their *Heart of Hope* resource guide, Carolyn Boyes-Watson and Kay Pranis (2010) outline in detail how to build healthy partnerships between families, communities and systems, especially Child Protection Services, through the power of family-workers' Circles, which focus on the family's strengths and the support services needed for them thrive. The safe structure of a Circle, as a form of family group decision making and empowerment, has immense potential.

Assuming that people have the power to make changes within their lives if there is a will and are given the right resources, sitting in a Circle meeting offers many opportunities for building inner capacities, developing social emotional literacy skills, and learning conflict management tools. For most, relating in a Circle meeting has its roots in our ancient ancestral traditions and, if appropriately structured and facilitated (as described by Pranis in *The Little Book of Circle Processes* (2005), and Boyes-Watson and Pranis (2010)), it can have a calming and stabilizing effect on the participants. Two successful models of Circle work used in addressing family domestic violence have already been introduced in Canada: we describe them below. We suggest that, for Charlotte and Joe, their participation in such a program could have increased opportunities and possibilities for Joe, the person who caused the harm, to be held accountable, accept responsibility for his actions, and to heal. For Charlotte and her children, the possibility of feeling safe, respected and supported as they recover and heal from the violence is increased.

## Two Promising Examples

### *Wikimanej Kikmanaq Family Group Circles and Family Group Decision Making*

Family group circles or more formally Family Group Conferencing (FGC) or Family Group Decision Making (FGDM) was initiated by the Mi'kmaw Family and Children's Services (MFCS) in Nova Scotia in 2001. Their promising model, entitled the Wikimanej Kikmanaq Family Group Circle Program, embodies Mi'kmaw customs, traditions and values, and it has been received well by both families and Child Protection Services. Typically, it goes through the following six phases:

1 Pre-conference preparation: this involves talking with the families and others (such as friends and supportive community members), deciding on participants, and explaining the process of Family Group Conferencing to all involved.
2 Opening the Circle with traditional ceremonies and establishing and getting agreement to the ground rules.
3 Describing the situation that has occurred, discussing the issues and alternative courses of action.
4 Supporting a family caucus with family members, allowing them the option to decide their own course of action.
5 A family member reporting to the larger group about the responsibilities and timelines they have established with the agency's approval.
6 Establishing follow-up meetings to monitor implementation and adjust any plans as required.

*(Wien & Gloade, 2011)*

Pennell describes, in *A Restorative Approach to Family Violence. Feminist Kin-Making* (2023b), another successful family- and cultural-based model that helps end severe family violence. This conferencing model, known as Family Group Decision Making, was applied in three diverse Canadian communities, including Inuit, rural and urban. The model facilitates family empowerment by helping them recognize their own competence and will to survive as a family unit. Furthermore, because of its democratic structure and process, the Family Group Decision Making model reduced some of the profound societal distrust of families and their cultural networks' ability to provide ongoing support and care. By highlighting the capacity of families and communities to offer care, this model suggested the importance of prioritizing and empowering their engagement. Pennell (2023b) defines feminist kin-making as a feminist theory of change that emerged from women's movements and prioritizes principles of equity that are aligned with other emancipatory movements such as the labor, peace and environmental movements. She explains that "a restorative approach overturns intergenerational and gendered violation by making kinship" (Pennell, 2023b, p. 4) and, by doing so, renders that violence as unacceptable despite the family's intergenerational history. It celebrates and "frees energy and good will for wider change that flips gendered and intergenerational patterns of abuse to relationships of caring" (ibid., p. 4) Pennell's work, grounded in the theory of feminist kin-making, and the Basque's Mi'kmaw program, which recognizes the strength of extended family and community, are two restorative approaches that challenge carceral interventions and could serve as a guide for participants, practitioners, policymakers and researchers.

## Additional Reflections

Despite the promise and appeal of restorative justice we recognize this approach will not be chosen by all women who experience gender-based domestic violence, nor work equally well for all families. We need to anticipate how issues of safety, power, control and choice will be experienced by individual women. Just as they should not be coerced by the criminal justice system to press charges and prosecute when they do not choose to, we need to ensure that they do not feel coerced to participate in restorative justice when this is not their preference. The level of danger and violence, degree of conflict, and existing impact of economic and housing needs alongside the power of child welfare may impact women's choices. Regardless, those who use violence need support both to repair the harms of violence and to address their own needs. Similarly, women need to know that, if they want to leave a person being violent to them, they will have adequate housing and economic support and their children will not be removed, especially if these are the only reasons why they are considering staying with that person. There are likely to be many influences on women's choices. We also need to imagine hybrids of restorative justice and the criminal justice system that fit with the needs and safety of the woman being abused and the overall well-being of the family.

## Conclusion

Throughout this chapter, we have argued for the need to move beyond the mandatory pro-arrest, pro-charge and pro-prosecution policies to restorative just policies that demonstrate trauma- and violence-informed care to intimate partner violence. To address the concerns of safety and power in interpersonal violence, a restorative approach must be grounded in theories of trauma- and violence-informed care that include a feminist intersectional lens. This requires a paradigm shift toward viewing interpersonal violence through the lens of a family unit that might want to remain in relationship, and offering restorative approaches that could support the healing of the trauma the family has experienced. This shift in thinking moves from the punitive, adversarial model to a trauma- and violence-informed infrastructure that is well-resourced, timely and grounded in the intelligence and care of the community as exemplified by the Wikimanej Kikmanaq Family Group Circle Program. The families who participate in this program are all involved with Child Protection Services. This program has been successful as evidenced by reducing the number of children in provincial care significantly with 90 percent of children remaining in the care of their families or in the local community (Pennell, 2023a, 2023b). We conclude that Family Group Circles and the Family Group Decision Making approach are promising models that could help us chart a path forward, informed by feminist and trauma-based principles.

## Acknowledgment

We would like to acknowledge our appreciation for the review and feedback of Dr. Joan Pennell, which helped improve this chapter.

## References

Augusta-Scott, T., Harrison, P., & Singer, V. (2017). Creating safety, respect and equality for women. Lessons from the intimate partner violence and restorative justice movements. In T. Augusta-Scott, K. Scott, & L.M. Tutty (Eds.), *Innovations in interventions to address intimate partner violence. research and practice* (pp. 157–173). Taylor and Francis.

Augusta-Scott, T. (2023). *Safety and repair: A 3-phase approach to address gender-based violence. A practitioners guide.* Tod Augusta-Scott.

Barata, P.C., & Schneider, F. (2004). Battered women add their voices to the debate about the merits of mandatory arrest. *Women's Studies Quar*terly, 32(3–4), 148–163.

Bethell, C.D., Solloway, M.R., Guinossa S., Hassink, S., Srivastav, A., Ford D., & Simpson L.A. (2017). Prioritizing possibilities for child and family health: An agenda to address adverse childhood experiences and foster the social and emotional roots of well-being in pediatrics. *Academic Pediatrics*, 17(7S): S36–S50. doi: 10.1016/j.acap.2017.06.002.

Bombay, A., Matheson, K., & Anisman, H. (2014). The intergenerational effects of Indian Residential Schools: Implications for the concept of historical trauma. *Transcultural Psychiatry*, 51(3), 320–338.

Boulding, E. (2002) A journey into the future: Imagining a nonviolent world. *Peace and Conflict Studies*, 9(1), 51–56.

Boyes-Watson, C., & Pranis, K. (2010). *Heart of hope: A guide for using peacemaking circles to develop emotional literacy, promote healing and build healthy relationships* (pp. 253–271). Living Justice Press and the Institute for Restorative Initiatives.

Brown, C. (2021). Critical clinical social work and the neoliberal constraints on social justice in mental health. *Research on Social Work Practice*, 31(6), 644–652.

Burstow, B. (2003). Toward a radical understanding of trauma and trauma work. *Violence Against Women*, 19, 1293–1317.

Clark, N. (2016) Shock and awe: Trauma as the new colonial frontier. *Humanities*, 5(1), 14. https://doi.org/10.3390/h5010014.

Coker, D., Park, S., Goldscheid, J., Neal, T., & Halstead, V. (2015). Responses from the field: sexual assault, domestic violence, and policing. https://www.aclu.org/issues/womens-rights/violence-against-women/responses-field?redirect=responsesfromthefield. doi: 10.2139/ssrn.2709499.

Cravens, J.D., Whiting, J.B., & Aamar, R.O. (2015). Why I stayed/left: An analysis of voices of intimate partner violence on social media. *Contemporary Family Therapy*, 37(4), 372–385. https://doi. org/ 10. 1007/ s10591- 015- 9360-8.

Creative Interventions. (2021). *Creative interventions toolkit. A practical guide to stop interpersonal violence.* https://www.creative-interventions.org/toolkit/.

Curle, A. (1996) Violence and alienation: An issue of public mental health. *Medicine and War*, 12(1), 14–22.

Curle, A. (1999) *To tame the hydra: Undermining the culture of violence.* Jon Carpenter Publishing.

Davidson, C.L. (2004). *Protection orders, partner abuse and police liability: A socialist feminist analysis.* Publication No. 305200124. Master's thesis. Carleton University, ProQuest Dissertations and Theses Global.

Department of Justice. (2010). *Domestic violence action plan.* Nova Scotia.

Fallon, B., Van Wert, M., Trocmé, N., MacLaurin, B., Sinha, V., Lefebvre, R., & Rha, W. (2015). *Ontario incidence study of reported child abuse and neglect 2013.* Canadian Child Welfare Research Portal, Toronto.

Ellis, W., & Dietz, W. (2017). A new framework for addressing adverse childhood and community experiences: The building community resilience (BCR) model. *Academic Pediatrics,* 17, S86–S93.

Galtung, J. (1990). Cultural violence. *Journal of Peace Research,* 27(3), 291–305.

Galtung, J., & Webel, C. (2007) (Eds.), *Handbook of peace and conflict studies.* Routledge.

Government of Canada. (2021). Trauma- and violence-informed approaches to policy and practice. https://www.canada.ca/en/public-health/services/publications/health-risks-safety/trauma-violence informed-approaches-policy-practice.html.

Herman, J.L. (1992). *Trauma and recovery.* New York: Basic Books.

Herman J.L. (2015). *In Trauma and recovery. The aftermath of violence- from domestic abuse to political terror* (2nd ed.). Basic Books.

Hubl, T. (2020). *Healing collective trauma: A process for integrating our intergenerational and cultural wounds.* Sounds True.

Hughes, K., Bellis, M.A., Hardcastle, K.A., Sethi, D., Butchart A., Mikton, C., et al. (2017). The effect of multiple adverse childhood experiences on health: A systematic review and meta-analysis. *Lancet Public Health,* 2(8): e356–e366. https://doi.org/10.1016/S2468-2667(17)30118-4PMID:29253477.

*In plain sight: Addressing Indigenous-specific racism and discrimination in B.C. health care.* (2021). Camosun College, Victoria, British Columbia.

Johnstone, M., Brown, C., & Ross, N. (2022). The Mcdonaldization of social work: A critical analysis of mental health care services using the choice and partnership approach (CAPA) in Canada. *Journal of Progressive Social Services.* doi: 10.1080/10428232.2022.2050117.

Jülich, S. & Thorburn, N. (2017). Sexual violence and substantive equality: Can restorative justice deliver? *Journal of Human Rights and Social Work,* 2(1–2), 34–44. https://doi .org/10.1007/s41134-017-0029-0.

Koss, M. (2014). The RESTORE program of restorative justice for sex crimes: Vision, process, and outcomes. *Journal of Interpersonal Violence,* 29(9), 1623–1660. https://doi .org/10.1177/0886260513511537.

Kulkarni, S. (2019). Intersectional trauma-informed intimate partner violence services: Narrowing the gap between interpersonal violence service delivery and survivor needs. *Journal of Family Violence,* 34(1), 55–64. https:// doi. org/ 10.1007/s10896-018-0001-5.

Larkin, H., Felitti, V., & Anda, R. (2014). Social work and adverse childhood experiences research: Implications for practice and health policy. *Social Work in Public Health,* 29(1), 1–16.

Levenson, J. (2017). Trauma-informed social work practice. *Social Work,* 62(1) 105–113. doi: 10.1093/sw/swx001. PMID: 28339563.

Llewellyn, J. (2018) Realizing the full potential of restorative justice. *Policy Options.* http://policyoptions.irpp.org/magazines/may-2018/realizing-the-full-potential-of-restorative -justice/.

Maté, G. (2008). *In the realm of hungry ghosts: Close encounters with addiction.* Knopf.

Nova Scotia Advisory Council on the Status of Women (2022). *Making changes.* https:// women.novascotia.ca/sites/default/files/MC10_2022/MakingChanges_2022_July19 _Digital_FINAL.pdf.

Packer, H. (2021). *Restorative justice and intimate partner violence: A summary of findings from two reports.* New York, Center for Court Innovation, January 2021. https://www .innovatingjustice.org/sites/default/files/media/documents/2021-01/Monograph_RJ _Summaries_01292021.pdf.

Pennell, J. (2023a). Family group decision making (FGDM) example: A Newfoundland story. In J. Pennell, *A restorative approach to family violence: Feminist kin-making* (pp. 43–64). Taylor & Francis Group.

Pennell, J. (2023b). *A restorative approach to family violence: Feminist kin-making.* Taylor & Francis Group.

Pennell, J., Burford, G., Sasson, E., Packer, H., & Smith, E.L. (2021). Family and community approaches to intimate partner violence: Restorative programs in the United States. *Violence Against Women,* 27(10), 1608–1629. https://doi.org/10.1177 /1077801220945030.

Pranis, K. (2005). *The little book of circle processes: A new/old approach to peacemaking.* Good Books.

Public Health Agency of Canada. (2018a). *Family violence: How big is the problem in Canada?* Canada.ca/en/public-health/services/health-promotion/stop-family-violence/ problem-canada.html.

Public Health Agency of Canada. (2018b). *Trauma- and violence-informed approaches to policy and practice.* https://www.canada.ca/en/public-health/services/publications/ health-risks-safety/trauma-violence-informed-approaches-policy-practice.html.

Ross, N. (2017). Grassroots community peacebuilding in Lunenburg County, Nova Scotia, Canada. Identifying local perceptions of the causes of and means of preventing .interpersonal violence. University of Bradford. http://hdl.handle.net/10454/16060.

Ross, N., & Ryan, C. (2021). *A review of pro-arrest, pro-charge, and pro-prosecution policies: Redefining responses to domestic violence. A report.* https://dalspace.library .dal.ca//handle/10222/80242.

Ryan, C., Silvio, D., Borden, T., & Ross, N. (2022). A review of pro-arrest, pro-charge and pro-prosecution policies as a response to domestic violence in Canada. *Journal of Social Work,* 22(1), 211–238.

RYSE Center (n.d.). https://rysecenter.org/.

Substance Abuse and Mental Health Services Administration. (2014). TIP 57: Trauma-based care in behavioral health services. http://store.samhsa.gov/shin/content//SMA14 -4816/SMA14-4816.pdf.

Thompson, J., & O Dea, J. (2011). *The social healing project report.* Available at: http:// jamesodea.com/wp-content/uploads/2012/09/The-Social-Healing-Project-Report.pdf.

Tseris, E. (2013). Trauma theory without feminism? Evaluating contemporary understandings of women. *Affilia: Journal of Women and Social Work,* 28(2), 153–164.

Vides, B., Middleton, J., Edwards, E.E., McCorkle, D., Crosby, S., Loftis, B.A., & Goggin, R. (2022). The trauma resilient communities (TRC) model: A theoretical framework for disrupting structural violence and healing communities. *Journal of Aggression, Maltreatment & Trauma,* 31(8), 1052–1070. https://doi.org/10.1080/10926771.2022 .2112344.

Wien, F., & Glode, J. (2011). Evaluating family group conferencing in a First Nation setting: An example of university-First Nation child welfare agency collaboration.

In S. Léveillé, N. Trocmé, I. Brown, & C. Chamberland (Eds.), *Research-community partnerships in child welfare* (pp. 139–154). Centre of Excellence for Child Welfare/ Centre d'excellence pour la protection et le bien-être des enfants, Toronto. www.cecw -cepb.ca.

Woodhouse, T., & Santiago, I. (2012). Elise Boulding: New voices in conflict resolution. *Journal of Conflictology*, 3(2), 3–12.

# 16

# MEN, TRAUMA AND GENDER

## The Safety and Repair Approach to Address Gender-Based Violence

*Tod Augusta-Scott*

## Introduction

*Safety and Repair* is an approach to addressing gender-based violence that I developed from community-based work in the field. The approach is primarily influenced by narrative therapy, trauma work and restorative justice. With the *Safety and Repair* approach, practitioners challenge both gender expectations and ideas that stem from past traumatic experiences. With this approach, practitioners support men not only to stop the abuse, but also to repair the harm they have caused. Clients are supported in repairing harm with both those who have hurt them and those whom they have hurt.

The *Safety and Repair* approach consists of three phases. Phase one involves establishing safety for both individuals involved. Phase two focuses on preparing each individual to repair harm with the person who hurt them and the person whom they hurt. In this phase, practitioners address how gender expectations and ideas that stem from traumatic experiences can impair people's ability to repair harm. Phase three involves supporting both individuals to repair harm without creating further harm. This approach seeks to empower both people to repair harm with the person who hurt them or whom they hurt, either independently or with the direct support of practitioners if appropriate.

Before entering Phase three, both clients must be assessed for their readiness to engage in direct communication. It's possible clients may not have the opportunity to repair harm with the person who initially brought them into the process. Nevertheless, the process builds people's capacity to repair harm with those who have hurt them and with those whom they have hurt in any relationship they may be in. This chapter provides an example of practitioner interventions at each phase of the *Safety and Repair* approach.

DOI: 10.4324/9781003379591-17

## Literature Review

Narrative therapy has made a significant impact on the field of work with men who have perpetrated intimate partner violence (Scott, Heslop, David, & Kelly, 2017; Wendt, Seymour, Buchanan, Dolman, & Greenland, 2019). The literature has shown that men can be invited to consider their desires for respectful, fair and safe relationships with their partners and children. While gender expectations can lead men to expect power and control over their partners, a narrative approach also recognizes that men also often want loving and caring relationships. Narrative therapy practices can draw on men's values for fairness and respect as a means of confronting their own use of violence and working to repair the harm they have done (Augusta-Scott, 2001, 2009, 2017, 2020; Brown, C. & Augusta-Scott, 2007; Jenkins, 1990, 2009; Jenkins, Joy, & Hall, 2002; White, 1995).

In addition to confronting gender expectations, there is a growing body of literature in the field of intimate partner violence that emphasizes the importance of challenging ideas that stem from men's own experiences of trauma (Augusta-Scott, 2020; Augusta-Scott & Maerz, 2017; LaMotte & Murphy, 2016; Taft, Murphy, & Creech, 2016; Webermann & Murphy, 2019). Similarly, advocates for women have long recognized that women's choices are often influenced by gender expectations and the effects of experiences of trauma (Herman, 2015; Tseris, 2019).

For the past 30 years, I have worked beside women's advocates in the domestic violence movement. Early in my career I focused solely on challenging the influence of gender expectations (Pence & Paymar, 1993). Over time, along with addressing gender expectations, I recognized the importance of also challenging ideas that stem from men's own experiences of trauma that influence their choices to abuse (Augusta-Scott, 2020; Augusta-Scott & Maerz, 2017; Baugher & Gazmararian, 2015). Men's experiences of trauma include being exposed to racism, homophobia, poverty and childhood violence (Ansara & Hindin, 2010; Augusta-Scott, 2007a; Slootmaeckers & Migerode, 2018, 2019; Sonkin & Dutton, 2003; Stosny, 1995; Williams, Oliver, & Pope, 2008). I was initially reluctant to focus on men's experiences of trauma. I was concerned that focusing on men's experiences of violence would shift attention away from the impact of gender expectations and their own use of violence (Pence & Paymar, 1993). I also acknowledge that many men experience abuse but do not perpetrate abuse. Many men's experiences of trauma are moderated by other factors that contribute to them not perpetrating abuse. Further, trauma is not the only factor influencing men's choices to abuse. I was also concerned this might allow men to justify and/or excuse their behavior (Bowker, Arbitell & McFerron, 1988). While some men men use their own experiences of victimization to excuse their present choices to abuse (Jenkins, 1990), I have found that by helping men to understand how their experiences of trauma have impacted their choices, I was better able to support them to take responsibility to challenge these ideas, work toward repairing the harm they have caused, and address their own experiences of trauma (Augusta-Scott, 2020, 2023).

There is also a growing body of literature in the intimate partner violence field that supports using restorative justice to repair harm (Augusta-Scott, 2023; Barocas, Avieli, & Shimizu, 2020; Goupillot & McConville, 2019; Hayden, Gelsthorpe, King, & Morris, 2014; Mills, Barocas, Butters & Ariel, 2019; Nettleton & Strang, 2018; Pennell, Burford, Sasson, Packer, & Smith, 2021; Ptacek, 2009, 2017). The practices and ideas informing this restorative approach overlap with practitioners who are creating safety and repair in the context of couples' counseling (Goldner, 1992; Goldner, Penn, Sheinberg, & Walker, 1990; Jenkins, 1990; Lipchik & Kubicki, 1996; Slootmaeckers & Migerode, 2019; Stith, Rosen, & McCollum, 2003; Stith, McCollum, Amanor-Boadu, & Smith, 2012; Strang & Braithwaite, 2002; Wendt, Buchanan, Dolman & Moss, 2018).

Along with being reluctant to address men's experiences of trauma, the field has traditionally been reluctant to consider that men could help women repair the harm. I, for instance, did not believe men would ever sincerely acknowledge to their partners that they, the men, were completely responsible for their own choices, they were wrong for perpetrating abuse, and that the partners were not to blame. Instead, I was trained in the Duluth model (see Pence & Paymar, 1993), which adopted a cynical view about the possibility of men stopping their violence. I never considered the possibility that not only can some men stop the violence, but also they can invest in understanding the impact their abuse has had on others and work to repair these effects. In part, I was unable to consider that repair might be possible because I saw men's efforts at repair as only being manipulative. I defined any signs of change that men exhibited as a manipulative "honeymoon stage" in a cycle of violence (Bancroft, 2002; Walker, 1979). I defined men's identities in terms of their bad choices, labelling them "batterers", "abusers" and so forth. Over the years, as I became more hopeful that not only can men stop the abuse but also they can participate in repairing the harm they caused, my work became more effective.

## Safety and Repair Approach

### Phase One: Safety

The objectives of Phase one are crucial for laying the foundation for the rest of the *Safety and Repair* approach (Augusta-Scott, 2022, 2023). Once these objectives are met in individual sessions, people may move into Phase two, which involves joining group sessions or continuing individual sessions or both. In Phase two people are prepared to repair harm. The objectives of the phase are:

1   People feel safe.
2   People are able to use skills to self-regulate and co-regulate their emotions/ nervous system.

3 People are clear about their values, what is important to them, and who is important to them.
4 People are able to resist unhelpful ideas that stem from trauma and gender expectations.
5 People are clear about the choices they are and are not responsible for.
6 People resist minimizing the seriousness of the abuse, denying it, or blaming others.

Grounded in narrative practice, re-authoring identity is a crucial part of the Safety and Repair approach as it helps clients to challenge negative self-concepts and beliefs that have resulted from their experiences of trauma and unhelpful gender ideas (Augusta-Scott, 2022, 2023; White, 2007). By doing so, it can contribute to creating a sense of safety for the client.

In re-authoring identity, the practitioner helps the client identify their values, skills and knowledge that support the life they want to lead. This process involves exploring how the client would prefer to be and who they would like to be, rather than focusing on the negative aspects of their identity that may have resulted from their experiences of trauma and gender expectations. By encouraging clients to focus on their strengths, values and resources, practitioners can help them create a new narrative for their lives, one that is empowering and allows for growth and change.

### Establishing Values

The process of re-authoring identity involves inviting people to consider their values (White, 2007). People are encouraged to identify what is important to them in relationships, the qualities they want their relationships to have, and what they care about in relation to their children and partners. While men often want power and control over their partners, they also often want more than just power and control in their relationships. Men often speak about wanting loving, caring, respectful, fair relationships. Naming these values and re-authoring identity around these values contributes to creating a foundation for men to stop abuse and repair harm (Augusta-Scott, 2001, 2023).

By identifying and clarifying their values, men can begin to recognize how their choices to abuse are incongruent with these values. This process can lead to a sense of cognitive dissonance and motivation to make choices to align with their values. Furthermore, identifying positive values can help men develop a sense of identity and self-efficacy, which can be undermined by experiences of trauma and unhelpful gender ideas. Re-authoring identity can help men develop a more positive self-concept, which can in turn contribute to stopping abuse and repairing harm with their children.

The process of re-authoriing identity includes explorations of vallues such as mutual respect and taking responsibility. The influence of these ideas that stem from trauma and gender expectations often distorts both values. Initially, I avoid inviting men to articulate the unhelpful ideas because I want to resist challenging and shaming them for being influenced by these ideas. In the past, I particiaped in this type of conversation and, as a result, I closed down many conversations. Instead, I now initiate conversations about these values and invite men to consider alternative ideas about them, from which they can challenge for themselves previous unhelpful assumptions they may have about respect and taking responsibility.

## *Respect*

As the practitioner inquires about their values and what is important in relationships with partners and children, they invite men to consider the importance of respect. Often men are initially only thinking about people respecting them. Rather than directly confronting and shaming men for being influenced by these ideas, I initiate a conversation about mutual respect. An example of this line of inquiry includes the following conversation between myself and a man named Frank who abused his partner:

> *Tod:* Some men say that "respect" is important to them in a relationship. Is respect important to you, Frank?
> *Frank:* Yes. She should respect me.
> *Tod:* Frank, when you say respect is important to you, do you mean mutual respect – her respecting you, you respecting her – or is the respect you are talking about just one way.
> *Frank:* Oh no, I want mutual respect. Me respecting her, her respecting me.
> *Tod:* That's interesting. So it sounds like mutual respect is important to you. How important is mutual respect in a relationship?
> *Frank:* Really important.

Often men are influenced by ideas such as "you disrespect me, so I disrespect you" and "you hurt me, so I hurt you." I also inquire about the importance of valuing being respectful even when others are not.

> *Tod:* Frank, I'm wondering if it is important to you even when your partner gets off track with her value for respect. If your partner goes down the disrespect path and starts yelling, do you think you could hang on to your value for respect then, even if she doesn't? Could you hang on to your own values in those moments, standing up for your own values, or would you just be okay to let go of your own values and follow her down the disrespect path?
> *Frank:* Oh, I want to hang on to my own values. I want to act respectfully even if she is not.

## Taking Responsibility

Practitioners also invite men to consider if they value taking responsibility for their choices. Many men define taking responsibility as simply admitting, "I did it". Often, however, many men do not have any template for taking responsibility. They do not know how to repair harm and make things better after making mistakes or bad choices. They often feel defeated about the harm they have caused, thinking there is nothing can be done about it so they might as well avoid thinking about it. Many men were abused as children when they were responsible for making mistakes, which contributed to them avoiding any responsibility and not having a template for how to take responsibility to repair harm they caused. Again, to avoid directly confronting and shaming men for being influenced by these ideas, I initiate a conversation where they consider expanding their ideas about taking responsibility. I continue the conversation with Frank:

*Tod:* Some men indicate that taking responsibility is important to them. Is it important to you?
*Frank:* Yes, it's important to me.
*Tod:* Is it important to you, Frank, that your children learn how to take responsibility when they make mistakes or bad choices?
*Frank:* Yes.
*Tod:* What does taking responsibility mean to you Frank?
*Frank:* Well, when my children make bad choices I want them to own up to it. I want them to learn from their mistakes and make sure they don't happen again.
*Tod:* And what do you mean by own up to it?
*Frank:* I want them to acknowledge what they did,
*Tod:* Why is that important to you Frank?
*Frank:* Well if they don't acknowledge what they have done, they can't do anything about it.

By asking men about what they want their children to learn about taking responsibility, they begin to build a template of how they could take responsibility themselves.

Often men think their partners or ex-partners are responsible for the men's abusive behavior. Ideas that stem from trauma and gender expectations contribute to men blaming their partners or ex-partners for their abusive actions or behaviors (Augusta-Scott, 2023). Again, to avoid directly confronting and shaming men for blaming their partners, before the men blame their partners, I ask men about who is responsible for an individual's choices.

*Tod:* Frank, if your partner is yelling, who is responsible for her choices to yell?
*Frank:* She is.
*Tod:* Frank if you are yelling, who is responsible for your choices to yell?
*Frank:* ... Me. I am responsible.

Furthermore, I also want to ensure that men value taking responsibility for their choices, even when others do not.

*Tod:* Frank, so I understand that taking responsibility for your choices is important to you, does that include times when your partner is not taking responsibility?

*Frank:* Yes. I want to live my values and take responsibility even if she is not.

*Tod:* Of course, my partner may be responsible for hurting my feelings, I'm responsible for how I choose to express my feelings in response. If I decide to start yelling out my feelings, I'm responsible for my choices to yell. What do you think of that idea?

*Frank:* I'm not sure. I guess I'm responsible.

Men often are influenced by the idea that "it takes two" or "I can't change if she doesn't change". Again, to avoid shaming the men for the influence of these ideas, I immediately ask:

*Tod:* Of course, it takes two people to make a relationship work. If either one of you decide to continue to not take responsibility by continuing to yell, the relationship may not survive. While it takes two people to make the relationship work, if I am yelling, it only takes me. If I am yelling, it's hard to do, but I can choose to stop even if she doesn't. It's true, by not yelling I alone cannot save the relationship. For the relationship to work she would also have to take responsibility to stop yelling. At the same time, the only choices I can make to save the relationship at that moment is to choose not to escalate, even if my partner is escalating.

*Frank:* Yeah.

Focusing on choices rather than actions and behavior helps men take ownership of their decision-making process and realize that they have agency in their relationships. Often past trauma contributes to men experiencing their (re-)actions and behaviors as involuntary, which often contributes to their confusion of who is responsible for their actions and behaviors. By focusing on *choices*, I invite men to begin to reclaim their agency over their choices. Men are better able to discern who is responsible if someone chooses abuse in a relationship.

Another line of inquiry addresses that many men have been violated by those who never took responsibility for the harm they caused. These experiences may include racism, homophobia, poverty and childhood violence. Men are often distracted by this double standard until it is acknowledged by the practitioners. I ask men about double standards that often get invoked with respect to taking responsibility.

*Tod:* What's it like, Frank, when people ask you to take responsibility for hurting others, when no one is taking responsibility for how you have been hurt?
*Frank:* It doesn't feel very good.

Through this line of questioning, I implicitly affirm the men's own victimization and the value that there is no excuse for abuse. The man is responsible for abusing others even if others have abused him. I also address the double standard that often exists when men are being asked to take responsibility while those hurting them are not (Jenkins, 2009). Acknowledging this double standard often allows men to let go of focusing on others' responsibility and proceed with living their own values – of taking responsibility – even when others are not.

By re-authoring identity with a man according to his own values and ethics, the foundation is established for the man to work at stopping the violence and preparing to repair the harm in Phase two. An important part of this process includes attending to the values of mutual respect and taking responsibility, values which have often been distorted by men's own experiences of trauma and gender expectations.

## Phase Two: Preparing to Repair Harm

Phase two is designed to support people to repair harm with the person who hurt them and with the person they hurt. The objectives for Phase two are:

1   People are able to repair harm done to themselves from past abuse.
2   People can repair harm with the other person without creating more harm.
3   People do not objectify themselves or the other person according to their bad choices or mistakes.
4   People do not objectify themselves or others as only victim or only perpetrator.
5   People can identify how ideas that stem from trauma and gender expectations can impair people's ability to repair harm.

### When people have been hurt:

1   People can identify how they were harmed in the present and separate it from past harm.
2   People are able to identify what they want to repair harm.
3   People are able to ask for what they want without creating harm.
4   People are able to express anger and resolve conflict without using abuse.
5   People are able to distinguish between self-defense and retaliation.
6   People are able to receive what they want.
7   People are able to resist automatic forgiveness.

### When people have hurt others:

1 People can face their shame without becoming self-absorbed and experience shame while also being compassionate toward those they harmed.
2 People respect themselves for taking responsibility/repairing harm.
3 People can acknowledge the abuse.
4 People have a plan for stopping the abuse.
5 People can acknowledge the effects of the abuse.
6 People have a plan to repair the effects of the abuse.

## People Repairing Harm with the Person Who Hurt Them

In the early stages of this process, men often think that taking responsibility simply means admitting to what they have done. Although acknowledging their actions is important, in Phase two men will further explore the meaning of taking responsibility and repairing the harm they caused. Practitioners assist men in reflecting on what else taking responsibility might entail by asking them what they would want from someone who has hurt them. For instance, by examining their partner or ex-partner's responsibility for her poor choices; for example, men can create a template for taking responsibility and repairing the harm, which they can follow themselves. I often follow this line of inquiry:

> *Tod:* Frank, I can see that others taking responsibility for the harm they did to you is important. I'm wondering Frank, are there any parts of taking responsibility that you want to use in relation to your own choices that have hurt others.
> *Frank:* Yes.
> *Tod:* Again, is taking responsibility important to you even when others do not? Do you want to be living up to your own values rather than other people's values?
> *Frank:* I want to live my own values even if others are not.

To define the meaning of taking responsibility and repairing harm, I ask men how they would want someone who hurt *them* to respond. This exploration draws on the work of restorative justice leader Howard Zehr (2015) and gender-based violence movement leader Judith Lewis Herman (2005; 2023), both of whom address what people want to repair after they have been hurt. Generally, repairing harm involves *four* components. Adult people who have been harmed through domestic violence often want: (1) an acknowledgment of the details of the abuse without minimizing them; (2) information about the plan to stop the abuse; (3) a full acknowledgment of the effects of the abuse; and (4) an explanation of how the other person intends to be accountable and repair the effects of the abuse. By considering what they themselves want from the people that harmed them, men are better able to consider what those they have hurt might want from them.

For men to repair harm without creating more harm, men need support to identify, ask for, and receive what they want from the person who hurt them. I spend time assisting men to clearly and respectfully ask for what they want from those that have hurt them, whether the person is their partner, ex-partner, parents or teachers when they were young.

### The Impact of Trauma and Gender on the Ability To Repair Harm

Men's ability to identify, ask for and receive what they want after they have been hurt is often impaired by ideas influenced by trauma and gender expectations. I support men to consider the ideas that make identifying what they want difficult, which may include "What I want is not important" and "I'm not worthy to get what I want" (Levine, 1997, 2015). Gender expectations reinforce these ideas by supporting the idea that men should not need help, men should not feel hurt and pain, and men should be able to solve their own problems. Additionally, men are often discouraged from making themselves vulnerable by identifying or asking for what they want in a relationship.

#### Asking for What They Want

I help men consider how their past experiences, including child abuse, may be affecting their ability to ask for what they want in a manner that will not create more harm. Men who have experienced abuse often learned as children that expressing their anger through yelling and aggression is the only way to be heard. Many men have no other template for expressing their anger and, therefore, are prone to create harm in their efforts to ask for what they want when they are hurt. Gender expectations contribute to men thinking that anger is the only emotion they can express, and that they need to avoid being vulnerable when asking for what they want when they are hurt. Furthermore, many men are often taught that conflict can only be resolved through violence. They often lack a template for resolving conflict that respects both people and leads to resolution. Gender expectations also reinforce the notion that men should rely on physical violence rather than dialogue to resolve conflicts.

Men's efforts to repair harm when they are hurt are also often influenced by the conflation of self-defense with revenge and retaliation (Augusta-Scott, 2020; Winslow & Hall, 2009). Men who have experienced abusive childhoods often learn that revenge is the same as self-defense. However, they may not learn that the intent of self-defense is to prevent further harm, while the intent of retaliation is to inflict harm (Augusta-Scott, 2020).

*Receiving What They Want*

Practitioners also help men to understand how ideas stemming from childhood trauma can hinder their ability to receive what they want from their partners. Often experiences of childhood trauma influence men's perceptions of themselves and others, leading them to reject partners who genuinely care for them. As children, many men learned to blame themselves for being abused, believing they were bad, disgusting, dirty and unworthy of love. When men bring these ideas into their adult intimate relationships, they often dismiss any positive feedback from their partners, which could help them heal from past traumas. Instead, they reject such feedback because they feel unworthy of it due to their experiences of childhood trauma (Levine, 1997, 2015).

Alternatively, men may reject positive feedback from their partners because they learned in childhood that they cannot trust others, particularly those who are close to them. This can lead them to reject positive feedback because they often assume their partners' intention is to harm them. Gender expectations reinforce these ideas such as: "Don't trust anyone", "Look out for number one", and "A dog is a man's best friend". These notions suggest that relationships are based on competition and the need to control others, and that vulnerability with others should be avoided.

Men who have experienced childhood abuse often confuse the past and the present. They confuse themselves with their younger self and they confuse their partners with either their abusive parents or past abusive partners. Practitioners can assist men separating their past experiences from their present reality, allowing them to receive what they want from their partner to repair harm in a manner that avoids further harm.

I become curious about how men may be struggling to distinguish between their past and present. When talking about an interaction with their partner, men are invited to separate their partner from their past:

*Tod:* Frank, what's it like when your partner gives you a compliment?
*Frank:* I don't believe her.
*Tod:* Why is that, do you think?
*Frank:* I was told by my Dad my whole life that I was no good.
*Tod:* So what is it like for her to say something different?
*Frank:* I think she just must be trying to manipulate me to get something?
*Tod:* Does that remind you of anything, Frank?
*Frank:* That's what my Mom use to do – she'd only compliment me if she wanted something from me.
*Tod:* What would it be like to accept a compliment from her?
*Frank:* I'd be scared of getting too close and that I could get hurt?

*Tod:* What do you think that might be about?

*Frank:* Whenever I was close to someone when I was young, I got hurt.

*Tod:* Frank, when you think about it, why is your partner actually complimenting you.

*Frank:* Well she probably appreciates me.

*Tod:* Do you think when your partner compliments you that you may be confusing your past with your present? That you may be confusing your partner with your Dad sometimes and your mother at other times?

*Frank:* Definitely.

*Tod:* Frank, how would you like to respond to your partner's compliments?

*Frank:* I'd like to be able to accept them?

*Tod:* To accept them Frank, what would you have to remind yourself about your partner?

*Frank:* She's not mother or father.

*Tod:* Frank, Is your partner trustworthy? Does she want to hurt you?

*Frank:* No

*Tod:* Frank what difference could it make if you were able to separate your partner from your Dad and Mom when she is complimenting you?

*Frank:* It might make a big difference.

*Tod:* Frank, what difference would it make for your own healing if you could receive the compliments you actually want from your partner rather than rejecting them?

Again, by exploring how men's own experience of trauma can negatively influence men's ability to identify, ask for and receive what they want from their partners. When they are hurt by their partners, they are able to separate past hurt from the present and, in turn, become better able to repair harm respectfully, in a manner that does not create more harm.

### People Repairing Harm with the Person They Hurt

After exploring how individuals who have hurt them could take responsibility and repair harm, I ask men whether they want to take responsibility for the harm they have caused in a similar manner (Augusta-Scott, 2007b). Men rarely argue for a double standard in which they hold others accountable for their choices but exempt themselves from taking responsibility for their choices. Instead, they emphasize the value of taking responsibility and repairing harm for their own choices, even if this value is not shared by others. Consequently, men are better able to explore how they want to take responsibility and work through the four components of repair in relation to harm they have caused others. Again, the four components of repair include: (1) acknowledging the details of the abuse; (2) creating a plan to stop the abuse; (3) acknowledging the effects of abuse; and (4) creating a plan to address the effects of the abuse.

Studying past incidents of abuse can help men prepare for engaging in the four components of repair with the person they hurt in Phase three. By doing so, they can acknowledge the details of their actions and address any details which they may have denied or forgotten. This allows them to communicate more effectively with their partners or ex-partners in Phase three, without becoming defensive due to the lack of consideration of the specifics of their behavior. Additionally, studying past incidents of abuse can help men become more open to hearing other details they may have forgotten.

### Agency

Studying past incidents of abuse in a deliberate and gradual manner can assist men in recognizing their agency. By doing so, they can become aware of the various choices available to them, whether to escalate a situation or not. Experiences of trauma can contribute to individuals habitually reacting to others based on past events (van der Kolk, 2014). Many men exhibit a trauma response of fight or flight, perceiving their abusive behavior as involuntary. Often men say to me, "I just lose it", "I get out of control" or "I go instantly from 0 to 100". In many cases, these reactions are habitual and are related to past experiences of being hurt, which are immediately apparent in the present moment. Often, men insist there are no "warning signs" preceding their abusive actions. Addressing the impact of trauma involves a process of slowing down and allowing men to examine their experiences, identify warning signs and reflect on their decisions to escalate situations. Through this process, men transition from perceiving themselves as involuntary actors to embracing their agency as voluntary actors. This transformative process helps to empower men by providing them the opportunity to make different choices. I may discuss this as shown:

*Tod:* Frank, some men say that they are going so fast they just go from "0 to 100".
*Frank: Nods in agreement.*
*Tod:* So does it make sense, Frank, that since the problem is the escalation is going fast, that the solution may be to slow it down? The solution might be to study the escalation so that you can notice your warning signs?
*Frank:* Yeah
*Tod:* Frank, I often hear guys say that after they are done yelling they say, "I don't know why I did that".
*Frank:* Yeah, I get that.
*Tod:* Does it make sense, Frank, that if part of the problem is not knowing why they did it, part of the solution would include actually studying an incident down to understand why they did do it?
*Frank:* I guess.

When a man is asked to describe a time when he abused his partner in the past, the practitioners underscore the man's agency. This process helps men to identify the various choices they made that escalated the situation. I encourage men to immerse themselves back into the scene and then begin to systematically ask them about their thoughts, feelings and decisions during this situation:

> *Tod:* Where were you when the escalation happened?
> *Frank:* The bedroom.
> *Tod:* Where were you?
> *Frank:* Beside the bed.
> *Tod:* Where was she?
> *Frank:* At the foot of the bed?
> *Tod:* What was she saying?
> *Frank:* She was accusing me of cheating on her.
> *Tod:* What were you thinking at that point?
> *Frank:* I was thinking she was attacking me.
> *Tod:* Then what were you feeling?
> *Frank:* Frustrated.
> *Tod:* Frank, then what did you *decide* to do?

This process of asking about a man's thoughts, feelings and decisions or choices continues until the end of the incident.

### Warning Signs

Studying past abuse also gives men the opportunity to develop a plan to prevent future abuse. By carefully examining previous incidents of abuse, men can identify warning signs that precede men's choices to abuse (Pence & Paymar, 1993). These warning signs can manifest themselves in the form of emotions, bodily sensations or ideas. For instance, men may recognize warning signs such as tension in the body, their partners starting to escalate, or feeling threatened. To begin this process, I ask about the following:

> *Tod:* What difference might it make if you could slow down and study the warning signs that precede the escalation?
> *Frank:* Well if I could spot the warning signs then I could do something different.

### Values

Many men report that when they notice warning signs preceding abuse, reminding themselves about who they care about and the costs of the abuse on them and their relationships is very helpful in interrupting the escalation. They often need to recall their values and what is important to them. For instance, they may reflect on the safety and security they want for their children or the love and respect they want with their partners.

Gender expectations tend to limit the range of ways men can contribute to their families, often reducing their role to providing financial security and possibly discipline for the children. The *Safety and Repair* approach challenges these gender expectations by inviting men to consider what else they care about in their family relationships.

### Effects

Practitioners not only help men to connect with their values, but also remind them of the costs of their abusive choices on what and who is important to them. When men reflect on past incidents of abuse, I encourage them to consider their partner's and children's feelings in each moment. Often, men think about the costs of their abusive choices after the fact. In the midst of being abusive, they are usually self-absorbed and believe that they do not care about anything. In this state of mind, they make decisions that can be very destructive to the people they actually care about. When men are able to recognize the warning signs, and remind themselves of their values and the associated costs, they are much better able to interrupt the escalation towards abuse. I ask the following:

> *Tod:* Frank, what difference would it make if you could remind yourself of the costs, the costs you are thinking right now, before you escalate rather than thinking about them afterward?
> *Frank:* If I could catch the warning signs and remind myself of the costs and think like I'm thinking now, I definitely wouldn't escalate.

Many men minimize or deny the seriousness of the effects of the abuse (Pence & Paymar, 1993). Part of the reason men continue to abuse is because they do not fully consider how the abuse affects their loved ones. The habit of minimizing and denying the abuse of their partners is often consistent with men denying and minimizing the seriousness of the abuse that was done to them. To challenge this practice and explore the effects of abuse on others, I invite men to consider the effects abuse has had on themselves:

> *Tod:* Frank, when you consider the effects of your yelling on your partner and children does it remind you of some of your own experiences growing up?
> *Frank:* Yes. I remember being scared in my bedroom when my dad was yelling and throwing things in the kitchen.

*Tod:* Frank, what difference would it make if you could remind yourself of these effects before you escalated to yelling?

*Frank:* It would help me put the brakes on.

### Separating Past from Present

Practitioners also invite men to notice when they are confusing their past experiences with the present. Often, men mistake their current partners with past partners who have hurt them or parents who have abused them (Slootmaeckers & Migerode, 2018, 2019). Due to their past experiences, men may feel threatened even when there is no threat. As men learn to notice their habitual reactions toward their partners, I invite men to consider how the present may feel the same as past experiences even when they are not the same. Because a situation feels the same, does not mean it is the same. Furthermore, practitioners can ask men to reflect on how their current partner is different from people they were close to in the past. Even if a man is being disrespected in the present, I invite them to consider how they are different from when they were children and, in turn, how they want to respond to being disrespected in the present compared to how they reacted to being disrespected in the past. I ask:

*Tod:* Frank, when you're describing feeling powerless to get your partner to listen to you, how old do you feel?

*Frank:* Age 10.

*Tod:* Frank, can you tell me how your parents responded to your ideas and feelings?

*Frank:* They'd yell and scream. They didn't listen to anything I said. I was to be seen and not heard.

*Tod:* Do you think that your partner Sally actually cares how you feel, Frank?

*Frank:* Yes.

*Tod:* Do you think you might be confusing her with your parents? Do you think you might be confusing the past and the present Frank?

*Frank:* I think I do that often.

### Fourth Component of Repair: Plan for Repairing Effects

The fourth component of preparing men to take responsibility for repairing the harm they caused involves considering what they can do to repair the effects of the abuse. Often, people's experiences of trauma – both when they are hurt and when they hurt others – result in painful feelings of shame and embarrassment. To get past these painful feelings, people often minimize or deny the effects of the abuse. For those who have perpetrated the abuse, the process of taking responsibility involves studying past incidents and their effects on both people and their relationship.

*Tod:* Is it important for someone to acknowledge the effects their choices have had on others?

*Frank: Nods in agreement.*

*Tod:* What difference would it make?

*Frank:* A big difference.

*Tod:* What would it be like if a person tried to apologize for something they did before they considered the effects on the other person?

*Frank:* It probably wouldn't feel like a real apology.

*Tod:* Who might the person who was hurt think the apology was really for?

*Frank:* For the person who was apologizing.

*Tod:* What's the difference between a sincere apology and hollow promises and apologies?

*Frank:* Well a sincere apology is when you make it for the other person and you have a plan to make the problem stop and to make things better.

In addition to considering apologies and acknowledging what happened, I also invite men to consider other ways of repairing the effects of the abuse. For instance, men may consider repairing damage to the family home, ensuring timely child care payments or renouncing the abuse in front of the children.

However, men who have experienced abuse throughout their childhood may not have a framework for repairing harm. Again, men often say, "What's done is done, there's nothing I can do about it now". This common phrase reveals the lack of a template for repairing harm after someone has made mistakes or bad choices. I often take the following line of questioning:

*Tod:* What did you learn about taking responsibility and the possibility of repairing harm?

*Frank:* Nothing.

*Tod:* What do you mean?

*Frank:* I learned that when you messed up and admitted it you deserved to be beaten. There was no step to take responsibility or repair harm. There was no redemption. It was just, "you did bad, you are bad".

*Tod:* And how does that idea affect a person's ability to take responsibility and repair harm over time?

*Frank:* I didn't learn anything. I just thought, what's done is done. There's nothing you can do about it now. I never considered repairing the harm or making things better was an option. I just thought, ignore it and keep going.

Gender expectations also contribute to men not taking responsibility to repair harm. For men to take responsibility for mistakes and bad choices, I challenge these gender expectations:

*Tod:* What are some of the social expectations that are put on men when they make a mistake?

*Frank:* Men aren't supposed to make mistakes.

*Tod:* And what if they are having problems?

*Frank:* Don't show it to anyone. You need to solve everything yourself, don't ask for help. Pretend you always have everything under control.

*Tod:* How would these ideas about being a man influence a man's ability to take responsibility and repair harm?

*Frank:* He never would. He would just blame other people for his mistakes. He would never repair any harm because he would never admit to creating any.

Practitioners often have to challenge ideas that limit the possibility of repair, before men can consider that value of considering practical ideas about how they may repair harm.

## Phase Three: Repairing Harm

The objectives of Phase three are for practitioners to support people in repairing harm with the person they have hurt or who has hurt them. This can occur between two people on their own and/or with practitioners present for support. In either situation, practitioners ensure that both individuals have met the objectives of Phase one (Safety) and Phase two (Preparation) before they are invited to consider opening communication to engage in the practice of repairing harm in Phase three.

During Phase three, individuals are encouraged to practice repairing harm with the person who hurt them or whom they hurt, without the practitioner being present. However, if people require support, practitioners may be directly involved in facilitating this communication between the two people. In this phase, both individuals are prepared to discuss the four components of repair. One partner can ask the other to acknowledge the abuse that they inflicted. The partner who caused the harm is prepared to describe their abuse without minimizing or denying it. Partners or ex-partners can also ask to hear the proposed plan for ensuring the abuse stops. Through this process, partners can hear about the distorted ideas, justifications and excuses that men now know were contributing to their choice to abuse. Additionally, partners can also request that their partners or ex-partners acknowledge the effects of the abuse. Finally, partners can ask about men's plan to be accountable to repair the effects over time.

## Conclusion

The *Safety and Repair* approach to addressing gender-based violence contributes to various developments in the field. The approach focuses on re-authoriing identity in a manner that makes men's efforts to stop their abuse and repair harm possible. The approach also engages in non-confrontational ways of challenging the unhelpful ideas that may be influencing men's ideas about the values of respect and taking responsibility. The approach challenges ideas that stem from men's experiences of trauma, as well as the gender expectations that impair their ability to both stop the abuse and repair the harm they caused. Moreover, the approach offers a vision for work in the gender-based violence sector in which men not only can stop the abuse and help create safety for partners or ex-partners, but also support women's efforts to repair harm from the effects of the men's abuse on the partners, their children and their relationships.

## References

Ansara, D.L., & Hindin, M.J. (2010). Exploring gender differences in the patterns of intimate partner violence in Canada: A latent class approach. *Journal of Epidemiology and Community Health*, 64(10), 849–854. https://doi.org/10.1136/jech.2009.095208.

Augusta-Scott, T. (2001). Dichotomies in the power and control story: Exploring multiple stories about men who choose abuse in intimate relationships. *Gecko*, 2, 31–68. Reprinted in D. Denborough (Ed.), (2003), *Responding to violence: A Collection of papers relating to child sexual abuse and violence in intimate relationships* (pp. 204–224.). Dulwich Centre Publications.

Augusta-Scott, T. (2007a). Challenging anti-oppressive discourse: Uniting against racism and sexism. In C. Brown & T. Augusta-Scott (Eds.), *Narrative therapy: Making meaning, making lives* (pp. 211–228). Sage.

Augusta-Scott, T. (2007b). Conversations with men about women's violence: Ending men's violence by challenging gender essentialism. In C. Brown & T. Augusta-Scott (Eds.), *Narrative therapy: Making meaning, making lives* (pp. 197–210). Sage.

Augusta-Scott, T. (2009). A narrative therapy approach to conversations with men about perpetrating abuse. In P. Lehmann & C. Simmons (Eds.), *Strengths based batterers intervention: A new paradigm in ending family violence* (pp. 113–136). Springer.

Augusta-Scott, T. (2017). Preparing men to help the women they abused achieve just outcomes: A restorative approach. In T. Augusta-Scott, K. Scott, and L. Tutty (Eds.), *Innovations in interventions to address intimate partner violence: Research and practice* (pp. 191–204).)Routledge.

Augusta-Scott, T. (2020). Exploring trauma and masculinity among men who perpetrate intimate partner violence. In C. Brown & J. MacDonald (Eds.), *Critical clinical social work: Counterstorying for social justice* (pp. 127–149). Canadian Scholars Press.

Augusta-Scott, T. (2022). *Safety and repair: A manual for individual, group and family conversations to address gender-based violence.* Tod Augusta-Scott.

Augusta-Scott, T. (2023). Safety and repair: A three phase approach to address gender-based violence. In C. Holtmann, S. O'Donnell, & L. Neilson (Eds.), *Ending gender-based violence: Harnessing research for social change* (pp. 147–171). Captus.

Augusta-Scott, T., & Maerz, L. (2017). Complex trauma and dominant masculinity: A narrative therapy approach with men who choose to abuse their female partners. In T. Augusta-Scott, K. Scott, & L. Tutty (Eds.), *Innovations in interventions to address intimate partner violence: Research and practice* (pp. 75–92). Routledge.

Bancroft, L. (2002). *Why does he do that? Inside the minds of angry and controlling men.* Berkley.

Barocas, B., Avieli, H., & Shimizu, R. (2020). Restorative justice approaches to intimate partner violence: A review of interventions. *Partner Abuse*, 11(3), 318–349.

Baugher, A.R., & Gazmararian, J.A. (2015). Masculine gender role stress and violence: A literature review and future directions. *Aggression & Violent Behavior*, 24, 107–112.

Bowker, L., Arbitell, M., & McFerron, R. (1988). Rethinking clinical approaches. Treatment models of men who batter: A profeminist analysis. In K. Yello & M. Bograd (Eds.), *Feminist perspectives on wife abuse* (pp. 176–199). Sage.

Brown, C., & Augusta-Scott, T. (2007). *Narrative therapy: Making meaning, making lives.* Sage.

Goldner, V. (1992). Making room for both/and. *The Family Therapy Networker*, 16(2), 55–61.

Goldner, V., Penn, P., Sheinberg, M., & Walker, G. (1990). Love and violence: Gender paradoxes in volatile attachments. *Family Process*, 29, 343–364.

Goupillot, B., & McConville, T. (2019). Developing restorative relationship therapy: Towards working safely with couples where there is abuse. *Couple and Family Psychoanalysis*, 9(1), 36–54.

Hayden, A., Gelsthorpe, L., King, V.C., & Morris, A. (Eds.). (2014). *A restorative approach to family violence: Changing tack.* Ashgate.

Herman, J.L. (2005). Justice from the victim's perspective. *Violence Against Women*, 11(5), 571–602.

Herman, J.L. (2015). *Trauma and recovery: The aftermath of violence – from domestic abuse to political terror* (2nd ed.). Basic Books.

Herman, J.L. (2023). *Truth and repair: How trauma survivors envision justice.* Basic Books.

Jenkins, A. (1990). *Invitations to responsibility: The therapeutic engagement of men who are violent and abusive.* Dulwich Centre Publications.

Jenkins, A. (2009). *Becoming ethical: A parallel, political journey with men who have abused.* Russell House.

Jenkins, A., Joy, M., & Hall, R. (2002). Forgiveness and child sexual abuse: A matrix of meanings. *International Journal of Narrative Therapy and Community Work*, 1(1), 35–51.

LaMotte, A.D., & Murphy, C.M. (2016). Trauma, posttraumatic stress disorder symptoms, and dissociative experiences during men's intimate partner violence perpetration. *Psychological Trauma: Theory, Research, Practice, and Policy*, 9, 567–574.

Levine P.A. (1997). *Waking the tiger: Healing trauma: The innate capacity to transform overwhelming experiences.* North Atlantic Books.

Levine, P. (2015). *Trauma and memory: Brain and body in a search for the living past: A practical guide for understanding and working with traumatic memory.* North Atlantic Books.

Lipchik, E., & Kubicki, A.D. (1996). Solution-focused domestic violence views: Bridges toward a new reality in couples therapy. In S.D. Miller, M.A. Hubble, & B.L. Duncan (Eds.), *Handbook of solution-focused brief therapy* (pp. 65–99). Jossey-Bass.

Mills, L.G., Barocas, B., Butters, R.P., & Ariel, B. (2019). A randomized controlled trial of restorative justice-informed treatment for domestic violence crimes. *Nature Human Behaviour*, 3, 1284–1294.

Nettleton, C., & Strang, H. (2018). Face-to-face restorative justice conferences for intimate partner abuse: An exploratory study of victim and offender views. *Cambridge Journal of Evidence-Based Policing*, 2, 125–138.

Pence, E., & Paymar, M. (1993). *Education groups for men who batter: The Duluth model.* Springer.

Pennell, J., Burford, G., Sasson, E., Packer, H., & Smith, E.L. (2021). Family and community approaches to intimate partner violence: Restorative programs in the United States. *Violence Against Women*, 27(10), 1608–1629.

Ptacek, J. (Ed.). (2009). *Restorative justice and violence against women*. Oxford University Press.

Ptacek, J. (2017). Research on restorative justice in cases of intimate partner violence. In C.M. Renzetti, D.R. Follingstad, & A.L. Coker (Eds.), *Preventing intimate partner violence: Interdisciplinary perspectives* (pp.159–184). University of Chicago Press.

Scott, K., Heslop, L., David, R., & Kelly, T. (2017). Justice-linked domestic violence intervention services: Description and analysis of practices across Canada. In T. Augusta-Scott, K. Scott, & L. Tutty (Eds.), *Innovations in interventions to address intimate partner violence: Research and practice* (pp. 53–74). Routledge.

Slootmaeckers, J., & Migerode, L. (2018). Fighting for connection: Patterns of intimate partner violence. *Journal of Couple & Relationship Therapy: Innovations in Clinical and Educational Interventions*, 17(1), 1–19.

Slootmaeckers, J., & Migerode, L. (2019). EFT and intimate partner violence: A roadmap to de-escalating violent patterns. *Family Process*, 59(2), 328–345.

Sonkin, D.J., & Dutton, D. (2003). Treating assaultive men from an attachment perspective. *Journal of Aggression, Maltreatment & Trauma*, 7(1–2), 105–133.

Stith, S.M., McCollum, E., Amanor-Boadu, Y., & Smith, D. (2012). Systemic perspectives on intimate partner violence treatment. *Journal of Marital and Family Therapy*, 38(1), 220–240.

Stith, S., Rosen, K., & McCollum, E. (2003). Effectiveness of couple treatment for spouse abuse. *Journal of Marital and Family Therapy*, 29, 407–426.

Stosny, S. (1995). *Treating attachment abuse: A compassionate approach*. Springer.

Strang, H. & Braithwaite, J. (2002). *Restorative justice and family violence*. Cambridge University Press.

Taft, C.T., Murphy, C.M., & Creech, S.K. (2016). *Trauma-informed treatment and prevention of intimate partner violence*. American Psychological Association.

Tseris, E. (2019). *Trauma, women's mental health, and social justice: Pitfalls and possibilities*. Routledge.

van der Kolk, B.A. (2014). *The body keeps the score: Brain, mind, and body in the healing of trauma*. Viking.

Walker, L. (1979). *The battered woman*. Harper and Row.

Webermann, A.R., & Murphy C.M. (2019). Childhood trauma and dissociative intimate partner violence. *Violence Against Women*, 25(2), 148–166.

Wendt, S., Buchanan, F., Dolman, C., & Moss, D. (2018). Engagement: Narrative ways of working with men when domestic violence is noticed in couple counselling. *Journal of Social Work*, 20(2), 234–256.

Wendt, S., Seymour, K., Buchanan, F., Dolman, C., & Greenland, N. (2019). Engaging men who use violence: Invitational narrative approaches. Australia's National Research Organization for Women's Safety. https://anrowsdev.wpenginepowered.com/wp-content/uploads/2019/10/PI.17.12-Wendt-Invitational-Narrative-Therapies-ANROWS-RtPP.pdf.

White, M. (1995). A conversation about accountability. In *Re-authoring lives: Interviews and essays* (pp.155–170). Dulwich Centre Publications.

White, M. (2007). *Maps of narrative practice*. W.W. Norton.

Williams, O.J., Oliver, W., & Pope, M. (2008). Domestic violence in the African American community. *Journal of Aggression, Maltreatment, & Trauma*, 16(3), 229–237.

Winslow, S., & Hall, S. (2009). Retaliate first: Memory, humiliation and male violence. *Crime, Media, Culture*, 5, 285–304.

Zehr, H. (2015). *The little book of restorative justice*. Revised and updated. Good Books.

# 17

# MALE CHILDHOOD SEXUAL TRAUMA

## Challenging, Deconstructing and Re-Storying Dominant Discourses

*Colin James Morrison*

### Introduction

Cultural myths and lack of discourse surrounding the sexual trauma experiences of boys and men pose a serious risk to our clinical understanding of the phenomena and can serve to disrupt and obstruct healing processes. Unfortunately, there exists a profound silence that renders the plight of male survivors invisible in several ways: through an absence of public discourse, a lack of available male-centered treatments and support, and an inherent bias in clinicians that fails to recognize traumatic histories in their male clients. Not acknowledging the significant issue of male childhood sexual abuse and its impact is problematic because it minimizes survivors' experiences and diverts them from needed resources. The absence of discourse, therefore, leads to a lack of support and a scarcity of professional knowledge, leading to sexually traumatized males struggling to heal, while left silenced and invisible to mental health care systems that are ill-equipped and poorly prepared to support them.

Because of beliefs embedded in masculinity that men and boys cannot be victims, male survivors struggle with feeling vulnerable and weak. They equate their abusive experience to female experience, something that only happens to girls and women (Alaggia, 2010; Kia-Keating, Grossman, Sorsoli, & Epstein, 2005). Victimization is a transgression of masculine identity influenced by a patriarchal, heteronormative and misogynistic culture that devalues women (Fisher & Goodwin, 2008; Kia-Keating, Grossman, Sorsoli, & Epstein, 2005). Survivors also fear being perceived as homosexual or gay as the result of queer biases in culture and the enormity of pressures in heteronormative society to conform to dominant ways of being a man (Alaggia, 2005; Gartner, 2017; Lisak, 2007). As a researcher, I critically examined the experiences of male sexual trauma survivors

DOI: 10.4324/9781003379591-18

through the perspectives of mental health clinical therapists, those who counsel and provide therapeutic interventions to this population. My research explored gaps in current knowledge regarding the unique needs of survivors while highlighting the importance of engagement through a gendered, male-centric lens. My work as a clinician with youth in an emergency mental health setting positions me in front of males who have endured trauma regularly, where I address their pain and witness their struggle with the terrible knowledge of the scarcity of support and the limited understanding available. I recognize, however, that females are statistically much more likely to experience sexual trauma in early childhood (Collin-Vézina et al., 2015; Herman, 2015). So, while I argue for more attention and focus on male experiences of childhood sexual trauma, this is not meant to detract attention or focus from the significant societal issues we face with violence and abuse toward women. This chapter will critically explore the most troublesome impact of male sexual trauma. In particular, it will address how misogynistic and homophobic attitudes and cultural biases resulting from a heteronormative/patriarchal society that subordinates all things considered feminine serve to emasculate male survivors and sever them from healing processes.

## Male Childhood Sexual Abuse and the Dangers of Disclosure

As many as one in six men are survivors of early childhood sexual trauma histories ("1 in 6", 2023; Dube et al., 2005; Fisher & Goodwin, 2008). However, many clinicians believe this number is a gross underestimate of those affected. A strong relationship exists, irrespective of gender, between childhood sexual abuse and several adverse health, behavioral and social outcomes among survivors, such as severe mental health issues, depression and anxiety, suicidality, substance-use problems, chronic health issues and high-risk sexualized behaviors (Dube et al., 2005; Fisher & Goodwin, 2008; Kia-Keating, Grossman, Sorsoli, & Epstein, 2005). In the aftermath of abuse, delayed disclosure and avoidance coping are common behaviors among boys and girls with a history of sexual abuse (Alaggia, 2005; Filipas & Ullman, 2006). Despite evidence, children may deny the abuse or recant an initial disclosure (Alaggia, 2005; Easton, Saltzman, & Willis, 2014). Research broadly suggests that children struggle with disclosure for many reasons, including fear of not being believed, risk of further harm, worries related to family disruption, mistrust of law enforcement and child protective services, and a desire to protect the abuser (Alaggia, 2005; Easton, 2014; Easton, Saltzman, & Willis, 2014; Herman, 2015; van der Kolk, 2014).

Retrospective studies of adults with histories of child sexual abuse found some significant gender differences in disclosure rates, with males purposefully disclosing much less frequently than females (Alaggia, 2005; Easton, Saltzman, & Willis, 2014). O'Leary and Barber (2008) evaluated disclosure patterns in a sample of 296 child sexual abuse survivors (151 women, 145 men), where only

26 percent of male respondents, compared to 63.6 percent of female respondents, told someone in the immediate aftermath of the sexual abuse. Other studies have found statistically significantly lower disclosure rates during childhood for male survivors than female survivors (Alaggia, 2010; Easton, Saltzman, & Willis, 2014).

When males do disclose, they take longer and make fewer, more selective disclosures (Cashmore & Shackel, 2014). Men and boys also withhold, for years and even decades, disclosing their experiences to others, initiating help-seeking behaviors and seeking appropriate resources (Easton, Saltzman, & Willis, 2014; Fisher & Goodwin, 2008; van der Kolk, 2014). Because boys are reluctant to disclose in the aftermath of the abuse, much of what we know about the immediate impacts of victimization is through self-reports of adult males regarding their childhood experiences, which may involve gaps in memories filtered through present-day difficulties, which have a potential to skew recall (Cashmore & Shackel, 2014; Easton, Saltzman, & Willis, 2014). However, post-traumatic responses for any trauma survivor may often involve a degree of uncertainty and ambivalence in telling a trauma narrative (Brown, C., 2013). C. Brown (2018) notes how disclosing trauma can be perceived as dangerous by the survivor, exposing them to uncomfortable emotions and fears of being blamed or untrusted. This danger may, therefore, "shape the storytelling, and caution and self-surveillance may render invisible or disqualify aspects of the story" (Brown, C., 2018, p. 46). Furthermore, survivors are left to make sense of their trauma through dominant social narratives that provide inadequate accounts of their experiences and tend to reify and leave unchallenged oppressive dominant discourse (Brown, C., 2013; McKenzie-Mohr & LaFrance, 2011). Ultimately, male childhood sexual trauma is much more common than we had assumed, grossly underrecognized and often left undertreated (Denov, 2004; Fisher & Goodwin, 2008; Lisak, 1994) and the high degree of lack of discourse around it continues to contribute to its invisibility.

## Hegemonic/Dominant Masculinity

Our current understanding of hegemonic or dominant masculinity was first conceptualized in the mid-1980s by Raewyn Connell (1995) as a form of masculinity relative to historical and societal influences and settings. Hegemonic masculinity validates and co-exists with men's dominant societal position. It legitimizes patriarchal power and unequal gender relations between men and women, masculinity and femininity, and among other types of masculinity, such as those subordinated (2SLGBTQIA+ persons) and those marginalized (men who are racialized or of lower socioeconomic status). Although not assumed, hegemonic masculinity is viewed as normative through its enactment while embodying a time-honored and traditional way of being a man, requiring other men to position themselves according to it by performing gender in a preferred way (Connell & Messerschmidt,

2005; Courtenay, 2000). Men may adhere to or reject and resist hegemonic masculinity through their own formulation of masculine identity.

Guiding beliefs about hegemonic masculinity exist alongside hegemonic femininity, which serves to essentialize, naturalize and totalize the social construction of gender. These hegemonic constructions view men and women as inherently different, fitting strictly into gender boxes, often problematically constructed as binary opposites. Though not all men – perhaps only a minority (Connell & Messerschmidt, 2005) – subscribe to or enact hegemonic masculinity, all men stand to benefit from its social privileges and be policed or punished for deviating from its boundaries (Pascoe, 2007). Socially gendered characterizations of sexual trauma as "feminine" and the influence of hegemonic masculinity can, therefore, impact men's responses to their own victimization and support providers' responses to them (Javid, 2017).

Numerous scholars have critiqued hegemonic masculinity as being too structuralist and deterministic, too derived from a heteronormative construction of gender and too problematizing of masculinity as a whole (Beasley, 2015; Connell & Messerschmidt, 2005; Waling, 2019). As such, there have been notable attempts to rework the theory to account for men's experiences of masculinity and the broader systemic social structures and discourses that work to shape it. Hegemonic masculinity attends to and focuses on broader discourses regarding power relations and systemic structures but does not consider how agency is produced and negotiated within these discussions (Beasley, 2015; Waling, 2019).

bell hooks (2005) said that in order "to indoctrinate boys into the rules of patriarchy, we force them to feel pain and to deny their feelings" (p. 22). Men are meant to endure their pain as a testament to their strength. hooks argues that traditional masculinity constrains men emotionally and relationally and that a more equitable gender framework can liberate everyone, irrespective of gender (hooks, 2005). Hegemonic masculinity equates stoicism with strength, even in the face of danger; and gender socialization of boys appears to teach boys to minimize the emotional experience of pain or powerlessness that may be associated with abuse. As noted earlier, a disconnect often exists between existing frameworks and experiences of abuse, violence and trauma. They often blame and minimize, making it difficult to tell one's story.

Ultimately, any expectations of masculine performance are shaped by the institutional structures and broader social contexts in which they are situated. These socially constructed ideals of manhood are restrictive and repressive, and men increasingly reject and challenge these notions today. However, a young male impacted by trauma that forces him to question his masculine identity and sexual orientation can quickly become entrenched in a belief system that tells him that he has failed at masculinity because of his victimization. Even though this achievement of hegemonic masculinity is unrealistic, failure to embody these rules creates pain and confusion for many.

## Toxic Masculinity

The Good Men Project (2020) describes toxic masculinity as a narrow, repressive description of manhood, reducing masculinity to a cultural ideal of manliness, emotions as weakness, and sexual pursuits and forced aggression as measures of success while so-called "feminine" traits – ranging from emotional vulnerability to simply not being hypersexual – indicate how your status as a man is taken away or negated. While not explicitly using the term "toxic", the American Psychological Association (APA), in their *Guidelines for Psychological Practice with Men and Boys* (APA, 2018), warns that extreme forms of certain "traditional" masculine traits are linked to aggression, misogyny and adverse health outcomes.

As noted earlier, women are often much more impacted by sexual violence, with the everyday threat of violence and sexual assault a part of female existence. Stereotypes related to cultural expectations placed on males can lead to problematic or toxic behavior for some. To be sure, masculinity itself is not innately or inherently evil. However, how certain boys are socialized in our culture has the potential to be dangerous and harmful for themselves and for others. For example, independence, self-reliance and stoicism can be admirable traditional male traits, but when a man is unable to ask for help, feels incapable of relying on others, or struggles in the expression of vulnerable emotions, those once admirable traits become increasingly problematic or troublesome (Augusta-Scott, 2020; Fisher & Goodwin, 2008). Ironically, male trauma remains unresolved and all-consuming due to *not* acknowledging victimization and needing to prove invulnerability (Augusta-Scott, 2020).

While hegemonic masculinity shares many similar characteristics, I believe that the term "toxic masculine culture" is helpful because it helps to delineate and differentiate between those aspects of hegemonic masculinity that are most harmful or destructive, such as misogyny, homophobia and transphobia, and those that are most honored or valued, such as courageousness, self-reliance and the desire to protect others. However, this also implies a binary of toxic versus healthy masculinity, which can appear unhelpful. Waling (2019) and Salter (2019) both encourage a move away from categorizations such as "toxic masculinity" as the only explanation for particular social, political, cultural and economic issues experienced in social life. While toxic masculine culture can play a role in perpetuating sexual violence against women and men's reluctance to engage in help-seeking, they are not the sole reasons. To claim violence against women as just an effect of "toxic masculinity" disembodies men from their actions while denying a long-standing history of women being consciously and systematically marginalized and oppressed and also ignoring how masculinity has changed and evolved over time and space (Beasley, 2015; Kimmel, 2008; Salter (2019; Waling, 2019).

## Discourses of Gender and Sexuality

In his work, "The History of Sexuality," Foucault (1991) argued that ideas and norms around sexuality and desire are not fixed or natural but the result of discourse about "sexuality", with heterosexuality positioned as the point of reference for "socially acceptable" behavior. Foucault (1980) tells us, "[w]e are subjected to the production of truth through power, and we cannot exercise power except through the production of truth" (Foucault, 1980, p. 93). For Foucault (1991), knowledge and power are joined through discourses, which are social "practices that systematically form the objects of which they speak" (p. 49). Foucault (1991) argued that while in pre-industrial times power was exercised in society through sovereignty, this gradually shifted to disciplinary power, which regulates the beliefs and actions of members of society much more subtly through established regulations or by conditioning people to survey themselves and others. This disciplinary power permeates various institutions in which we interact within society – from schools, workplaces and hospitals to prisons and militaries. Through self-surveillance, we learn to control ourselves by constantly monitoring our thinking, behavior, lifestyles and appearances. Our ideas about gender, and in this case masculinity, are shaped by these discursive formations that determine what is accepted and what is not.

Butler (1999) follows Foucault's ideas that subject positions are not natural but are, in fact, discursive products of modern power. Like Foucault, Butler argues that gender is not a biological fact or a state of "being" but an enacted performance and way of "doing" that makes us believe in its existence. Butler (1999) claims that "acts of gender create the idea of gender, and without those acts, there would be no gender at all" (p. 521). Therefore, gender is entirely performative, and cultural norms and societal expectations dictate what is considered masculine and feminine, and these ideas become so ingrained and normalized that they seem natural but are constructed. According to Butler (1999), gender is always performed within a limiting and highly rigid regulatory frame, yet there are always possibilities to destabilize and resist this order. In this view, masculinity is not an innate or static identity but rather an ongoing series of acts and gestures that individuals engage in, one that conforms to societal norms and expectations. By revealing the performative nature of gender, Butler (1999) implies that these performances can be disrupted, resisted, challenged and reinterpreted.

## Misogyny/Homophobia

Sexual abuse perpetrated by a male against another male can raise questions about one's sexual orientation and sexual identity (Corbett, 2016; Fisher & Goodwin., 2008). Survivors often struggle with heightened issues related to homophobia, shame and stigma (Lew, 2004), an outcome of being raised and socialized in a heteronormative society that reifies and privileges heterosexuality. Challenges in reconciling membership as masculine within a heteronormative and predominantly homophobic society for some survivors can result in a hypermasculine persona that displays problematic attitudes and behaviors involving threats, violence, aggression, homophobia/transphobia and misogyny (Dorais, 2002; Kia-Keating, Grossman, Sorsoli, & Epstein, 2005).

Hegemonic masculinity, influenced by a heterosexist society, communicates to young males that, in sexual situations, they can expect to be the one who desires another and initiates sex (Corbett, 2016; Kimmel, 2013). Sexual abuse of men and boys therefore subverts dominant expectations of masculinity so profoundly that it is experienced as an attack on the male self (Corbett, 2016). If we accept that hegemonic masculinity and those who subscribe to it pride themselves on notions of sexual conquest and prowess, we must acknowledge that male survivors are sometimes actively encouraged to recognize experiences initiated by female perpetrators as rites of passage or healthy exploration and to refuse an offer denies one's prowess (Denov, 2004; Lisak, 1994). This widely accepted myth is dangerous in that it limits the ability of a survivor to speak of his abuse, because to do so could result in ridicule and, in rejecting these advances, call into question his manhood.

For 2SLGBTQIA+ youth, experiences of sexual trauma raise concern that abuse happened because they were perceived as gay or that the experience was somehow contrived to "make" them gay (Cassese, 2000; Corbett, 2016). Male survivors may also feel compelled to sexually pursue female partners to re-establish or reclaim their heterosexual identity or to replay or remodel what was enacted upon them. In addition, they can feel hurried into identifying their sexual orientation and associate their sexual identity and sexual activity with feelings of betrayal, exploitation and secrecy (Gartner, 2017; Lew, 2004). In early adolescence, self-concepts of both sexual orientation and gender identity have yet to coalesce fully. Fear, prejudice and misinformation regarding identity and orientation can be particularly prominent and problematic within the developing adolescent (Gartner, 1999). Dominant masculinity excludes 2SLGBTQIA+ males because they violate fundamental criteria for being considered masculine due to their sexual attraction or engagement with other men (Sanchez, Westefeld, Liu, & Vilain, 2010). Gay males who value or subscribe to traditional masculine norms may experience shame or guilt because being truly "masculine" is unattainable due to their same-sex attraction (Bockting, Benner, & Coleman, 2009). From childhood abuse to homophobic jokes that shame and ridicule to hate crimes, queer men and boys can often experience dominant culture as traumatic. Experiences of childhood sexual abuse only compound these issues further and exacerbate trauma. Much research has also detailed the role of masculinity in homophobic and transphobic violence and aggression against those who do not conform to strict gender rules or narratives. Daily media coverage details horrific violent assaults and often fatal hate crimes against transgender and gender-non-conforming people worldwide, with threats and challenges to the perpetrator's masculinity as the root cause (Gruenewald & Kelley, 2014; Kimmel, 2013). Male sexual trauma survivors "confront a set of stigmatizing cultural narratives that contribute to a unique sense of shame. Male sexual victimhood is incomprehensible because it contradicts cultural ideas of

316 Colin James Morrison

being a man – strong, powerful, self-sufficient, and impenetrable" (Hlavka, 2017, p. 483).

Manne (2015) proposes a definition of misogyny that provides a conceptual distinction between what she calls a naive conception and a feminist account of misogyny. The former refers to those who may generally feel hatred or hostility toward women simply because they are women. A feminist account of misogyny denotes the "system which operates within a patriarchal social order to police and enforce women's subordination and to uphold men's dominance' (Manne, 2015, p. 2). It also emphasizes the role of social structures in producing misogynistic attitudes that serve a patriarchal ideology. It is the discourse, attitudes and values that uphold patriarchal power and the valuing of masculinity and devaluing of femininity that are both constructed and created in opposition to each other. However, we must consider the evolving nature of masculinity, how men and boys navigate modern societal expectations, and how these are constantly shifting (Pascoe & Bridges, 2016). Connell (1995) states that while certain forms of masculinity might perpetuate domination over femininities, other expressions do not, and masculinities can and do co-exist harmoniously with various forms of femininity.

Homophobia – the culturally produced fear of and prejudice against gay people – is a central principle of a cultural definition of manhood (Kimmel, 2015). Homophobia is more than an irrational fear of gay men and more than the fear that one might be perceived as gay. The word "faggot" has nothing to do with the homosexual experience or even with the fears of homosexuals. Instead, it comes out of the depths of manhood: a label of ultimate contempt for anyone who seems sissy, effeminate, untough, or not brave (ibid.). Homophobia is the fear that others will unmask and emasculate men, revealing that they do not measure up to manhood. Fear leads to shame because, in acknowledging that fear of not measuring up, men find proof of the limits of their masculinity (Kimmel, 2008).

A common challenge facing many sexual trauma survivors is the myth of complicity, wherein survivors struggle with deep feelings of shame centered around the physiological response and sexual arousal they may have experienced during the abuse (Alaggia & Millington, 2008; Fisher & Goodwin, 2008). Developing an erection or experiencing ejaculation during a sexually abusive experience is a confusing and distressing aspect of male sexual trauma. Trauma, confusion and arousal can leave men and boys with shame and disgust at themselves and their perceived body betrayal. Among many gay and bisexual male survivors, a shared discourse persists that the experience is responsible for influencing their sexual orientation, for some leading to issues related to internalized homophobia or fear of becoming an abuser (Alaggia & Millington, 2008; Gartner, 2017; Lisak, 1994).

Myths and cultural delusions about male sexual victimization are generated in the intersection between the traditional male code and the reality of male sexual victimization. Because the latter is utterly incompatible with the former, "the delusions either deny or minimize the abuse or portray it as a failure of masculinity" (Fisher & Goodwin, 2008, p. 56). Misogyny and homophobia can serve to silence male survivors. It is a silence centered on a fear of reprisal from other men that allows men to walk past a woman harassed in the street and not call it out or listen to a sexist rant or a gay-bashing joke and not challenge it. These fears serve as the source of men's silences, and men's silence keeps the patriarchal systems running and dominates the cultural hegemonic definition of manhood.

## Conclusion

Male sexual trauma survivors "confront a set of stigmatizing cultural narratives that contribute to a unique sense of shame. Male sexual victimhood is incomprehensible because it contradicts cultural ideas of what it means to be a man – strong, powerful, self-sufficient and impenetrable" (Hlavka, 2017, p. 483). These cultural narratives continue to permeate society and exacerbate survivors' difficulties in disclosing their experiences, which can increase stigma, hinder the development and provision of appropriate services, and impact further research on the phenomenon (Stermac, Cabral, Clarke, & Toner, 2014). A crucial dimension of survivors' recovery "is finding a way to 'make sense' of what happened to them in the past, and to make some kind of meaning of the place the abuse has in their current lives" (Grossman, Sorsoli, & Kia-Keating, 2006, p. 44). Gender socialization strongly influences how males construct meaning from their abuse (Gartner, 1999, 2017; Grossman, Sorsoli, & Kia-Keating, 2006; Kia-Keating, Grossman, Sorsoli, & Epstein, 2005). When men and boys attempt to process their trauma, they are walking a fine line between a need as a survivor to be vulnerable while at the same time navigating pain or discomfort they might feel through a violation of perceived heteronormative and hegemonic masculine norms. As David Lisak so eloquently tells us, the path to recovery from childhood sexual trauma "winds straight through masculinity's forbidden territory: the conscious experience of those intense, overwhelming emotional states of fear, vulnerability, and helplessness" (Lisak, 1994, p. 262).

Herman (2015) believes the construction of a "truthful" narrative is crucial to healing. It helps survivors recall detailed traumatic memories, to process and transform their recollections, and to mourn their traumatic losses. As C. Brown and Augusta-Scott (2007) tell us, all stories about social life and subjective experience involve interpretation and meaning-making, which are impacted by cultural and historical influences. If we do not question or unpack these stories through the therapeutic process, we can inadvertently reproduce unchallenged problematic stories and reinforce damaging dominant discourses (Brown, C., 2007). However, disclosure and a subsequent narrative for survivors often come years after their initial abuse experiences. As a result, they are challenged by the passing of time and the trouble with memory, which can further cloud a male survivor's recollection and make the entire process more complicated and uncertain as a result (Alaggia, 2010; Kia-Keating, Grossman, Sorsoli, & Epstein, 2005; Kimmel, 2008).

Sexual trauma survivors may try to make sense of their experiences within dominant social narratives, often providing inadequate or unhelpful accounts of their experiences, while reifying oppressive dominant discourses (Brown, C., 2007). Much like female survivors, the stories men and boys are often left with are unhelpful and full of self-blame and uncertainty. However, their experiences are not separate from more powerful social stories that are accepted as truth and remain largely unquestioned (ibid.). Therefore, challenging discourses, making meaning and re-storying the trauma narrative remain crucial in promoting healing, recovery and future wellness. Unfortunately, while many boys are survivors of sexual abuse, they often grow up in a culture of masculine expectations that can amplify their trauma and move them away from the capacities they need to heal. This is because toxic notions of masculinity tell boys to discourage expressing thoughts and emotions, accepting help from others, and acknowledging the pain and hurt.

Masculinity is not innately evil or inherently harmful, but male survivors of sexual trauma suffer in its shadow. As mental health professionals, we need to adapt services to meet the needs of men and boys who experience sexual trauma, and we should not make harmful assumptions regarding their capacity to understand and explore emotions that might preclude them from therapy (Addis & Mahalik, 2003; Lisak, 2007). We need to support gender-based adaptations for work with men and boys – shorter therapeutic sessions, movement breaks, incorporation of art or musical instruments as components of therapy – and consider the possibility of moving to more informal or outdoor settings like parks and hiking trails (Addis & Mahalik, 2003; Englar-Carlson & Kiselica, 2013). We need to be cautious how we interpret acting out or externalizing behavior, and consider it as possible signs of challenge such as anxiety or depression, often within the context of past trauma (Gartner, 2017; Lisak, 2007). We need to recognize an internet bias in clinicians that fails to recognize symptoms of traumatic history in male clients (Alaggia, 2005; Fisher & Goodwin, 2008; Kia-Keating, Grossman, Sorsoli, & Epstein, 2005; Lisak, 2007). We need to recognize that for many boys and men, if we do not ask about their trauma they will not tell. We must respond to the needs of male sexual trauma survivors through an understanding of complex trauma and an awareness of the pervasive influence of masculine gender construction. We must look at a male survivor's history of trauma through a gendered lens, unpack harmful discourses, and consider treatment approaches with men and boys as a uniquely gendered experience.

## References

1 in 6. (March 30, 2023). Sexual abuse & assault of boys & men | Confidential support for men. Retrieved February 2019 from https://1in6.org/.
Addis, M.E., & Mahalik, J.R. (2003). Men, masculinity, and the contexts of help seeking. *The American Psychologist*, 58(1), 5–14. https://doi.org/10.1037/0003-066X.58.1.5.

Alaggia, R. (2005). Disclosing the trauma of child sexual abuse: A gender analysis. *Journal of Loss and Trauma*, 10(5), 453–470. https://doi.org/10.1080/15325020500193895.

Alaggia R. (2010). An ecological analysis of child sexual abuse disclosure: Considerations for child and adolescent mental health. *Journal of the Canadian Academy of Child and Adolescent Psychiatry*, 19(1), 32–39.

Alaggia, R., & Millington, G. (2008). Male child sexual abuse: A phenomenology of betrayal. *Clinical Social Work Journal*, 36(3), 265–275.

American Psychological Association, Boys and Men Guidelines Group (APA). (2018). *APA guidelines for psychological practice with boys and men.* APA.

Augusta-Scott, T. (2020). Exploring trauma and masculinity among men who perpetrate intimate partner violence. In C. Brown & J. MacDonald (Eds.), *Critical clinical social work. Counterstorying for social justice* (pp. 127–149.) Canadian Scholars Press.

Beasley, C. (2015). Caution! Hazards ahead: Considering the potential gap between feminist thinking and men/masculinities theory and practice. *Journal of Sociology*, 51, 566–581.

Bockting, W., Benner, A., & Coleman, E. (2009). Gay and bisexual identity development among female-to-male transsexuals in North America: Emergence of transgender sexuality. *Archives of Sexual Behavior*, 38(5), 688–701.

Brown, C. (2007). Situating knowledge and power in the therapeutic alliance. In C. Brown & T. Augusta-Scott (Eds.), *Narrative therapy. Making meaning, making lives* (pp. 3–22). Sage.

Brown, C. (2013). Women's narratives of trauma: (Re)storying uncertainty, minimization and self-blame. *Narrative Works: Issues, Investigations & Interventions*, 3(1), 1–30.

Brown, C. (2018). The dangers of trauma talk: Counterstorying co-occurring strategies for coping with trauma. *Journal of Systemic Therapies*, 37(3), 42–60.

Brown, C., & Augusta-Scott, T. (2007). *Narrative therapy: Making meaning, making lives.* Sage.

Butler, J. (1999). *Gender trouble: Feminism and the subversion of identity.* Routledge.

Cashmore, J., & Shackel, R. (2014). Responding to historical child sexual abuse and the needs of survivors. *Current Issues in Criminal Justice*, 26(1), 1–4. https://doi.org/10.1080/10345329.2014.12036003.

Cassese, J. (2000). *Gay men and childhood sexual trauma: Integrating the shattered self.* Haworth Press.

Collin-Vézina, D., De La Sablonnière-Griffin, M., Palmer, A.M., & Milne, L. (2015). A preliminary mapping of individual, relational, and social factors that impede disclosure of childhood sexual abuse. *Child Abuse & Neglect*, 43, 123–134. https://doi.org/10.1016/j.chiabu.2015.03.010.

Connell, R. (1995). *Masculinities.* Polity.

Connell, R.W., & Messerschmidt, J.W. (2005). Hegemonic masculinity: Rethinking the concept. *Gender & Society*, 19(6), 829–859. https://doi.org/10.1177/0891243205278639.

Corbett, A. (2016). *Psychotherapy with male survivors of sexual abuse: The invisible men.* Karnac Books.

Courtenay, W.H. (2000). Constructions of masculinity and their influence on men's well-being: A theory of gender and health. *Social Science & Medicine*, 50(10), 1385–1401. https://doi.org/10.1016/S0277-9536(99)00390-1.

Denov, M.S. (2004). The long-term effects of child sexual abuse by female perpetrators. *Journal of Interpersonal Violence*, 19(10), 1137–1156.

Dorais, M. (2002). *Don't tell: The sexual abuse of boys* (2nd ed.). McGill-Queen's Press.

Dube, S., Anda, R., Whitfield, C., Brown, D., Felitti, V., Dong, M., & Giles, W. (2005). Long-term consequences of childhood sexual abuse by gender of victim. *American Journal of Preventive Medicine*, 28(5), 430–438.

Easton, S.D. (2014). Masculine norms, disclosure, and childhood adversities predict long-term mental distress among men with histories of child sexual abuse. *Child Abuse & Neglect*, 38(2), 243–251. https://doi.org/10.1016/j.chiabu.2013.08.020.

Easton, S.D., Saltzman, L.Y., & Willis, D.G. (2014). "Would you tell under circumstances like that?": Barriers to disclosure of child sexual abuse for men. *Psychology of Men & Masculinity*, 15(4), 460–469. https://doi.org/10.1037/a0034223.

Englar-Carlson, M., & Kiselica, M.S. (2013). Affirming the strengths in men: A positive masculinity approach to assisting male clients. *Journal of Counseling and Development*, 91(4), 399–409. https://doi.org/10.1002/j.1556-6676.2013.00111.x.

Filipas, H.H., & Ullman, S.E. (2006). Child sexual abuse, coping responses, self-blame, posttraumatic stress disorder, and adult sexual revictimization. *Journal of Interpersonal Violence*, 21(5), 652–672. https://doi.org/10.1177/0886260506286879.

Fisher, A., & Goodwin, R. (2008). *Men and healing: Theory, research, and practice in working with male survivors of childhood sexual abuse.* Report prepared for the Cornwall Public Inquiry at The Men's Project, Ottawa, Canada.

Foucault, M. (1980). *Power/knowledge: Selected interviews and other writings, 1972–1977.* Pantheon.

Foucault, M. (1991). *The Foucault reader.* P. Rabinow (Ed.). Pantheon.

Gartner, R.B. (1999). *Betrayed as boys: Psychodynamic treatment of sexually abused men.* Guilford.

Gartner, R.B. (2017). *Healing sexually betrayed men and boys: Treatment for sexual abuse, assault, and trauma.* Routledge.

The Good Men Project. (2020). https://goodmenproject.com/

Grossman, F.K., Sorsoli, L., & Kia-Keating, M. (2006). A gale force wind: Meaning making by male survivors of childhood sexual abuse. *American Journal of Orthopsychiatry*, 76(4), 434–443. https://doi.org/10.1037/0002-9432.76.4.434.

Gruenewald, J., & Kelley, K. (2014). Exploring anti-LGBT homicide by mode of victim selection. *Criminal Justice and Behavior*, 41(9), 1130–1152.

Herman J.L. (2015). *Trauma and recovery: The aftermath of violence – from domestic abuse to political terror* (2nd ed.). Basic Books.

Hlavka, H.R. (2017). Speaking of stigma and the silence of shame. *Men and Masculinities*, 20(4), 482–505.

hooks, b. (2005). *The will to change: Men, masculinity, and love.* Washington Square Press.

Javid, A. (2017). The unknown victims: Hegemonic masculinity, masculinities, and male sexual victimisation. *Sociological Research Online*, 22(1), 28–47. https://doi.org/10.5153/sro.4155.

Kia-Keating, M., Grossman, F.K., Sorsoli, L., & Epstein, M. (2005). Containing and resisting masculinity: Narratives of renegotiation among resilient male survivors of childhood sexual abuse. *Psychology of Men & Masculinity*, 6(3), 169–185.

Kimmel, M. (2008). Masculinity as homophobia: Fear, shame and silence in the construction of gender identity. In H. Brod & M. Kaufman (Eds.), *Theorizing Masculinities* (2nd ed.). Sage.

Kimmel, M.S. (2013). Guyland: Gendering the transition to adulthood. In M.S. Kimmel & M.A. Messner (Eds.), *Men's lives* (8th ed.) (pp. 119–133). Pearson.

Kimmel, M. (2015). *The gendered society reader* (3rd ed.). Oxford University Press.

Lew, M. (2004). *Victims no longer: The classic guide for men recovering from sexual child abuse* (2nd ed.). HarperCollins.

Lisak, D. (1994). The psychological impact of sexual abuse: Content analysis of interviews with male survivors. *Journal of Traumatic Stress*, 7(4), 525–548.

Lisak, D. (2007). Male gender socialization and the perpetration of sexual abuse. In G. Handel, S. Cahill, & F. Elkin (Eds.), *Children and society: The sociology of children and childhood socialization*. Oxford University Press.

McKenzie-Mohr, S., & LaFrance, M.N. (2011). Telling stories without the words: "Tightrope talk" in women's accounts of coming to live well after rape or depression. *Feminism & Psychology*, 21(1), 49–73.

Manne, K. (2015). *Ameliorating misogyny*. Oxford Scholarship Online.

O'Leary, P.J., & Barber, J. (2008). Gender differences in silencing following childhood sexual abuse. *Journal of Child Sexual Abuse*, 17(2), 133–143. https://doi.org/10.1080/10538710801916416.

Pascoe, C.J. (2007). *Dude, you're a fag: Masculinity and sexuality in high school*. University of California Press.

Pascoe, C.J., & Bridges, T. (2016). *Exploring masculinities: Identity, inequality, continuity and change*. Oxford University Press.

Salter, M. (2019). The problem with a fight against toxic masculinity. *The Atlantic*. https://www.theatlantic.com/health/archive/2019/02/toxic-masculinity-history/583411/.

Sánchez, F.J., Westefeld, J.S., Liu, W.M., & Vilain, E. (2010). Masculine gender role conflict and negative feelings about being gay. *Professional Psychology: Research and Practice*, 41(2), 104–111.

Stermac, L., Cabral, C.M., Clarke, A.K., & Toner, B. (2014). Mediators of posttraumatic mental health in sexual assault survivors. *Journal of Aggression, Maltreatment & Trauma*, 23(3), 301–317. https://doi.org/10.1080/10926771.2014.881948.

van der Kolk, B. (2014). *The body keeps the score: Brain, mind, and body in the healing of trauma*. Penguin.

Waling, A. (2019). Problematizing "toxic" and "healthy" masculinity for addressing gender inequalities. *Australian Feminist Studies*, 34(101), 362–375.

# 18

## HOW CRITICAL PERFORMANCE PEDAGOGY REINVIGORATES FEMINIST SOCIAL WORK IN THE CONTEXT OF GENDERED VIOLENCE

*Jean Carruthers*

### Introduction

This chapter outlines the seemingly neutral yet dominant use of neoliberal, medicalized and traditional epistemologies in social work education and practice, which are commonly prioritized over feminist responses to trauma as a result of gendered violence (see Morley, MacFarlane, & Ablett, 2019). It seeks to demonstrate how, fundamentally, these approaches reinforce discourses that seek to individualize, medicalize, and depoliticize social work approaches (Ferguson, 2008; Morley, MacFarlane, & Ablett, 2017). In addition, I highlight how these approaches are consistent in their uncritical administration of techniques, as opposed to praxis (i.e., the linking of theory and practice) and void of any analysis of the broader structures, discourses and power relations that implicate victim/survivors of gendered violence (Morley, Macfarlane, & Ablett, 2019). Critical performance pedagogy is a counter-hegemonic approach that offers a critical and creative response to gendered violence. It seeks to support students to engage in critically reflexive practice. As such, it encourages students to think critically and work collaboratively to foster a more relevant, socially just and emancipatory response (Carruthers, 2020). I will showcase a performative assessment that demonstrates how social work education can reinvigorate the value and importance of critical social work (in this example, a feminist response to domestic and family violence) through the development of students' capacity for critical praxis. This will then help to develop students' ability to think critically when applying theories to practice situations as a form of embodied, transformative education.

The way we view and respond to trauma has changed over time, shaped by social and political shifts in both society and social work. There is, however, no clear global definition of trauma in social work and definitions are often drawn

DOI: 10.4324/9781003379591-19

from mental health and psychiatric definitions from the United States, such as the Substance Abuse and Mental Health Services Administration (SAMHSA) (SAMHSA, 2014, p. 7) which defines trauma as:

[a]n event, series of events, or set of circumstances that is experienced by an individual as physically or emotionally harmful or life threatening and that has lasting adverse effects on the individual's functioning and mental, physical, social, emotional, or spiritual well-being.

The Australian Institute of Health and Welfare (AIHW) (2022, p. 1, section 3) defines trauma as:

[a]ny event that involves exposure to actual or threatened death, serious injury, or sexual violence [that] has the potential to be traumatic. The trauma experienced can be physical, and/or mental and not everyone will respond in the same way.

Trauma can also be described as a traumatic injury or wound that can be experienced as physical, emotional and/or cognitive. Traumatic injury can result in a sense of isolation and powerlessness, causing personal, social, cultural, spiritual and political disruption (Brown, C. & Macdonald, 2020; Shah & Muffeed, 2023).

The International Federation of Social Workers (IFSW) does not use the word trauma in its definition of social work, instead referring to issues of global and local inequity and social justice, juxtaposed with language on mental health and illness. In its knowledge statement it draws on theoretical perspectives informed by social work as well as other epistemologies, including those rooted in psychiatry and psychology. Although trauma is not specifically mentioned, the IFSW (2014) knowledge statement reminds us of the fundamental social justice worldview of social work that should guide our practice:

[e]ngages people and structures to address life challenges and enhance wellbeing … From an emancipatory perspective, this definition supports social work strategies that are aimed at increasing people's hope, self-esteem and creative potential to confront and challenge oppressive power dynamics and structural sources of injustices, thus incorporating into a coherent whole the micro-macro, personal-political dimension of intervention.

The prevailing influence of neoliberalism in social work has, however, shifted away from social justice, resulting in social concerns (such as responding to the impact of trauma), becoming more about upholding the values of the market economy and developing personal responsibility than the social context of trauma and appropriately addressing the impact on people's well-being (see Ferguson, 2008; Morley, Macfarlane, & Ablett, 2017). As a result, approaches in social work education and practice have become predominantly individualized, pathologized, universalized and technicized (Macfarlane, 2016). According to Morley and Ablett (2017a, p. 7) "official statements that claim social work is committed to promoting 'social change ... and the empowerment and liberation of people' are often reduced to rhetoric, when much of social work practice reflects an individualised, and increasingly psychologised understanding of social problems that reproduce inequality". The popularity of the term mental illness/health and the dominance of medicalized and psychologized approaches that seek to generalize the impacts of trauma to specific symptoms, diagnosis as a mental illness and treatment interventions that prioritize medication are evidence of this dominance (Morley & Stenhouse, 2021). This is evidenced when the response to gendered violence (e.g., intimate partner violence, domestic and family violence, sexual-based violence) (Morley & Dunstan, 2016) shifts to a diagnosis of post-traumatic stress disorder (PTSD).

Burstow (cited in Brown, C., 2020, p. 88) asserts "trauma is not a disorder but a reaction to a kind of wound". It is a reaction to profoundly injurious events and situations in the real world and, indeed, to a world in which people are routinely wounded. Influenced by early feminist thinkers in the 1970s and 1980s, contemporary trauma theory, the foundation for trauma-informed approaches to social work, agree that trauma is not an illness or deficiency but is a common phenomenon experienced by most people that, once experienced, often reshapes their worldview (Anyikwa, 2016; Goodwin & Tiderington, 2022). This view suggests that practitioners should employ "universal trauma precautions" when seeking support in the social work context (Anyikwa, 2016; Goodwin & Tiderington, 2022).

Trauma-informed approaches have gained popularity across all areas of practice (most specifically in medicalized settings). While trauma-informed discourse is not universal it is somewhat progressive, given that trauma-informed practice claims to promote the assumption that trauma is likely to be part of a service user's experience and is not aiming to "fix the problem", rather, to seek to build a safe, transparent and collaborative environment to foster trust and empowerment (Levenson, 2020). Despite perhaps progressive intent, in medicalized settings, with increased focus on diagnoses and locating traumatic injury in the individual and the body, it is difficult to argue most trauma work is occurring in safe, transparent and collaborative environments. Feminist, social justice leaning social work practices often seek to acknowledge and reduce power disparities within the helping relationship and recognize cultural, historical and gender-based analyses to avoid stigmatization (ibid.). However, simply claiming to be trauma-informed does not in fact mean one is acknowledging power in the helping relationship or the social inequities and discourses in which trauma is often situated. Nor does it mean individuals are not blamed, shamed and harmed in the process of seeking help. Indeed, the growing fiscal constraints of neoliberalism mean that service provision is underfunded, underdeveloped, reductive, oversimplified, decontextualized and medicalized. Short term, these approaches tend to generalize trauma and responses to trauma become one-size-fits-all, short-term approaches, revoking the desire for any contextual analysis (Anyikwa, 2016).

Furthermore, in its efforts to avoid specialization it depoliticizes the issue by administering a technicist response to support coping based on strengths-based practices, whereby strategies are implemented that prioritize creating comfort and resilience over responding to social injustice and developing a broader social, political and contextual analysis of gendered violence (Levenson, 2020; MacFarlane, 2016). Despite critiques pertaining to the lack of social and political analysis, trauma-informed work seems to have chosen to adopt technicist interventions that focus on coping strategies and behavior change (MacFarlane, 2016), without any recognition of the systems and structures that create and perpetuate gendered violence or the implications of uncritically administering conservative approaches to practice (Pease & Nipperess, 2016).

As a starting point, trauma-informed practice had potential to delegitimize a more medicalized approach, however, it seems to have largely become an approach that is seen to minimize harm rather than respond to trauma (Brown, C., 2020). While the current popularization of "trauma-informed" care is not unhelpful, especially when compared to more medicalized, diagnostic and pathological approaches, the approach has become increasingly, however unwittingly, conflated. Often, lacking adequate training and knowledge, and seeking to feel equipped to work with trauma, social workers have been vulnerable to co-optation to approaches that claim to be evidence-based. By being able to use diagnostic language or, having learned about the biological impact of trauma on body such as "polyvagal theory", they feel more equipped while becoming more and more distant from the social justice lens that early feminist practitioners adopted in their empowerment-based approaches to rape, sexual abuse, incest and domestic violence. As a result, the value of feminism is diluted and rendered insignificant. This is dangerous when responding to gendered violence, considering the potential for victim-blaming if, for example, the intervention was to seek family counseling in domestic and family violence disputes or restorative justice processes without recognition of the structures of patriarchy that perpetuate oppression for women (including non-binary people assigned as woman at birth and trans women) who are predominantly victim/survivors of gendered violence (Brown, C. & MacDonald, 2022; Morley & Dunstan, 2016).

A feminist approach challenges the neutralizing of trauma in response to gendered violence. In addition, a feminist approach to trauma would suggest that gender and a critique of patriarchy should be at the forefront of the goals, policy, research, practices and institutions addressing trauma as a result of gendered violence (Messing, 2020). C. Brown (2020, p. 88) proposes "the 'personal is political' approach seeks to make sense of, rather than pathologize women's responses to trauma and violence by listening to and hearing women's stories and having an impact on policy and law". Furthermore, for men who have experienced trauma and, as a result of this mistreatment and betrayal, have adopted patriarchal societal norms leading to perpetration of gendered violence, a trauma-informed approach on its own is not adequately equipped to redress these human rights violations (Augusta-Scott, 2020). From a social justice perspective, when responding to gendered violence, an approach to trauma needs to contextually recognize the personal, social, cultural and political implications of personal suffering (Morley & Dunstan, 2016). Feminist theory has been recognized as the most relevant response since its inception into social work in the early 1970s and 1980s and it is still just as relevant today.

As an educator, I have witnessed the enticement of dominant conservative approaches (e.g., psychodynamic, cognitive behavior therapy (CBT), systems theory and trauma-informed practice) as a benchmark for "best practice". To uphold the social justice values espoused by social work and maintain a vision for emancipatory change, it is argued that creative approaches to social work education are required. Encouraging students and practitioners to prioritize critical and reflexive analysis (e.g., critical praxis) when responding to trauma is important if socially just practice is the aim (see Carruthers, 2020). The importance of understanding the ways that social work approaches are positioned differently offers emerging practitioners a means for critically reflexive evaluation. Social work education has a crucial role in supporting emerging practitioners to conceptualize nuances and potential for harm as a result of adopting uncritical responses when using theory in practice. Critical performance pedagogy is an approach that enables critical and reflexive conceptualization of theory and practice. A performance play titled *Sittina's Insight* that was developed and delivered by students in a first-year introductory unit (as an assessment piece) will be used as an example. This example will demonstrate how critical performance pedagogy invigorates the crucial role feminist theory plays in equipping students with a gendered analysis and practices to critically respond to issues of gendered violence as a form of emancipatory practice.

## Critical Performance Pedagogy

Critical performance pedagogy is a process of teaching and learning that positions social justice at the forefront of education practice in social work. This pedagogical approach draws on critical (i.e., critical theory and critical pedagogy), performative (i.e., performing arts) and collaborative practices to facilitate transformative learning and encourage critically reflective education practices in social work (Carruthers & Ablett, 2020).

Critical performance pedagogy is a collective approach informed by the following key assumptions outlined by Carruthers (2020, p. 245):

1 Critical performance pedagogy assumes a counter-hegemonic stance that resists the dominance of mainstream social work education (e.g., neoliberal,

technical-rational, narrowly evidence-based), rather, drawing on subordinated traditions (e.g., critical, artistic, Indigenous, sociological and philosophical knowledges) that promote other ways of knowing and being.

2   The performative and political aspects are intersectional and philosophically aligned with social justice principles.

3   Critical theory and critical pedagogy are central to critical performance pedagogy as a democratic and transformative strategy that encourages students to become social and political actors for emancipatory social change (Morley, Macfarlane & Ablett, 2019).

4   Critical performance pedagogy is intentionally collaborative in practice and assessment.

Critical performance pedagogy is an embodied learning approach that seeks to develop students' capacity for critical thinking and action through the development of critical praxis (e.g., the ability to think critically when applying theory to practice situations). As a transformative strategy for critical education, critical performance pedagogy acknowledges the task of educating students as becoming:

> critical agents who actively question and negotiate the relationships between theory and practice, critical analysis and common sense, and learning and social change.
>
> *(Giroux, 2007, p. 1)*

Mezirow (2003, p. 62) proposes the investment of the educator in the process of transformative learning can "foster the development of skills, insights and especially dispositions", which are essential for students to critically reflect on their own deeply held, taken-for-granted assumptions. Through participation in embodied performative practices alongside "critical-dialectical discourse", students are able to develop knowledge and skills in critical analysis and critical reflection (Carruthers, 2020; Mezirow, 2003, p. 62). The performance assessment shown below demonstrates the ways critical performance pedagogy is a strategy for students to become critically reflexive in their practice when responding to gendered violence.

## Performance Assessment Based on the Play *Sittina's Insight*

The performance assessment is a part of the curriculum in an introductory social work program (Carruthers, 2020; Carruthers & Ablett, 2020; Morley & Ablett, 2017b). The purpose of the assessment is to assist students to think critically about the ways they analyse and respond to a social justice issue related to social work practice. Students are tasked to develop and deliver a performance play that showcases three practice-related critical and conservative theories (e.g., feminist, critical, postmodern, psychodynamic, cognitive behavioral, systems theory) and how these theories would support students to analyse and respond to a case situation.

There are three stages in the process: (1) collaborative development of a case study; (2) small theory group presentations; and (3) the development and delivery of the performance play. The first stage, developing a case study, involves students working together to choose a social justice issue and to construct a case scenario they can work with to explore the theories' key assumptions and practice methods. Developing the case study as a tutorial group "enables the group to start a process of being able to work together, identify common interests, particular issues that they would really like to pursue but also assumptions that are embedded in 'ooh who is this client going to be that we work with?'" (Carruthers, 2020, p. 111).

For stage two, students are tasked to divide into small groups (approximately six to eight per group) and choose a theory. They then research and present the chosen theory in their tutorial as a way to describe, apply and critique it, particularly from a social justice perspective (Carruthers, 2020, p. 115).

Stage three requires students to work collaboratively as a whole tutorial group to develop a performance play (approximately 20 minutes in duration) to showcase their analysis of three theories (a mix of conservative and critical) from those they researched earlier. They then use an existing creative narrative (e.g., a fairytale, game show, reality television, political debate, etc.) to shape the story of the theories and their application to practice. As part of a performance showcase, the groups creatively share this knowledge by performing the play to the entire cohort of students in the course. According to Morley and Ablett (2017b, p. 5) the process supports students to "devise innovative ways to present their material creatively in order to engage their peers from other tutorials". The tutorial group decides what theories and creative frame they will use to showcase their learning in the performance presentation (Carruthers, 2020; Morley & Ablett, 2017b, p. 5).

The performance *Sittina's Insight* was based on an existing talk show narrative using a Special Broadcasting Service (SBS) television program called *Insight* (see Carruthers, 2020). The theme was an enactment of a fictional character's lived experience of domestic violence as the topic of the program, which was drawn from a case scenario. The story was about a Sudanese woman who was a victim/survivor of domestic and family violence (see Carruthers, 2020). The group explains:

> [T]he case study was a young mother [named Sittina] ... She was an immigrant to Australia [and was] in a domestic violence situation ... [W]e looked at critical [theory], CBT and systems [theory] ... It was basically an interviewer and he interviewed each of the "theorists" [representing the three theories] to say "what is your theory?" and then that person went into what CBT was and how it was going to benefit the client and how systems theory worked and how that would benefit the client and then the same with critical theory and how that would benefit the client as well ... [T]here were people who offered

support and told her [Sittina] about what networks were available to her. We had people who came on as experts [representing different theories] and then we had people in the audience who were just adding [theoretical insights and critiques] as well.

*(Carruthers, 2020, pp. 109–110)*

The platform explores not only different theories but also concepts and discourses from a range of identity groups associated with social work, such as helping professionals (e.g., experts, activists, therapists) and people representing public opinion through enactments of politically targeted social media feeds on a projector screen reflecting a range of diverse perspectives from highly right-wing conservative views to radical feminist views. The talk show host's facilitation role was highlighted as they guided the theoretical discussions and provoked opportunities for critique of the different perspectives. The educator's role is to support students to develop their capacity to think critically, work together ethically and to share knowledge relevant to critical praxis whereby social justice is positioned as central to students' analysis and responses (Carruthers, 2020). Structurally, the performance assessment process has been described as synonymous to working in a multidisciplinary environment and mobilizing for social change. Performances are assessed using collaborative methods (e.g., team teaching approach and self/peer evaluation) (ibid.).

One of the significant outcomes of this performance was the reinvigoration of feminist theory as the most relevant approach for analyzing and responding to domestic and family violence in the performance *Sittina's Insight*. Students espoused a critical approach, drawing on radical and postmodern feminism to support a comprehensive and nuanced recognition of feminist theory's role in equipping the social worker with a gendered analysis and socially just action. The performance models language a feminist social worker might use, an understanding of the impact of patriarchy and a critique of the conservative theories that, in this instance, have fallen short of the emancipatory aims of social work. As highlighted in the play script, students acknowledge the courage it takes for victim/survivors to voice their experiences of domestic and family violence. Students utilize a feminist analysis and critical skills for social work practice as a means to validate Sittina's experience and universalize the issue of domestic and family violence as one face by many women (Morley, Macfarlane & Ablett, 2019). as shown in the following excerpt from the play script.

Hello Sittina, before I begin, I would like to thank you for your brave decision to speak so publicly about what you are going through. It is incredibly important to share experiences such as yours so that women suffering domestic violence know that they are not alone.

*(Carruthers, 2020)*

The play offers a critique of the more conservative theories that are informed by assumptions of linear intervention toward a progressive outcome (e.g., to fix the problem or change the person). In this instance, the tendency for conservative approaches to unintentionally blame the victim/survivor for their situation is recognized and the skill of "deguilting" (see Morley, Macfarlane & Ablett, 2019) is demonstrated. Feminist assumptions of solidarity and building a therapeutic alliance (also recognized in trauma-informed practice) and practice methods to support this are highlighted.

> Unlike my colleagues [CBT and systems theorists], I am not here to try and change or fix you and I believe it is important for you to understand that you are not to blame for the abuse you have suffered. Were we to work together, and working "together" is the key term, as I believe our relationship should be one of mutual respect and learning. I would begin by seeking to understand how you feel and what you wish to gain from our time together ... This could possibly be achieved through counselling and group work with other women that have had similar experiences, and hopefully this will also help provide the support missing from your friends and family.
>
> *(Carruthers, 2020)*

The excerpt below recognizes the role feminist theory plays in offering a broader social and political analysis, acknowledging patriarchy as influential in the perpetuation of domestic violence and the practice methods of advocacy and activism to combat this:

> I hope in our time together you would be able to gain a greater understanding of how societal forces such as patriarchy enable domestic violence to flourish so that you can see your own blamelessness ... Unlike my systems theory colleague, I do not believe domestic abuse to be a relationship problem but a severe humans right abuse that needs to be addressed at societal levels through advocacy and community development ... I can also assist you by putting you in contact with a number of women's advocacy and domestic abuse survivors' groups who may be able to assist you in feeling supported and not alone and in time you may even choose to participate in supporting other women and further direct action.
>
> *(Carruthers, 2020)*

This speaks to the well-regarded feminist concept "the personal as political" (Hanisch, 1969) by positioning domestic violence as a social concern, not simply an individual problem, as such resisting any desire to blame or pathologize Sittina and taking action for social and emancipatory change.

The final excerpt recognizes that gender also plays a significant role in the service user/worker relationship whereby some women might not feel comfortable working with a male, however recognizing the importance of male practitioners having a feminist analysis:

> I also understand that as a male you may not be completely comfortable working with me, so I can provide you with a list of fantastic female colleagues who may be better able to assist you, however it is your decision.
>
> *(Carruthers, 2020)*

This analysis recognizes the influence of patriarchy in matters of domestic violence. There is a strong misconception that feminist theory is only for women and, therefore, not relevant if you are a male practitioner or working with men. This assumption can result in male students and practitioners not adopting an adequate response to violence against women or addressing their own patriarchal conditioning. This was evident in the performance, whereby the male student playing the role of the feminist theorist did not appear entirely comfortable in the role. The written analysis in and of itself was well developed and cleverly nuanced, however when delivered in the actual performance the essence and value of the feminist analysis was stifled (Carruthers, 2020). Despite there being a vast body of literature that espouses a pro-feminist approach to gendered violence (Augusta-Scott, 2020; Pease, 2016), it was evident the male student who verbally delivered the excerpt above had no investment in pro-feminist ideas and assumptions and, as such, he stumbled over words and spoke in a matter-of-fact tone that lacked warmth and empathy. The delivery appeared more technicist than feminist. This could have been partly due to nerves, however the student's inability to embody the theory and apply this to practice in a reflexive manner was noteworthy and speaks to the uncritical assumption that men do not need feminist theory in their framework for practice. This is a myth that requires debunking.

The influence of patriarchy also extends to the cultural implications of patriarchal discourse, whereby women from Sudanese cultural backgrounds such as Sittina are likely to be shamed if they leave a domestically violent relationship as a form of victim-blaming. The performance was able to explicitly demonstrate this point through the embodied visualization of Sittina's mother judging Sittina for leaving due to her patriarchal conditioning. A postmodern feminist response, provided by the characterization of two feminist practitioners (planted in the audience) was provided as a counterargument to Sittina's mother's narrative, which reflected internalized assumptions of cultural shame:

**Sittina**'s *mother:* I am very upset by Sittina, a marriage is between a husband and a wife. Sittina has bought shame to her family and shame to her culture!! She is no daughter of mine.

*Counter argument from a planted feminist practitioner:* I would just really like to commend Sittina in coming forward to seek help. It was courageous of her to do so, and through more community awareness we can raise people's consciousness surrounding domestic violence. We should be enabling women to come forward and break their silence by acknowledging it for what it is. We need to dispel myths and ideas that feed into her sense of self blame and shame.

*(Carruthers, 2020, p. 176)*

In the narrative from Sittina's mother, it is evident that patriarchal constructions in this instance have intersected with cultural traditions, which highlights how patriarchal discourses can be compounded by cultural dominance and can be held by the people they oppress (Poynting & Briskman, 2018). This speaks to the ways that gendered oppression can be intersectional and the important role both intersectional and postmodern feminism play in recognizing that not all women's experience of oppression is the same and that gender is fluid, not fixed (Messing, 2020). The dialogue supports recognition of victim-blaming attitudes as espoused by Sittina's mother, however this was delivered carefully and sensitively to avoid oppositionalizing or placing blame on Sittina's mother. who has likely been a victim of the same treatment and would want to protect her daughter from experiencing further trauma as a result of her resistance.

Feminist theory offers the most relevant analysis and practice for social justice work, regardless of the practitioner's gender, when responding to gendered violence with women. This includes trans women, non-binary people assigned as woman at birth, Black women and women with (dis)Ability. Reflective spaces to challenge hegemonic assumptions about gender would be beneficial to students. The critical pedagogic approach supports educators to encourage students to choose contextually relevant theories when responding to particularly contexts, as suggested by one educator:

There were only a couple of times where I gave some suggestions around a choice of theory that [students] were going to leave out that I thought was important to use. One example was a domestic violence scenario and they were not going to use feminist theory. So, my influence made sure that feminist theory was one of the theories included in their theory exploration. Because feminist movements and feminist theory has been where a lot of our understanding and public appreciation around the issue of domestic violence has come from… it is incredibly important in practice.

*(Carruthers, 2020, pp. 125–126)*

Consequently, the performance became a catalyst for transformative learning through recognition of the dominant discourses that may play out in students' deeply held assumptions and an opportunity to redress these uncritical actions through critical dialogical praxis with the educator and the rest of the group.

Using a performative approach there is a risk of trivializing, stereotyping and disembodying knowledge due to uncritical assumptions about some theories (usually critical theories). In addition, students sometimes have a tendency to choose a "best" theory, like a winner. This is not unrealistic considering the push for "best" practice, which is a common discourse in Australian social work. This assumption, however, downplays the benefits of the theories that were dismissed and can travel through their course work in later semesters (Carruthers, 2020). What this highlights is the importance of educators to be well versed in critical theory and critical pedagogy in order to pick up on these sometimes subtle assumptions and make an educated point about the importance of embodying the values of social work to support ethically informed emancipatory responses as a form of critically reflexive practice.

## Conclusion

When responding to trauma in social work, a social justice perspective is required if the aim is emancipatory practice. As shown in this chapter, this is not an easy task when neoliberal, medicalized and universalizing responses have resulted in the depoliticizing of social justice concerns such as gendered violence. Critical performance pedagogy is one strategy that has been successful in supporting the reinvigoration of a feminist approach as demonstrated in the performance play *Sittina's Insight*. Through this demonstration with the support of their educator (informed by a critical pedagogical approach) students were able to recognize feminist theory as the most contextually relevant response to a situation of domestic and family violence. Critical performance pedagogy is an embodied, transformative approach in social work education that assist students to develop the capacity and confidence for critical praxis and reflexivity in their emerging social work practice.

## References

Anyikwa, V.A. (2016). Trauma-informed approach to survivors of intimate partner violence. *Journal of Evidence Informed Social Work, 13*(5), 484–491.https://doi.org/10.1080/23761407.2016.1166824.

Augusta-Scott, T. (2020). Exploring trauma and masculinity among men who perpetuate intimate partner violence. In C. Brown & J. Macdonald (Eds.), *Critical clinical social work: Counterstorying for social justice* (pp. 127–140). Canadian Scholars Press.

Australian Institute of Health and Welfare (AIHW). (2022). *Stress and trauma.* Retrieved from https://www.aihw.gov.au/reports/mental-health-services/stress-and-trauma.

Brown, C. (2020). Feminist narrative therapy and complex trauma: Critical clinical work with women diagnosed as "Borderline". In C. Brown and J. Macdonald (Eds.), *Critical clinical social work: Counterstorying for social justice* (pp. 82–109). Canadian Scholars Press.

Brown, C., & MacDonald, J. (2022). *Critical clinical social work: Counterstorying for social justice.* Canadian Scholars Press.

Carruthers, J.C. (2020). *Performance as a platform for critical pedagogy in social work education.* Doctoral dissertation, Queensland University of Technology. https://qut.primo.exlibrisgroup.com/permalink/61QUT_INST/1g7tbfa/alma99101000225 7604001.

Carruthers, J., & Ablett, P. (2020). Boal and Gadamer: A complimentary relationship towards critical performance pedagogy. In C. Morley, P. Ablett, C. Noble, and S. Cowden (Eds.), *Routledge handbook of critical pedagogies* (pp. 477–488). Routledge. https://doi.org/10.4324/9781351002042-39.

Ferguson, I. (2008). *Reclaiming social work: Challenging neo-liberalism and promoting social justice.* Sage. https://doi.org/10.4135/9781446212110.

Giroux, H.A. (2007). Democracy, education, and the politics of critical pedagogy. *Counterpoints*, 1–5.

Goodwin, J., & Tiderington, E. (2022). Building trauma-informed research competencies in social work education. *Social Work Education*, 41(2), 143–156. https://doi.org/10.1080/02615479.2020.1820977.

Hanisch, C. (1969). The personal is political. In A.K. Shulman & H. Moore (2021) (Eds.), *Women's liberation! Feminist writings that inspired a revolution & still can* (pp. 134–138). The Library of America.

International Federation of Social Workers (IFSW). (2014). *Global definition of social work.* https://www.ifsw.org/what-is-social-work/global-definition-of-social-work/.

Levenson, J. (2020). Translating trauma-informed principles into social work practice. *Social Work*, 65(3), 288–298. https://doi.org/10.1093/sw/swaa020.

Macfarlane, S. (2016). Education for critical social work: Being true to a worthy project. In B. Pease, S. Goldingay, N. Hosken, & S. Nipperess (Eds.), *Doing critical social work: Transformative practices for social justice* (pp. 326–338). Allen & Unwin. https://doi.org/10.4324/9781003115380-27.

Messing, J.T. (2020). Mainstreaming gender: An intersectional feminist approach to the grand challenges for social work. *Social Work*, 65(4), 313–315. https://doi.org/10.1093/sw/swaa042.

Mezirow, J. (2003). Transformative learning as discourse. *Journal of Transformative Education*, 1(1), 58–63. https://doi.org/10.1177/1541344603252172.

Morley, C., & Ablett, P. (2017a). Rising wealth and income inequality: A radical social work critique and response. *Aotearoa New Zealand Social* Work, 29(2), 6–18. https://qut.primo.exlibrisgroup.com/permalink/61QUT_INST/1fes5bt/cdi_rmit_collectionsjats_search_informit_org_doi_abs_10_3316_informit_337715362090337.

Morley, C., & Ablett, P. (2017b). Designing assessment to promote engagement among first year social work students. *Journal of Business, Education and Scholarship*, 11(2), 1–14. https://eprints.qut.edu.au/116369/.

Morley, C., & Dunstan, J. (2016). Putting gender back on the agenda in domestic and family violence policy: Using critical reflection to create cultural change. *Social Alternatives*, 35(4), 43–48. https://eprints.qut.edu.au/107631/.

Morley, C., Macfarlane, S., & Ablett, P. (2017). The neoliberal colonisation of social work education: A critical analysis and practices of resistance. *Advances in Social Work and Welfare Education*, 19(2), 25–40.

Morley, C., Macfarlane, S., & Ablett, P. (2019). *Engaging with social work: A critical introduction* (2nd ed.). Cambridge University Press. https://doi.org/10.1017/9781108681094.

Morley, C., & Stenhouse, K. (2021). Educating for critical social work practice in mental health. *Social Work Education*, 40(1), 80–94. https://doi.org/10.1080/02615479.2020.1774535.

Pease, B. (2016). Engaging men in feminist social work: Theory, politics and practice. In S. Wendt & N. Moulding (Eds.), *Contemporary feminisms in social work practice* (pp. 287–302). Routledge Advances in Social Work.

Pease, B., & Nipperess, S. (2016). Doing critical social working the neoliberal context: Working on the contradictions. In B. Pease, S. Goldingay, N. Hosken, & S. Nipperess (Eds.), *Doing critical social work: Transformative practices for social justice* (pp. 3–25). Allen & Unwin. https://doi.org/ 10.4324/9781003115380-2.

Poynting, S., & Briskman, L. (2018). Islamophobia in Australia: From far-right deplorables to respectable liberals. *Social Sciences*, 7(11), 213. https://doi.org/10.3390/socsci7110213.

Shah, S.S., & Mufeed, S.A. (2023). Urgency and relevance of feminist social work to curb domestic violence amid Covid-19. *International Social Work*, 66(1), 88–92.

Substance Abuse and Mental Health Services Administration (SAMHSA). (2014). *SAMHSA's concept of trauma and guidance for a trauma-informed approach.* https://www.samhsa.gov/trauma-violence.

# INDEX

Locators in *italic* indicate figures and in **bold** tables.

50, 188, 225–226; institutional, systemic violence 224–225; intergenerational trauma 182–183, 190, 274; male childhood sexual trauma 10, 309–318 (*see also under own heading*); mandatory pediatric assessment 273; parental substance-use 274

Choice and Partnership Approach (CAPA) 71, 74–76, 77, 78–79, 83

chronic pain; *see* (dis)Ability and chronic pain

chronic regional pain syndrome (CRPS) 134–139, **137–138**

Chung, D. 64

Coates, L. 168, 171

coercion: continuum of coercion 4; gender and psychiatric coercion project 59, 67; gender, violence 58, 61, 63, 64, 66–67; psychiatric, medicalized 4, 29, 58–59, 60, 61, 63, 65, 67

cognitive behavior therapy (CBT) 48, 328–329, 330

collective care 8–9, 235–246; as ancestral practice 236–237; collective trauma 8, 235, 238–240; as liberation tool 240–241, 242; practical barriers 246; as societal neglect alternative, marginalized communities 238, 240; theoretical framework 242–246 (*see also* theoretical framework, collective care); in trauma intervention work 240

collective trauma 8, 235, 238–240

Collins, B. 136

colonialization / decolonization 73, 186; anti-Black racism 239–240; case study: colonialization, generational trauma and healing in Indigenous Australia 49–54; collective care 8–9, 235–246 (*see also under own heading*); as collective trauma 8, 235, 238–240; decolonialization framework 8; First Nations people trauma work (*see* indigeneity, colonization and trauma work (First Nations, Australia)); historical and intergenerational trauma components 7–8 (*see also* intergenerational trauma); impact, intergenerational trauma

7–8; indigeneity, colonization and trauma work 219–231 (*see also under own heading*); and intergenerational trauma 180–195; phases 49; silencing effects (testimonial quieting / smothering) 211–212; psychiatrization of global mental health 82; trauma legacy 73, 82; structural and cultural violences 275, *276*

community care; *see* collective care

community trauma 49, 53, 235; *see also* collective trauma; intergenerational trauma

complex trauma 5, 103–124, 225–226, 235, 239, 318; adequate service access difficulties 3, 119; case example: Rosa 104, 110, 111–117, 119–123, 124n2; components 20; co-occurrences (socio-economic, mental health) 30, 134; healing requirements (safety, healing) 118; as intergenerational trauma 194; therapeutic shortfalls (pathologization, negation) 20, 104, 119

Connell, Raewyn W. 252, 256, 257, 311, 316

constriction 112–113

contributory epistemic injustice 45, 50, 52

contributory injustice 45, 47, 50

co-occurring mental health issues 30, 103, 112

co-occurring trauma 3, 19–20, 30, 103, 112, 134

coping strategies 2, 6, 16, 100, 105, 111, 184; case example: Rosa 104, 110, 111–117, 119–123, 124n2; constriction 112–113; as entry points to trauma stories 105; function 110; interpersonal violence 274; metaphors 104; self-harm / cutting 111, 112–113, 121, 122, 124n3, 274; substance use 2, 20, 164–165, 169, 274

counterstorying as discursive resistance 17, 29–31, 94, 100–101, 123, 203–204, 207, 243

counterviewing 3, 17, 100–101, 105–106, 109, 110; coping behavior 17; dominant stories / discursive influences 29, 105, 110; injurious speech 29, 109; as therapy entry, connection making 29, 105–106

intimate partner / interpersonal violence
219, 250–253; cognitive-behavioral
research approach 249, 250, 253,
254–256; prevalence, Indigenous
vs non-Indigenous women 219,
223–224; trauma-informed
research approach 249, 253, 254;
*see also violence, domestic /*
*family*
Intimate Partner Violence Movement 278
involuntary mental health treatment 63
Ireland, J. 136

Jabr, S. 65
James, William 48
Jeffery, D. 134
Jewish identity hiding, self-silencing 8,
182, 201
Joe, case example 268, 270
Johnstone, Lucy 79, 81
Johnstone, Marjorie 3–4, 43–54
Jovey, R. 128
Jülich, S. 279

Kafer, A. 130
Karabanow, Jeff 7, 161–174
Khan, S. 188
kin making 53, 281
knowledge, knowing, as constituent part of
human identity 44
Kristeva, Julia 259

Lafrance, M. 22
Lawrie, R. 223
Lawthom, R. 130
"Leave the Light On" (Hart) 124n3
Lee, Bandy 47–48
Lees, Eunjung 3–4, 43–54
Lewis, Daurene 203
Liasidou, A. 133
Liegghio, Maria 78
linguistic incongruence 106
*The Little Book of Circle Processes*
(Boyes-Watson, Pranis) 280
love ethic 8, 235, 237, 241; ethics 8, 235,
237, 241

MacDonald, Judy E. 6, 128–140
Mackelprang, R. 132
male childhood sexual trauma 10,
309–318; disclosure (rates,
gender differences, dangers)
310–311; discourse oppression
/ lack, consequences 309, 311,

313–314; hegemonic masculinity
252, 255, 256, 259, 260, 311–312,
313, 315; misogyny/homophobia
314–317; prevalence estimates 310;
stigmatizing cultural narratives
316; toxic masculinity 313;
victimization as transgression of
masculine identity 309–310
Manne 316
Marcus, G. 223
masculinities research 251–253, 256
masculinity: hegemonic 252, 255, 256,
259, 260, 311–312, 313, 315;
toxic 313
Matheson, K. 187
Matthews, W. 223
McClintock, J. 130
McDonaldization of social work 76
McKenzie-Mohr, S. 168, 171
meaning making, trauma/violence
experiences 5–6, 16; as collective
trauma 109; counterviewing
/ counterstorying 29, 109,
110; de-contextualization,
individualization 74, 76–77;
emotions essentialism and
social regulatory influence 28;
hermeneutic justice / epistemic
injustice 48–49, 52, 54, 190; and
identity forming 19; "irrational"
260; narratives, storytelling as
ancestral tools 245; neurocentric
perspectives 19; polyvagal theory
23, 325; social shaping 190
men: male childhood sexual trauma
(*see under own heading*); trauma
and gender: Safety and Repair
Approach (*see* Safety and Repair
Manual, approach to gendered
violence);
mental health / mental health services:
biomedical mental health service
and intergenerational trauma
74, 76–77, 184, 185–187, 193;
colonization/decolonialization,
psychiatrization of global mental
health 82; community mental
health 89, 90, 92, 93, 97, 100; as
complex trauma co-occurrences
30, 134; determinants 72, 109, 184,
189–190, 193, 202; Diagnostic
and Statistical Manual of Mental
Disorders (*see* DSM); epistemic
and institutional violence 71–83;

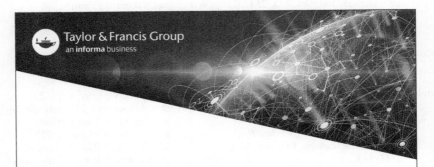

For Product Safety Concerns and Information please contact our EU
representative GPSR@taylorandfrancis.com Taylor & Francis Verlag GmbH,
Kaufingerstraße 24, 80331 München, Germany

Printed and bound by CPI Group (UK) Ltd, Croydon, CR0 4YY

08/06/2025
01897008-0016